Register
Access

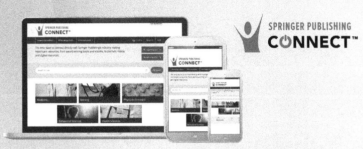

SPRINGER PUBLISHING
C🔅NNECT™

Your print purchase of *Handbook of Hematologic Malignancies,*
Second Edition, **includes online access to the contents of your**
book—increasing accessibility, portability, and searchability!

Access today at:
http://connect.springerpub.com/content/book/978-0-8261-4977-0
or scan the QR code at the right with your smartphone
and enter the access code below.

N0W3TMY8

Scan here for
quick access.

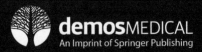

demosMEDICAL
An Imprint of Springer Publishing

View all our products at springerpub.com/demosmedical

MW00837039

Handbook of
Hematologic Malignancies

This resource is provided by Sobi, Inc.

Sobi, Inc. (Sobi) does not control the content of this textbook, and the book may describe uses for products that may not be approved or cleared by the U.S. Food and Drug Administration (FDA). Before prescribing any product, please consult the full Prescribing Information for that product. In addition, Sobi has not conducted an analysis to determine whether any of the authors of this text have any financial interest in Sobi or its products; therefore, one or more of the authors may have a financial interest in Sobi or its products.

Sobi reports payments and transfers of value made to healthcare providers in accordance with federal and state laws, regulations, and related obligations. Please be advised that information such as your name, type of item, and the retail value (including tax and shipping) of such items you receive from Sobi will be publicly disclosed and reported to governmental agencies, as required.

In addition, several states and U.S. federal agencies impose restrictions on receiving in-kind benefits such as textbooks. Certain healthcare providers, including but not limited to prescribers licensed in Minnesota or prescribers employed by the U.S. Department of Defense, are not eligible to receive a resource through this program. This does not constitute a comprehensive list of healthcare providers who are excluded from receiving transfers of value. Sobi will refer to all applicable state and federal regulations when determining a healthcare provider's eligibility to receive a resource under this program.

Handbook of Hematologic Malignancies

Second Edition

Editors

David A. Sallman, MD
Assistant Member, Department of Malignant Hematology
H. Lee Moffitt Cancer Center & Research Institute
University of South Florida Morsani College of Medicine
Tampa, Florida

Ateefa Chaudhury, MD
Hematologist, New Mexico Cancer Center
Albuquerque, New Mexico

Johnny Nguyen, MD
Assistant Professor, Anatomic Pathology Lab
Johns Hopkins All Children's Hospital
Baltimore, Maryland

Ling Zhang, MD
Senior Member, Professor, Department of Pathology
H. Lee Moffitt Cancer Center & Research Institute
Tampa, Florida

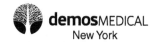
demosMEDICAL
New York

Springer Publishing Company, LLC
11 West 42nd Street, New York, NY 10036
www.springerpub.com
connect.springerpub.com/

Acquisitions Editor: David D'Addona
Compositor: Transforma

ISBN: 978-0-8261-4976-3
e-book ISBN: 978-0-8261-4977-0
DOI: 10.1891/9780826149770

Supplemental Clinical Cases are available from **https://connect.springerpub.com/content/
book/978-0-8261-4977-0**.

Clinical Case Material ISBN: 978-0-8261-4978-7

Printed by LSI

Medicine is an ever-changing science. Research and clinical experience are continually expanding our
knowledge, in particular our understanding of proper treatment and drug therapy. The authors,
editors, and publisher have made every effort to ensure that all information in this book is in
accordance with the state of knowledge at the time of production of the book. Nevertheless, the
authors, editors, and publisher are not responsible for any errors or omissions or for any conse-
quence from application of the information in this book and make no warranty, expressed or implied,
with respect to the content of this publication. Every reader should examine carefully the package
inserts accompanying each drug and should carefully check whether the dosage schedules therein or
the contraindications stated by the manufacturer differ from the statements made in this book. Such
examination is particularly important with drugs that are either rarely used or have been newly
released on the market.

Library of Congress Cataloging-in-Publication Data

Names: Sallman, David A., editor. | Chaudhury, Ateefa, editor. | Nguyen, Johnny, editor. |
   Zhang, Ling, MD editor.
Title: Handbook of hematologic malignancies / editors, David A. Sallman, Ateefa Chaudhury,
   Johnny Nguyen, Ling Zhang.
Description: Second edition. | New York, NY : Springer Publishing Company, LLC, [2021] |
   Includes bibliographical references and index. | Summary: "The 2nd edition of Handbook
   of Hematologic Malignancies encompasses the hard work and effort of many fellows and
   residents, working under the mentorship and guidance of attending staff physicians at
   world-renowned cancer centers throughout the country, not only at Moffitt Cancer
   Center, but also many others including Harvard, Mayo Clinic, and Memorial Sloan Kettering
   Cancer Center. Specifically, the editors would like acknowledge Dr. Kenian Liu from
   the Cytogenetic Laboratory (Moffitt) for providing FISH images and Drs. Lugen Chen
   (Tampa General Hospital), Wilfredo Chamizo (All Children Hospital at St Petersburg),
   Haipeng Shao (Moffitt), Xiaohui Zhang (Moffitt), and Jane Messina (Moffitt) for sharing
   unique cases to the book. The quality of their work and their willingness to contribute to
   make this textbook one that can serve the needs of readers across disciplines, made
   working on this project a rewarding experience for us all"-- Provided by publisher.
Identifiers: LCCN 2020038913 (print) | LCCN 2020038914 (ebook) | ISBN 9780826149763 (paperback) |
   ISBN 9780826149770 (ebook)
Subjects: MESH: Hematologic Neoplasms | Handbook
Classification: LCC RC280.H47 (print) | LCC RC280.H47 (ebook) | NLM WH 39
   | DDC 616.99/418--dc23
LC record available at https://lccn.loc.gov/2020038913
LC ebook record available at https://lccn.loc.gov/2020038914

Contact us to receive discount rates on bulk purchases. We can also customize our books to meet
your needs.
For more information please contact: sales@springerpub.com

Publisher's Note: New and used products purchased from third-party sellers are not guaranteed for
quality, authenticity, or access to any included digital components.

Printed in the United States of America.

Contents

Part XII. MATURE B-CELL LYMPHOMA

Very Aggressive

Aggressive

Indolent

Part XIII. MATURE T- AND NK-CELL LYMPHOMA

Part XIV. HISTIOCYTIC/DENDRITIC CELL NEOPLASMS

Part XV. BONE MARROW TRANSPLANTATION

Part XVI. NEW CELLULAR IMMUNOTHERAPY

Part XVII. EMERGENCIES IN HEMATOLOGY

Part XVIII. NEW CLINICAL CASES IN MALIGNANT HEMATOLOGY

Contributors

Omar Abdel-Wahab, MD   Associate Professor, Department of Medicine, Leukemia Service, Memorial Sloan Kettering Cancer Center, New York, New York

Sameem Abedin, MD   Assistant Professor, Department of Medicine, Medical College of Wisconsin, Milwaukee, Wisconsin

Jeremy S. Abramson, MD, MMSc   Associate Professor of Medicine, Harvard Medical School, Boston, Massachusetts

Utkarsh Acharya, DO, FACP   Attending Physician, Department of Medical Oncology, Dana-Farber Cancer Institute, Harvard Medical School, Boston, Massachusetts

Hannah Asghari, MD   Fellow, Department of Hematology/Oncology, H. Lee Moffitt Cancer Center & Research Institute, University of South Florida, Tampa, Florida

Ehab Atallah, MD   Professor of Medicine, Medical College of Wisconsin, Milwaukee, Wisconsin

Christina A. Bachmeier, PharmD   Clinical Pharmacist, Department of Blood and Marrow Transplant and Cellular Immunotherapy, H. Lee Moffitt Cancer Center & Research Institute, Tampa, Florida

Pukhraz Basra, MD   Hematopathology Fellow, H. Lee Moffitt Cancer Center & Research Institute, Tampa, Florida

Rachid Baz, MD   Senior Member, Director of Clinical Research, Myeloma Section Head, Department of Malignant Hematology, H. Lee Moffitt Cancer Center & Research Institute, Tampa, Florida

Celeste Bello, MD   Hematologist and Oncologist, Department of Malignant Hematology, H. Lee Moffitt Cancer Center & Research Institute, Tampa, Florida

Carmelo J. Blanquicett, MD, PhD, FACP   Fellow, Department of Hematology and Medical Oncology, H. Lee Moffitt Cancer Center & Research Institute, Tampa, Florida

Brandon Blue, MD Clinical Instructor, Department of Malignant Hematology, H. Lee Moffitt Cancer Center & Research Institute, Tampa, Florida

Brigett D. Brandjes, PA-C BMT-CI Physician Assistant, H. Lee Moffitt Cancer Center & Research Institute, Tampa, Florida

Silvia Tse Bunting, MD Director for Hematopathology and Hematology, Cleveland Clinic Florida, Weston, Florida

Liliana Bustamante, MD Hematologist & Oncologist, Florida Cancer Specialists, Fort Myers, Florida

Estelle Cervantes Medical Student, University of South Florida Morsani College of Medicine, Tampa, Florida

Onyee Chan, MD Assistant Member, Department of Malignant Hematology, H. Lee Moffitt Cancer Center & Research Institute, Tampa, Florida

Julio C. Chavez, MD Associate Professor, Department of Malignant Hematology, H. Lee Moffitt Cancer Center & Research Institute, Tampa, Florida

Jae Chung, MD Fellow, Department of Hematology/Oncology, H. Lee Moffitt Cancer Center & Research Institute, Tampa, Florida

Joseph Clara, MD Clinical Fellow, National Cancer Institute, National Heart, Lung, and Blood Institute, Bethesda, Maryland

Marco L. Davila, MD, PhD Associate Member, Department of Blood and Marrow Transplant and Cellular Immunotherapy, H. Lee Moffitt Cancer Center & Research Institute, Tampa, Florida

Jonathan R. Day, MD, PharmD Department of Internal Medicine, University of Iowa, Iowa City, Iowa; Division of Hematology/Oncology, Department of Internal Medicine, Simmons Cancer Institute at SIU School of Medicine, Springfield, Illinois

Poorvi Desai, MD Fellow, Department of Hematology/Oncology, H. Lee Moffitt Cancer Center & Research Institute, University of South Florida, Tampa, Florida

Ruchi Desai, MD Assistant Professor, Division of Hematology, Oncology, and Palliative Care, Virginia Commonwealth University Medical Center, Massey Cancer Center, Richmond, Virginia

Yehuda Deutsch, MD Assistant Member, Department of Malignant Hematology and Cellular Therapy, Moffitt Cancer Center at Memorial Healthcare System, Pembroke Pines, Florida

Hilda Ding, MD, MS   Physician, Assistant Clinical Professor, Department of Pediatric Hematology Oncology, University of California San Diego, Rady Children's Hospital, San Diego, California

Ning Dong, MD MS   Clinical Fellow, Department of Hematology and Oncology, H. Lee Moffitt Cancer Center & Research Institute, Tampa, Florida

Narendranath Epperla, MD, MS   Assistant Professor of Medicine, Division of Hematology, Department of Internal Medicine, The Ohio State University, Columbus, Ohio

Jennifer Eatrides, MD   Assistant Member, Department of Hematology and Oncology, H. Lee Moffitt Cancer Center & Research Institute, Tampa, Florida

Karen Feghali, MD, MSc   Resident, Department of Internal Medicine, St. Elizabeth's Medical Center, Boston, Massachusetts

Peter Forsyth, MD   Department Chair, Department of Neuro Oncology, H. Lee Moffitt Cancer Center & Research Institute, Tampa, Florida

Morie A. Gertz, MD   Professor of Medicine, Division of Hematology, Mayo Clinic, Rochester, Minnesota

Lucy A. Godley, MD, PhD   Professor, Section of Hematology/Oncology, Departments of Medicine and Human Genetics, The University of Chicago, Chicago, Illinois

Ruchika Goel, MD, MPH   Assistant Professor of Internal Medicine and Pediatrics, Division of Hematology/Oncology, Department of Internal Medicine, Simmons Cancer Institute at SIU School of Medicine, Springfield, Illinois; Adjunct Assistant Professor, Division of Transfusion Medicine, Department of Pathology, Johns Hopkins University, Baltimore, Maryland

Alexandra Gomez-Arteaga, MD   Assistant Professor of Medicine, Division of Hematology and Medical Oncology, Weill Cornell Medicine, New York, New York

Kristen Gonter-Aubin, DO   Fellow, Department of Hematology and Oncology, H. Lee Moffitt Cancer Center & Research Institute, Tampa, Florida

Ariel Grajales-Cruz, MD   Fellow, Department of Malignant Hematology, H. Lee Moffitt Cancer Center & Research Institute, Tampa, Florida

Patrick Griffin, MD   Physician, Hematology and Medical Oncology, Texas Oncology, Fort Worth, Texas

Mintallah Haider, MD Attending Physician, Department of Hematology/
Medical Oncology, H. Lee Moffitt Cancer Center & Research Institute,
Tampa, Florida

Walter Hanel, MD, PhD Fellow, Division of Hematology/Oncology,
Department of Internal Medicine, The Ohio State University,
Columbus, Ohio

Anthony M. Hunter, MD Hematology and Medical Oncology Fellow,
H. Lee Moffitt Cancer Center & Research Institute, Tampa, Florida

Michael Jaglal, MD Attending Physician, Department of Hematology/
Medical Oncology, H. Lee Moffitt Cancer Center & Research Institute,
Tampa, Florida

Michael D. Jain, MD, PhD Assistant Member, Department of Blood and
Marrow Transplant and Cellular Immunotherapy, H. Lee Moffitt Cancer
Center & Research Institute, Tampa, Florida

Arun Kadamkulam Syriac, MD Fellow, Division of Hematology-
Oncology, St. Elizabeth's Medical Center, Boston, Massachusetts

Jori Kaplan, MD Fellow, Department of Hematology/Oncology,
H. Lee Moffitt Cancer Center & Research Institute, Tampa, Florida

Mohamed A. Kharfan-Dabaja, MD Professor of Medicine,
Vice-Chair, Division of Hematology/Oncology, Mayo Clinic Florida,
Jacksonville, Florida

Rami Komrokji, MD Senior Member, Department of Malignant
Hematology, H. Lee Moffitt Cancer Center & Research Institute,
Tampa, Florida

Sophia C. Korotev Undergraduate Student, Section of Hematology/
Oncology, Department of Medicine, The University of Chicago,
Chicago, Illinois

Taxiarchis Kourelis, MD Assistant Professor of Medicine, Division of
Hematology, Mayo Clinic, Rochester, Minnesota

Ravitharan Krishnadasan, MD Associate Professor, Department of
Medicine, University of Arizona Cancer Center, Tucson, Arizona

Abhijeet Kumar, MD Assistant Professor, Division of Hematology
Oncology, University of Arizona Cancer Center, Tucson, Arizona

Tony Kurian, MD Fellow, Department of Hematology & Oncology,
H. Lee Moffitt Cancer Center & Research Institute, University of South
Florida, Tampa, Florida

Andrew Kuykendall, MD   Assistant Member, Department of Malignant Hematology, H. Lee Moffitt Cancer Center & Research Institute, Tampa, Florida

Jeffrey E. Lancet, MD   Senior Member, Chair, Department of Malignant Hematology, H. Lee Moffitt Cancer Center & Research Institute, Tampa, Florida

Andrew A. Lane, MD, PhD   Associate Professor, Department of Medical Oncology, Dana-Farber Cancer Institute, Harvard Medical School, Boston, Massachusetts

Dasom Caroline Lee, MD   Resident Physician, Department of Internal Medicine, University of South Florida, Tampa, Florida

Frederick L. Locke   Vice Chair and Associate Member, Department of Blood and Marrow Transplant and Cellular Immunotherapy, Co-Leader Moffitt Immunology Program, H. Lee Moffitt Cancer Center & Research Institute, Tampa, Florida

Jennifer M. Logue, MD   Fellow, Department of Hematology and Oncology, H. Lee Moffitt Cancer Center & Research Institute, Tampa, Florida

Keri Maher, DO, MS   Assistant Professor, Department of Medicine, University of Arizona Cancer Center, Tucson, Arizona

Shonali Midha, MD   Fellow, Department of Hematology and Oncology, H Lee Moffitt Cancer Center & Research Institute, Tampa, Florida

Yenny Alejandra Moreno Vanegas, MD   Resident, Internal Medicine, St. Elizabeth's Medical Center, Boston, Massachusetts

Nikhil Mukhi, MD   Attending Physician, Saint Francis Cancer Center, Tulsa, Oklahoma

Hemant S. Murthy, MD   Assistant Professor of Medicine, Division of Hematology/Oncology, Mayo Clinic Florida, Jacksonville, Florida

Anju Nair, MD   Oncologist/Hematologist, Texas Oncology, Dallas, Texas

Danny Nguyen, MD   Physician, Pacific Shores Medical Group, Long Beach, California

Taiga Nishihori, MD Associate Member, Department of Blood & Marrow Transplantation and Cellular Immunotherapy, H. Lee Moffitt Cancer Center & Research Institute, University of South Florida, Tampa, Florida

Eric Padron, MD Scientific Director, Associate Member, Department of Malignant Hematology, H. Lee Moffitt Cancer Center & Research Institute, University of South Florida, Tampa, Florida

Vania Phuoc, MD Assistant Member, Department of Medical Oncology, H. Lee Moffitt Cancer Center & Research Institute, Tampa, Florida

Javier Pinilla-Ibarz, MD, PhD Senior Member, Department of Malignant Hematology, H. Lee Moffitt Cancer Center & Research Institute, Tampa, Florida

Cristian I. Rodriguez Arocho, MD Fellow, Department of Blood and Marrow Transplantation and Cellular Immunotherapy, H. Lee Moffitt Cancer Center & Research Institute, Tampa, Florida

Hayder Saeed, MD Assistant Member, Department of Malignant Hematology, H. Lee Moffitt Cancer Center & Research Institute; Assistant Professor, Department of Oncologic Sciences, University of South Florida, Tampa, Florida

Solmaz Sahebjam, MD Leader Moffitt Phase 1 Program, Director of Clinical Research Unit, H. Lee Moffitt Cancer Center & Research Institute, Tampa, Florida

Andreas Saltos, MD Assistant Member, Department of Thoracic Oncology, H. Lee Moffitt Cancer Center & Research Institute, Tampa, Florida

Jose D. Sandoval-Sus, MD, FACP Assistant Member, Department of Malignant Hematology and Cellular therapy, Moffitt Cancer Center at Memorial Healthcare System, Pembroke Pines, Florida

Muhammad Sardar, MD Resident, College of Medicine, University of Arizona, Tucson, Arizona

Bijal Shah, MD, MS Associate Professor, Department of Malignant Hematology, H. Lee Moffitt Cancer Center & Research Institute, Tampa, Florida

Nikesh N. Shah, MD Fellow, Department of Hematology/Oncology, H. Lee Moffitt Cancer Center & Research Institute, Tampa, Florida

Haipeng Shao, MD, PhD Assistant Member, Department of Hematopathology and Laboratory Medicine, H. Lee Moffitt Cancer Center & Research Institute, Tampa, Florida

Rohit Sharma, MD Fellow, Department of Pathology, Memorial Sloan Kettering Cancer Center, New York, New York

Misty Dawn Shields, MD, PhD Fellow, Department of Hematology/Oncology, H. Lee Moffitt Cancer Center & Research Institute, Tampa, Florida

Lubomir Sokol, MD, PhD Senior Member, Leader, T-Cell Lymphoma/Leukemia Program, Department of Malignant Hematology, H. Lee Moffitt Cancer Center & Research Institute; Professor, Department of Oncologic Sciences, University of South Florida, Tampa, Florida

Kendra Sweet, MD Associate Member, Department of Malignant Hematology, H. Lee Moffitt Cancer Center & Research Institute, Tampa, Florida

David M. Swoboda, MD Hematology/Oncology Fellow, Department of Hematology and Oncology, H. Lee Moffitt Cancer Center & Research Institute, Tampa, Florida

Chetasi Talati, MD Assistant Member, Department of Malignant Hematology, H. Lee Moffitt Cancer Center & Research Institute, Tampa, Florida

Justin Taylor, MD Assistant Professor, Division of Hematology, Department of Medicine, Sylvester Comprehensive Cancer Center, University of Miami Miller School of Medicine, Miami, Florida

Nishan Tchekmedyian, MD Medical Director, Pacific Shores Medical Group, Huntington Beach, California

Amy M. Trottier, MD, MSc Assistant Professor, Division of Hematology, Department of Medicine, QEII Health Sciences Centre, Dalhousie University, Halifax, Nova Scotia, Canada

Magali Van den Bergh, MD Oncologist, Florida Cancer Specialist, Fort Myers, Florida

Fernando Vargas, MD Assistant Member, Department of Malignant Hematology and Cellular Therapy, Moffitt Cancer Center at Memorial Healthcare System, Pembroke Pines, Florida

Ljiljana V. Vasovic, MD Assistant Professor of Pathology and Laboratory Medicine, Department of Pathology, New York-Presbyterian Hospital, Weill Cornell Medical College, New York, New York

Virginia O. Volpe, MD Hematology/Oncology Fellow, Department of Hematology Oncology, H. Lee Moffitt Cancer Center & Research Institute, Tampa, Florida

Emilie Wang, MD   Hematology/Oncology Fellow, Department of Malignant Hematology, H. Lee Moffitt Cancer Center & Research Institute, Tampa, Florida

Justin M. Watts, MD   Assistant Professor of Medicine, University of Miami, Miami, Florida

Seongseok Yun, MD, PhD   Assistant Member, Department of Malignant Hematology, H. Lee Moffitt Cancer Center & Research Institute, Tampa, Florida

Pei Zhang, MD   Fellow, Division of Hematology Oncology, University of Arizona Cancer Center, Tucson, Arizona

Kenneth S. Zuckerman, MD   Senior Member Emeritus, Department of Malignant Hematology, H. Lee Moffitt Cancer Center & Research Institute, Tampa, Florida

Preface

Hematologic malignancies and their treatment have witnessed many changes in this past decade. Innovations from improved diagnostics to therapeutics have reshaped the ways in which these diseases are characterized and managed. The advent of molecular techniques, such as next-generation sequencing, has brought forth a paradigm shift not only in regard to diagnosis but also in refining prognostication, monitoring residual disease burden, and identifying novel therapeutic strategies. Now more than ever before, we as clinicians are able to apply mutational data to individualize treatment strategies through access to novel pharmaceuticals and clinical trials for patients who previously had limited options. As medical professionals, these are a few of the important clinical questions we would often discuss with fellow trainees, nurse practitioners, physician assistants, attending physicians, and pharmacists at Moffitt Cancer Center. These discussions served as the backbone to the creation of this handbook.

Our goal was to create a pocket-sized practical guide that could be used by trainees in malignant hematology, internal medicine, and pathology as well as pharmacists, advanced practice professionals, and attending physicians not only to provide the basic information on diagnosis and treatment but to go a step beyond what previous resource books have offered. This resource highlights critical differential diagnoses to consider as well as provides the most current prognostication tables for each disease in order to facilitate direct extension of this information to your patients. In addition, we have included full-color pathology images that have been selected for their exceptional clarity to help the reader elucidate subtle morphologic differences between disease entities. We have created relevant clinical cases not only in the book but also in accessible online cases. A benefit of these online cases is that the reader can test the unknown and try to diagnose cases before referring to the text (in order to do so, the reader is encouraged to view the supplemental online cases by accessing them at https://connect.springerpub.com/content/book/978-0-8261-4977-0). Together, these resources represent an innovative design in board preparation for practitioners in hematologic malignancies. Evidence-based algorithms guiding treatment recommendations are provided for both frontline and salvage settings, with key references supporting each recommendation. Our intention was to create a reference textbook that is concise and easy to read, serving the needs of the medical professional dealing with hematologic malignancies. We also highlight current clinical trials that may alter our future practice decisions. Notably, in this second edition, we have not only provided major updates and insight into future practice-changing clinical trials but added numerous chapters, particularly those focused on novel cellular immunotherapy, which has been the most exciting revolution in the clinical care of patients with hematologic malignancies.

The second edition of *Handbook of Hematologic Malignancies* encompasses the hard work and effort of many fellows and residents, working under the mentorship and guidance of attending staff physicians at world-renowned cancer centers throughout the country, not only Moffitt Cancer Center but also many others, including Harvard, Mayo Clinic, and Memorial Sloan Kettering Cancer Center. Specifically, the editors would like acknowledge Dr. Kenian Liu from the Cytogenetic Laboratory (Moffitt) for providing FISH images and Drs. Lugen Chen (Tampa General Hospital), Wilfredo Chamizo (All Children Hospital at St. Petersburg), Haipeng Shao (Moffitt), Xiaohui Zhang (Moffitt), and Jane Messina (Moffitt) for sharing unique cases in the book. The quality of their work and their willingness to contribute to make this textbook one that can serve the needs of readers across disciplines made working on this project a rewarding experience for us all.

Lastly, this textbook would not have been realized without the tireless commitment and outstanding contributions of our entire clinical and pathology editorial team. Drs. David Sallman and Ateefa Chaudhury directed the innovational chapter design and gave editorial oversight throughout the completion of this product. The high-quality images produced by Drs. Ling Zhang and Johnny Nguyen were critical to the exceptional hematopathology content. Moreover, we would like to give thanks to Dr. Alan List, who has been a world leader in the fight against hematologic malignancy. His passion to prevent and cure cancer through collaborative research was instrumental in the design and concept of the first edition. Our editorial team and chapter authors truly hope that this handbook helps improve your understanding of hematologic malignancies and enhances your approach to patient care.

David A. Sallman, MD
Ateefa Chaudhury, MD
Johnny Nguyen, MD
Ling Zhang, MD

Abbreviations

aCML	Atypical Chronic Myelogenous Leukemia
AFB Stain	Acid-Fast Bacilli Stain
AIDS	Acquired Immunodeficiency Syndrome
AITL	Angioimmunoblastic T-Cell Lymphoma
ALCL	Anaplastic Large Cell Lymphoma
ALK	Anaplastic Lymphoma Kinase
ALP	Alkaline Phosphatase
ALT	Alanine Transaminase
AML	Acute Myeloid Leukemia
AMML	Acute Myelomonocytic Leukemia
ANC	Absolute Neutrophil Count
APL	Acute Promyelocytic Leukemia
AST	Aspartate Transaminase
ATLL	Adult T-Cell Leukemia/Lymphoma
B-ALL	B-Acute Lymphoblastic Leukemia
BM	Bone Marrow
BMT	Bone Marrow Transplant
BMP	Basic Metabolic Panel
BPDCN	Blastic Plasmacytoid Dendritic Cell Neoplasm
BSA	Body Surface Area
BX	Biopsy
CBC	Complete Blood Count
CCUS	Clonal Cytopenia of Undetermined Significance
CD	Cluster of Differentiation
CHIP	Clonal Hematopoiesis of Indeterminate Potential
CHL	Classical Hodgkin Lymphoma
CLL/SLL	Chronic Lymphocytic Leukemia/Small Lymphocytic Lymphoma
CML	Chronic Myelogenous Leukemia
CMML	Chronic Myelomonocytic Leukemia
CMP	Complete Metabolic Panel
CNL	Chronic Neutrophilic Leukemia
CNS	Central Nervous System
Cr	Creatinine
CR	Complete Response
CRi	Complete Remission With Incomplete Blood Count Recovery
CRP	C Reactive Protein
CSF	Cerebrospinal Fluid

CT Scan	Computerized (or Computed) Tomography Scan
CTX	Chemotherapy
Del(5q)	Deletion of 5q
DFS	Disease-Free Survival
DIC	Disseminated Intravascular Coagulopathy
Diff	Differential
DLBCL	Diffuse Large B-Cell Lymphoma
DVT	Deep Vein Thrombosis
EBV	Epstein–Barr Virus
EBER	Epstein–Barr Virus Encoded RNA
eGFR	Estimated Glomerular Filtration Rate
EMH	Extramedullary Hematopoiesis
ESR	Erythrocyte Sedimentation Rate
ET	Essential Thrombocythemia
FDC	Follicular Dendritic Cell
FGFR1	Fibroblast Growth Factor Receptor 1
FISH	Fluorescence In Situ Hybridization
FL	Follicular Lymphoma
FNA	Fine Needle Aspirate
GI	Gastrointestinal
GMS	Grocott-Gomori's Methenamine Silver Stain
H&E	Hematoxylin and Eosin
HCL	Hairy Cell Leukemia
HCT	Hematopoietic Cell Transplantation
HGB	Hemoglobin
HGBL	High-Grade B-Cell Lymphoma
HHV8	Human Herpes Virus 8
HIV	Human Immunodeficiency Virus
HL	Hodgkin Lymphoma
HLH	Hemophagocytic Lymphohistiocytosis
HRS	Hodgkin Reed-Sternberg Cells
HSCT	Hematopoietic Stem Cell Transplantation
HSTCL	Hepatosplenic T-Cell Lymphoma
I-PIG	International PNH Interest Group
ICUS	Idiopathic Cytopenia of Undetermined Significance
IHC	Immunohistochemistry
INR	International Normalized Ratio
IOL	Intraocular Lymphoma
IPI	Internal Prognostic Index
IPS	International Prognostic Score
IPSS	International Prognostic Scoring System
ISCL	International Society for Cutaneous Lymphomas
ISH	In Situ Hybridization
ISM	Indolent Systemic Mastocytosis
ISRT	Involved Site Radiation Therapy
ISSWM	International Prognostic Scoring System for WM
IST	Immunosuppressive therapy
IT	Intrathecal
ITP	Immune Thrombocytopenic Purpura

IVIG	Intravenous Immunoglobulin
JMML	Juvenile Myelomonocytic Leukemia
KPI	Korean Prognostic Index
LBCL	Large B-Cell Lymphoma
LCH	Langerhans Cell Histiocytosis
LDH	Lactate Dehydrogenase
LDHL	Lymphocyte Depleted cHL
LFT	Liver Function Test
LGL	Large Granular Lymphocyte
LN	Lymph Node
LOH	Loss of Heterozygosity
LP	Lymphocyte Predominant
LPD	Lymphoproliferative Disorder
LPL	Lymphoplasmacytic Lymphoma
M-Spike	Monoclonal Spike
MALT	Mucosa-Associated Lymphoid Tissue
MCL	Mantle Cell Lymphoma
MCV	Mean Cell Volume
MDS	Myelodysplastic Syndromes
MDS/MPN	Myelodysplastic/Myeloproliferative Neoplasm
MDS-U	Myelodysplastic Syndrome, Unclassifiable
MF	Mycosis Fungoides
MGUS	Monoclonal Gammopathy of Undetermined Significance
MLL	Mixed Lineage Leukemia
MM	Multiple Myeloma (Plasma Cell Myeloma)
MMUD	Mismatched Unrelated Donor
MPAL	Mixed Phenotype Acute Leukemia
MPD	Myeloproliferative Disorders
MPN	Myeloproliferative Neoplasms
MPO	Myeloperoxidase
MR	Minor Response
MRD	Minimal Residual Disease; Matched Related Donor
mTOR	Mammalian Target of Rapamycin
MTX	Methotrexate
MUD	Matched Unrelated Donor
MUGA Scan	Multigated Acquisition Scan
MZL	Marginal Zone Lymphoma
NCCN	National Comprehensive Cancer Network
NCI	National Cancer Institute
NF-κB	Nuclear Factor-κB
NGS	Next-Generation Sequencing
NHL	Non-Hodgkin Lymphoma
NK	Natural Killer
NKPI	NK-/T-Cell Lymphoma Prognostic Index
NLPHL	Nodular Lymphocyte Predominant Hodgkin Lymphoma
NMZL	Nodal Marginal Zone Lymphoma
NOS	Not Otherwise Specified
OS	Overall Survival

PAS Stain	Periodic Acid–Schiff–Diastase Stain
PB	Peripheral Blood
PBL	Plasmablastic Lymphoma
PBS	Peripheral Blood Smear
PCR	Polymerase Chain Reaction
PDGFRA	Platelet-Derived Growth Factor Receptor, Alpha
PDGFRB	Platelet-Derived Growth Factor Receptor, Beta
PET/CT	Positron Emission Tomography/Computed Tomography
PFS	Progression-Free Survival
Ph+	Philadelphia Chromosome Positive
PIT	Prognostic Index for T-Cell
PLT	Platelet
PMBL	Primary Mediastinal B-Cell Lymphoma
PMF	Primary Myelofibrosis
PMLBCL	Primary Mediastinal Large B-Cell Lymphoma
PNH	Paroxysmal Nocturnal Hemoglobinuria
PR	Partial Response
PS	Performance Status
PT	Prothrombin Time
PTCL	Peripheral T-Cell Lymphoma
PTGC	Progressive Transformation of Germinal Centers
PTLD	Post-Transplant Lymphoproliferative Disorder
PTT	Partial Thromboplastin Time
PUVA	Psoralen-UV-A
PV	Plasma Volume; Polycythemia Vera
RA	Refractory Anemia (MDS Subtype)
RAEB	Refractory Anemia With Excess Blasts (MDS Subtype)
RARS	Refractory Anemia With Ring Sideroblasts (MDS Subtype)
RBC	Red Blood Cell
RCMD	Refractory Cytopenia With Multilineage Dysplasia (MDS Subtype)
RCMD-RS	Refractory Cytopenia With Multilineage Dysplasia and Ring Sideroblasts (MDS Subtype)
RS	Ring Sideroblasts
SM	Systemic Mastocytosis
SM-AHN	Systemic Mastocytosis With an Associated Hematologic Neoplasm (Formerly SM-AHNMD—Systemic Mastocytosis With Associated Hematologic Non-Mast Cell Lineage Disease)
SMZL	Splenic Marginal Zone Lymphoma
SVT	Superficial Venous Thrombosis
T-ALL	T-Lymphoblastic Leukemia
t-AML	Therapy-Related Acute Myeloid Leukemia
T-LBL	T-Lymphoblastic Lymphoma
t-MDS	Therapy-Related Myelodysplastic Syndrome
t-MN	Therapy-Related Myeloid Neoplasms
T-PLL	T-Cell Prolymphocytic Leukemia

TdT	Terminal Deoxynucleotidyl Transferase
THRLBCL	T-Cell/Histiocyte Rich Large B-Cell Lymphoma
TTP	Thrombotic Thrombocytopenic Purpura
VTE	Venous Thromboembolism
XRT	Radiation Therapy
WBC	White Blood Cell
WHO	World Health Organization
WM	Waldenström Macroglobulinemia

1

Normal Hematopoiesis and Diagnosis Algorithms for Cytopenias and Cytoses

Onyee Chan and Ling Zhang

▪ NORMAL HEMATOPOIESIS

ORIGINS OF HEMATOPOIETIC CELLS AND EMBRYOGENESIS

Hematopoiesis is the formation of blood cellular components that are critical for oxygen delivery, coagulation, and immune responses in our bodies.[1] Blood development initially involves the primitive wave in which erythroid progenitors give rise to erythrocytes in the yolk sac to match the high oxygen demand of the rapidly growing embryo.[2] This transitory wave is replaced by definitive hematopoiesis, leading to the creation of hematopoietic stem cells (HSCs) first found in the aorta-gonad-mesonephros (AGM) region at 4 to 6 weeks of gestation. HSCs are multipotent and capable of differentiating into any hematopoietic cell lineages to replenish the entire blood system. During mid-gestation (8–28 weeks), the liver and spleen become the dominant sites of hematopoiesis as a result of HSCs' migration. Around the end of gestation, HSCs start to take up residence in the bone marrow (BM) of most of the bones through an active process that relies on its C-X-C chemokine receptor type 4 (CXCR4) receptors.[2] Hematopoiesis later concentrates in the BM of the axial skeleton, pelvis, and proximal femur as development progresses into adulthood.[2] Table 1.1 summarizes the location and timing of hematopoiesis.

HEMATOPOIETIC STEM CELLS AND THE RISE OF DIFFERENT BLOOD CELLS

HSCs are pluripotent undifferentiated cells that are capable of self-renewal. A small subset of HSCs, so-called high quality, is largely quiescent and rarely recruited into the cell cycle, which may contribute to its resistance to chemotherapy. In contrast, low-quality HSCs are slightly more differentiated and responsible for normal waves of hematopoiesis and are usually sensitive to cytotoxic therapies.[1] Farther down the continuum are hematopoietic progenitor cells (HPCs), giving rise to various cell types with different degrees of self-renewal and differentiation potential. As HPCs mature toward the precursor level, they become less capable of self-renewal and more committed to a specific lineage. Myelopoiesis occurs in the BM and is associated with the production of myeloid precursors;

Table 1.1 Sites and Timing of Hematopoiesis[2]

Time of Development	Site of Hematopoiesis
0–8 weeks of gestation	Yolk sac
4–6 weeks of gestation	AGM
8–28 weeks of gestation	Liver, spleen
20–36 weeks of gestation	BM (all bones)
Childhood	BM (most medullary space, including sternum, skull, and ribs)
Adult	BM (mainly axial skeleton, pelvis, and proximal femur)

AGM, aorta-gonad-mesonephros region; BM, bone marrow.

however, more generically, it includes erythropoiesis, granulopoiesis, and megakaryopoiesis. Early lymphopoiesis also occurs in the BM, but the lymphoid precursors later migrate to the thymus (T-cells) and peripheral lymph nodes (B-cells) for maturation. Figure 1.1 illustrates the hierarchy of hematopoiesis.

Normal Hematopoiesis

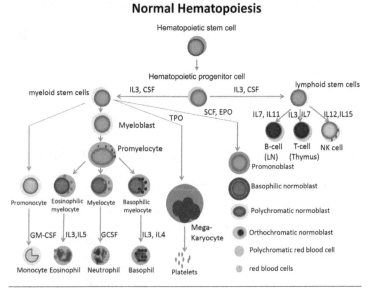

Figure 1.1 Hematopoiesis.

CSF, colony-stimulating factor; EPO, erythropoietin; G-CSF, granulocyte colony- stimulating factor; GM-CSF, granulocyte-monocyte colony-stimulating factor; IL, interleukin; LN, lymph node; SCF, stem cell factor; TPO, thrombopoietin.

Table 1.2 Natural Growth Factors and Recombinants in Hematopoiesis

Growth Factor	Source of Production	Target Cells
G-CSF – Filgrastim (Neupogen) Pegfilgrastim (Neulasta)	MSCs	Granulocytes
GM-CSF – Sargramostim (Leukine) – Molgramostim (Leucomax)	MSCs	Granulocytes, Macrophages
– Erythropoietin, epoetin alfa (Procrit, Epogen) – Darbepoetin (Aranesp)	Adult – kidney Fetus/Perinatal – liver	Erythrocyte progenitors
Thrombopoietin – Romiplostim (Nplate) – Eltrombopag (Promacta)	Liver, kidney, MSCs	Megakaryocyte progenitors

G-CSF, granulocyte–colony-stimulating factor; GM-CSF, granulocyte–macrophage–colony-stimulating factor; MSC, marrow stromal cells.

GROWTH FACTORS INVOLVED IN HEMATOPOIESIS

Of note, stromal cells in BM can produce growth factors and extracellular matrix proteins to help promote growth and tether the HSCs/HPCs while HSCs/HPCs express CXCR4 receptors, which is crucial for anchoring. These hematopoietic precursors can stay inside BM and sometimes mobilize out of BM into the systemic circulation, depending on hematopoietic stress. Armed with this understanding, it is intuitive to see why combining hematopoietic growth factors, such as granulocyte–colony-stimulating factor (G-CSF) (for mobilization) and plerixafor (a CXCR4 inhibitor), would be an effective strategy for stem-cell collection (*J Clin Oncol.* 2009;27(28):4767–4773). Besides targeting the granulocytes, there are other growth factors that can be given to target erythroid and megakaryocytic progenitors with clinical implications. Table 1.2 summarizes the major types of natural growth factors and their recombinants in hematopoiesis.

▓ CYTOPENIAS

Cytopenia is characterized by one or more cell lines being lower than normal. Depending on the etiology, it can be isolated to one cell line, such as leukopenia (low white blood count), anemia (low hemoglobin or hematocrit), or thrombocytopenia (low platelets). The differential for each of the single-lineage cytopenia is too extensive to be fully discussed herein. Table 1.3 summarizes the most common etiologies leading to isolated anemia, leukopenia, and thrombocytopenia.

Table 1.3 Etiology of Cytopenia

	Etiology		
	Impaired Production	**Peripheral Destruction/ Consumption**	**Others**
Anemia • (Normal reference range: for adult female, Hgb 12.0–15.5 g/dL; for adult male, 13.5–17.5 g/dL)	• Iron deficiency, vitamin B12/folate deficiency, hemoglobinopathy/ RBC membrane disorders, chronic renal failure, BM failure (inherited or acquired), or occupied disorders	• Bleeding, hemolysis (intrinsic or extratrinsic)	• Anemia of chronic disease, autoimmune disorders
Leukopenia • (Normal reference range: 4.5 × 10⁹/L to 11.0 × 10⁹/L)	• Cytoreduction • Iatogenic induced marrow suppression (e.g., ionizing radiation) • BM failure (inherited or acquired) or occupied disorders	• Drugs induced • Physical stress	• Infection • Autoim- mune • Stress • Unknown
Thrombocyto- penia • (Normal reference range: 150 × 10⁹/L to 450 × 10⁹/L)	• Iatogenic induced marrow suppression • BM failure (inherited or acquired) or occupied disorders	• Drugs • HIT • TTP • HELLP • Hypersplen- ism/liver cirrhosis	• Infection • Autoim- mune

HELLP, a syndrome consisting of hemolysis, elevated liver enzymes, and a low platelet count during pregnancy; HIT, heparin-induced thrombocytopenia; TTP, thrombotic thrombocytopenic purpura.

Note that for all reference ranges, there may be slight variation, depending on the laboratory.

In this section, we instead focus on the common and more critical problem of pancytopenia, which occurs when all three cell lines are low. The causes of pancytopenia can be broadly divided into three categories: impaired production, peripheral destruction, and combination of the two.[3] Some of the conditions related to impaired production leading to pancytopenia, such as aplastic anemia, could be congenital or acquired. Others are strictly congenital, including Fanconi's anemia, dyskeratosis congenita, Shwachman-Diamond syndrome, and amegakaryocytic thrombocytopenia.[3] Nutritional

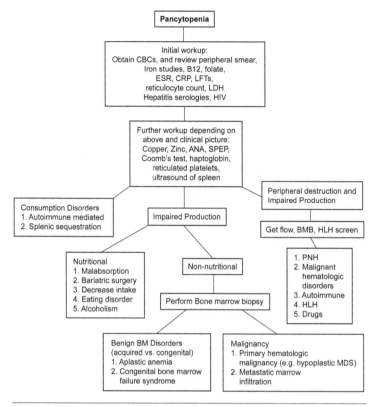

Figure 1.2 Diagnostic Algorithm for Pancytopenia.
ANA, antinuclear antibodies; BM, bone marrow; BMB, bone marrow biopsy; CRP, c-reactive protein; ESR, erythrocyte sedimentation rate; HIV, human immunodeficiency virus; HLH, hemophagocytic lymphohistiocytosis; LDH, lactate dehydrogenase; LFT, liver function tests; MDS, myelodysplastic syndrome; PNH, paroxysmal nocturnal hemoglobinuria; SPEP, serum protein electrophoresis.

deficiencies and primary or secondary BM disorders account for the majority of impaired-production etiology.[3] However, the former is more associated with lineage specific cytopenia, while the latter could often result in pancytopenia. Myelodysplastic syndrome (MDS), a clonal stem cell disease with ineffective hematopoiesis, is typically manifested by anemia and thrombocytopenia; however, pancytopenia can also occur. Recent molecular advances led to the recognition of novel entities, including idiopathic cytopenia of undetermined significance (ICUS) and clonal cytopenia of undetermined significance (CCUS), where patients with one or more unexplained cytopenias, including pancytopenia, did not meet the criteria for MDS

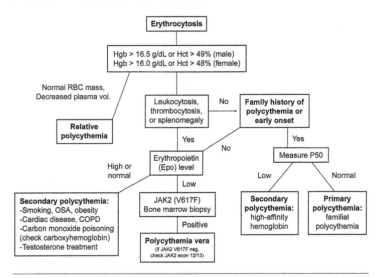

Figure 1.3 Diagnostic Algorithm for Erythrocytosis.

COPD, chronic obstructive pulmonary disease; Hct, hematocrit; Hgb, hemoglobin; OSA, obstructive sleep apnea; P50, oxygen tension at which hemoglobin is 50% saturated; RBC, red blood cell; Vol, volume.

or another hematologic disorder. Similar to ICUS, CCUS requires the presence of somatic mutations (variant allele frequency [VAF] ≥2%) of a leukemia-associated genes. The fibrotic stage of myeloproliferative neoplasms (MPN), such as primary myelofibrosis (PMF), can cause one, two, or all cell lines to be suppressed. In addition, marrow occupied by myeloma, lymphoma, and acute myeloid or lymphoblastic leukemias can all result in pancytopenia. Details of these primary BM malignancies are described in subsequent chapters. Furthermore, BM diffuse infiltration by solid tumor metastases or granulomatous diseases often causes pancytopenia. Another common cause of pancytopenia is peripheral destruction, usually from autoimmune-mediated diseases or splenic sequestration. Congenital conditions include common variable immunodeficiency disease (CVID), autoimmune neutropenia (AIN), and autoimmune lymphoproliferative syndrome (ALPS). The latter is a non-malignant condition, in which there is an uncontrolled proliferation of lymphocytes due to an overactive immune system, frequently caused by mutation of the Fas cell surface death receptor (*FAS*) gene. Besides autoimmune diseases, hypersplenism, which has many etiologies, including cirrhosis and congestive heart failure, can lead to pancytopenia via splenic sequestration. Figure 1.2 summarizes the differential diagnosis and diagnostic algorithm for evaluating patients with pancytopenia.

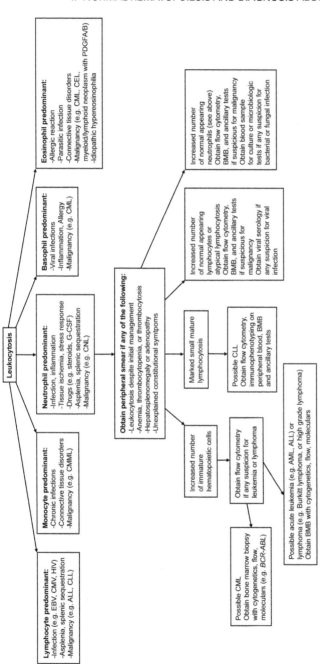

Figure 1.4 Diagnostic Algorithm for Leukocytosis. Adapted from Davis AS, Viera AJ, Mead MD. Leukemia: an overview for primary care. *Am Fam Physician.* 2014;89(9):731–738. e-pub ahead of print 2014/05/03.

AML, acute myeloid leukemia; ALL, acute lymphoblastic leukemia; BMB, bone marrow biopsy; CEL, chronic eosinophilic leukemia; CML, chronic myeloid leukemia; CMML, chronic myelomonocytic leukemia; CMV, cytomegalovirus; CLL, chronic lymphocytic leukemia; CNL, chronic neutrophilic leukemia; EBV, Epstein–Barr virus, G-CSF, granulocyte–colony–stimulating factor; HIV, human immunodeficiency virus; PDGFA/B, platelet-derived growth factor receptor alpha or beta.

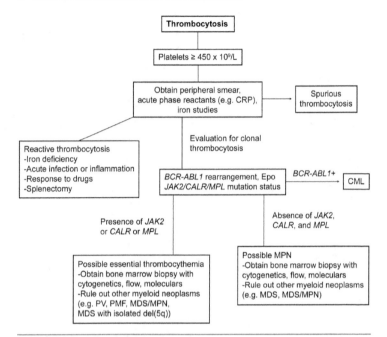

Figure 1.5 Diagnostic Algorithm for Thrombocytosis. Adapted from Rumi E, Cazzola M. How I treat essential thrombocythemia. *Blood.* 2016;128(20):2403–2414. Epub ahead of print 2016/08/27; doi: 10.1182/blood-2016-05-643346.

CML, chronic myeloid leukemia; CRP, c-reactive protein; EPO, erythropoietin; MDS, myelodysplastic syndromes; MPN, myeloproliferative neoplasms; PMF, primary myelofibrosis; PV, polycythemia vera.

▪ CYTOSES

Cytosis is an abnormal increase in the number of a specified type of cells. Erythrocytosis is defined as an increase in red cell mass. Polycythemia, sometimes used interchangeably with erythrocytosis, refers to an increase in red blood cells, hemoglobin, or hematocrit. The three major classes of erythrocytosis are primary, secondary, and relative polycythemia. Figure 1.3 summarizes the differential diagnosis and diagnostic algorithm for evaluating patients with erythrocytosis (*Int J Lab Hematol.* 2019;41 Suppl 1:142–150).

Leukocytosis is defined as an increase in white blood cells counts (normal range 4.5 × 10⁹/L to 11.0 × 10⁹/L for adult; note that there may be slight variation, depending on the laboratory). The predominant subtype (i.e., lymphocyte, monocyte, neutrophil, eosinophil, and basophil) helps guide diagnosis. In general, leukocytosis can be divided into primary/neoplastic and reactive. Figure 1.4 summarizes the differential diagnosis and diagnostic algorithm for evaluating patients with leukocytosis.[4]

Thrombocytosis is defined as an increase in platelet counts (normal range 150 × 10⁹/L to 450 × 10⁹/L). The most common cause is reactive (also known as secondary) from such conditions as iron deficiency, infection, and inflammation. Primary causes include a number of clonal myeloid neoplasms. Figure 1.5 summarizes the differential diagnosis and diagnostic algorithm for evaluating patients with thrombocytosis.[5]

■ CONCLUSION

Knowledge of normal hematopoiesis provides the foundation for understanding many of the disorders occurring in the BM, generally manifesting as cytopenia or cytosis. Pancytopenia can be caused by impair production, peripheral destruction, or both. Cytosis can be thought of as primary versus secondary. Taking a careful history and performing a physical along with appropriate testing are essential to make the correct diagnosis.

■ REFERENCES FOR SUPPLEMENTAL READING

1. Ghiaur G, Jones RJ. *Hematopoiesis*, 2nd ed. Springer Nature; 2019.

2. Jagannathan-Bogdan M, Zon LI. Hematopoiesis. *Development*. 2013; 140(12):2463–2467. Epub ahead of print 2013/05/30; doi: 10.1242/dev.083147

3. Gnanaraj J, Parnes A, Francis CW, et al. Approach to pancytopenia: diagnostic algorithm for clinical hematologists. *Blood Rev*. 2018;32(5):361–367. Epub ahead of print 2018/03/21; doi:10.1016/j.blre.2018.03.001

4. Davis AS, Viera AJ, Mead MD. Leukemia: an overview for primary care. *Am Fam Physician*. 2014;89(9):731–738. e-pub ahead of print 2014/05/03

5. Rumi E, Cazzola M. How I treat essential thrombocythemia. *Blood*. 2016; 128(20):2403–2414. Epub ahead of print 2016/08/27; doi: 10.1182/blood-2016-05-643346

2 Familial/Inherited Mutations and Risks of Hematologic Malignancies

Sophia C. Korotev, Lucy A. Godley,

and Amy M. Trottier

▦ INTRODUCTION

Germline mutations in many genes are becoming increasingly recognized as factors that predispose to hematologic malignancies (*Blood.* 2017;130(4):424–432). However, despite the increase in recognition, such mutations and their associated germline predisposition syndromes remain underdiagnosed and underreported. It is important to identify patients with these syndromes, because they can present with different clinical manifestations, bone marrow morphologies, and disease courses, and they may require additional assessments and/or adjustments to their management plans (*UpToDate* (2020): Familial acute leukemia and myelodysplastic syndromes). Depending on the particular gene involved, patients with germline predisposition may also be susceptible to solid cancers as well as organ and immune system dysfunctions. The latest World Health Organization (WHO) classification of hematologic malignancies includes a chapter that recognizes germline predisposition to myeloid malignancies (*IARC.* 2017;121–128), although there is emerging evidence for inherited susceptibility to lymphoid malignancies as well. For this handbook, we confine our remaining discussion to those patients with predisposition syndromes that increase risk for myeloid malignancies. These are divided into three categories within the WHO classification scheme: those without a preexisting disorder (e.g., *CEBPA* or *DDX41* mutations), those with preexisting thrombocytopenia (e.g., *RUNX1*, *ANKRD26*, or *ETV6* mutations), and those with other organ dysfunctions, such as myeloid neoplasms associated with bone marrow failure syndromes, telomere biology disorders, and immunodeficiency syndromes, as seen in *GATA2* deficiency.

▦ DIAGNOSIS

All patients diagnosed with a hematopoietic malignancy should be evaluated for a germline predisposition syndrome. Criteria that raise suspicion for an underlying germline predisposition mutation and should prompt further investigation include (i) a personal history of multiple cancers; (ii) a strong family history of cancer, defined as at least one additional case of hematologic malignancy and/or at least one solid tumor diagnosed earlier than at 50 years old within two generations of the proband; (iii) significantly younger age of onset than is typical for a given hematologic malignancy (i.e., diagnosis of myelodysplastic syndrome [MDS] below the age of 40); (iv) syndromic features or dysmorphology consistent with a germline predisposition syndrome; and/or (v) a deleterious mutation found in a known germline hematologic malignancy-associated gene upon molecular testing of tissue from an individual with cancer (*Blood.* 2016;128:1800–1813). Examples of syndromic features associated with a germline predisposition syndrome include pulmonary fibrosis with *TERT/TERC* mutations or lymphedema and warts seen with germline *GATA2* mutations (*Blood.* 2016;128:1800–1813). It is important to consider that although young age at diagnosis can be a red flag, diagnosis at an age typical for a particular disease does not preclude the presence of an underlying germline predisposition syndrome.

The diagnosis of a germline predisposition syndrome is confirmed through the identification of a deleterious germline mutation on genetic testing. When a patient undergoes clinical genetic testing for a germline predisposition, it is vital to avoid collection of tissues that may harbor somatic variants due to involvement with the patient's underlying disease, such as blood and bone marrow. For this reason, germline testing is commonly performed on DNA derived from cultured skin fibroblasts. Hair bulbs are another option for germline DNA isolation, although their low DNA yield can preclude some testing. Additionally, testing should be comprehensive for all types of mutations, including single nucleotide variants (SNVs) and copy number variants (CNVs), in all genes known to be associated with germline predisposition to hematologic malignancies. The American Society of Hematology is collaborating with ClinGen to develop standardized rules for the functional annotation of variants to provide consistency across laboratories in variant interpretation (*Blood Adv.* 2019;3(20):2962–2979). According to the American College of Medical Genetics and Genomics, variants can be classified as pathogenic, likely pathogenic, variant of uncertain significance, likely benign, or benign. Appropriate genetic counseling and cascade testing of relatives should be offered for patients with variants classified as pathogenic or likely pathogenic.

▓ KEY DIAGNOSTIC DILEMMA

It is important to recognize that not all patients with a germline predisposition syndrome have typical risk factors, such as a positive family history or younger age than would be expected at the time of diagnosis. A positive family history may be absent if the patient is adopted, if the family size is small, or if the inherited predisposition syndrome is caused by a *de novo* germline mutation. For example, *de novo* mutations are the most common cause of *GATA2* deficiency syndromes (*Blood.* 2016;127(11):1387–1397). Patients with mutations in certain genes, such as *DDX41*, develop MDS/leukemia at an average age of 65 years (*Int J Hematol*. 2017;106:163–174), no different than the population-based median age at diagnosis. Therefore, age cannot be used to rule out the possibility of an underlying germline predisposition.

Diagnosis can also be missed if incomplete testing is performed. Many clinical and commercial laboratories use next-generation sequencing (NGS) panels as the mainstay of testing. However, if the causative gene is not included in the panel, or if testing is only sensitive for SNV detection, such CNVs as deletion mutations will likely be missed. Selection of an appropriate and comprehensive panel that has the capabilities to detect SNVs and CNVs is essential. Table 2.1 shows a list of genes that should be incorporated if a familial workup is being completed, with the caveat that more genes are continually being discovered and may need to be included based on future research.

▓ PROGNOSIS

The penetrance of germline mutations can vary significantly, from 35% to 40% for *RUNX1* mutations to nearly 100% for pathogenic 5′-end *CEBPA* mutations (*Blood*. 2017;129(15):2070–2082, *Blood*. 2015;126(10):1214–1223). For many other germline mutations, the penetrance remains unknown.

Prognosis differs based on the particular gene that is mutated. Ten percent of acute myeloid leukemia (AML) patients with bi-allelic *CEBPA* mutations are found to have a germline variant as one of the mutations, typically the 5′-end mutation (*J Clin Oncol*. 2008;26(31):5088–5093). The second allele acquires a somatic *CEBPA* mutation, typically on the gene's 3′ end. In the case of bi-allelic *CEBPA* mutations, prognosis is favorable, particularly if one of the variants is germline (*Blood*. 2015;126(10):1214–1223). Germline *CEBPA* mutations predispose to second and even third primary leukemias, as evidenced by the acquisition of unique mutations, but the disease remains sensitive to induction chemotherapy (*Blood*. 2015;126(10):1214–1223). Germline mutations in other genes, such as *TERC* and *TERT,* are associated with a high risk of other life-threatening diseases, such as pulmonary fibrosis, hepatic cirrhosis, and head and neck cancers (*Genet Med*. 2010;12(12):753–764).

▓ TREATMENT

PATIENTS WITH A GERMLINE PREDISPOSITION MUTATION

Knowledge of a patient's germline mutational status has important implications for their treatment. Treatment with chemotherapy alone will not rid the patient of their germline mutation. As a result, they remain at risk of relapse and, in the case of germline *CEBPA*-mutated patients as noted above, at risk of second or third primary leukemias.

Table 2.1: List of Genes That Predispose to Hematologic Malignancy

Predisposition	Genes
Inherited syndromes associated with myeloid malignancies	*ANKRD26, ATG2B/GSKIP, ATM, BLM, BRCA1/2, CEBPA, CBL, CHEK2, CSF3R, DDX41, ETV6, GATA2, HRAS, IKZF1, KRAS, MBD4, MECOM/ EVI1, MEK1, MEK2, MLH1, MSH2, MSH6, NF1, NBN, NRAS, PAX5, PMS2, PTPN11, RAF1, RBBP6, RPL5, RPL11, RPS19, RTEL1, RUNX1, SAMD9, SAMD9L, SHOC2, SOS1, SRP72, TERC, TERT, TP53*
Inherited bone marrow failure syndromes	*ACD, ALAS2, BRCA1/2, BRIP1, CSF3R, CTC1, CXCR4, DDX41, DKC1, DNAJC21, ELANE, ERCC4, FANC genes, G6PC3, GATA1, GATA2, GFI1, HAX1, MPL, NAF1, NHP2, NOP10, PALB2, PARN, POT1, RAD51, RAD51C, RBM8A, RPL11, RPL15, RPL26, RPL35A, RPL5, RPS10, RPS19, RPS24, RPS26, RPS7, RTEL1, RUNX1, SAMD9, SAMD9L, SBDS, SLX4, SRP72, STN1, TERT, TERC, TINF2, UBE2T, USB1, VPS45, WAS, WRAP53, XRCC2*
Inherited syndromes associated with lymphoid malignancies	*ACD, ADA, ATM, BRCA1/2, CASP10, CD27, CHEK2, DOCK8, ETV6, FAS, FASLG, HCLS1, IKZF1, ITK, KLHDC8B, LAPTM5, MAGT1, MLH1, MSH2, MSH6, NBN, NBS1, NF1, NPAT, PAX5, PMS2, POT1, PRF1, RPL11, RPL5, RECQL3, SH2B3, SH2D1A, STXBP2, TERF2IP, TNFRSF13B, TP53, WAS/WASP*

Allogeneic stem cell transplantation offers the best chance of cure for many patients with hematologic malignancies, such as MDS and AML, and is the only way to replace germline mutation–carrying hematopoietic stem cells with normal stem cells. However, one must be very careful in the choice of allogeneic stem cell donor. Matched sibling donors have traditionally been the donor of choice, but in the case of a germline mutated patient, a sibling most often has a 50% chance of carrying the familial mutation. To avoid reintroducing the same disease-causing mutation, it is critical to test the related donor for the identified germline mutation prior to stem cell mobilization. There have been reports of severe complications when donors carrying a germline predisposition mutation have been used, including poor graft function, graft failure, donor-derived leukemias, and leukemia developing in the donor following stem cell mobilization (*Leukemia.* 2017;31(2):520–522). For these reasons, the current best practice is to use an human leukocyte antigen-matched related donor who lacks the familial mutation or, if unavailable, to select a matched unrelated donor with a low risk of having a germline mutation.

IMPLICATIONS FOR FAMILY MEMBERS

Patients identified as harboring a germline predisposition variant benefit from receiving a "family letter" written in lay terms that informs family members about the identified mutation, its associated risks, recommendations for disease and other cancer surveillance, and the option of pre-implantation genetic counseling/testing for those who seek family planning. This letter can be shared among the patient's relatives to facilitate genetic counseling and, if desired, targeted mutation-specific genetic testing. For family members found to carry a germline predisposition mutation but without hematologic malignancy, a baseline bone marrow biopsy and serial complete blood counts are recommended to assess the status of the bone marrow. Depending on the particular germline predisposition syndrome, there may be additional recommendations for enhanced screening to enable early detection of associated solid cancers and/or organ dysfunction. For example, *TERT* and *TERC* mutations predispose to pulmonary fibrosis, and in addition to myeloid malignancies, *DDX41* mutations may also predispose to numerous solid tumors, such as melanoma, breast, bladder, prostate, colon, stomach, and pancreatic cancer.

▓ POTENTIAL PRACTICE-CHANGING CLINICAL TRIALS

Much of what we know about inherited hematologic malignancies is based on case reports, case series, and expert recommendations. However, as more cases are recognized and followed, we will learn more about the natural history of cancer development, the mechanisms by which these germline mutations lead to malignancies, and interventions that can delay or possibly even prevent cancer or the development of other organ dysfunctions. For example, to characterize the etiology and natural history of patients with germline *RUNX1* mutations better, a large observational cohort study is being conducted (NCT03854318). An observational study using NGS to examine known germline mutations and to look for new ones in patients with familial AML and MDS is ongoing (NCT03058588). Similarly, research is ongoing to identify germline mutations that impart an increased risk of lymphoma (NCT00131014). We look forward to the results of these studies, which will improve our understanding of these diseases and lead to decreased morbidity and mortality for individuals and families with these mutations.

▓ REFERENCES FOR SUPPLEMENTAL READING

1. Godley LA, Shimamura A. Genetic predisposition to hematologic malignancies: management and surveillance. *Blood*. 2017;130:424–432. doi: 10.1182/blood-2017-02-735290

2. The University of Chicago Hematopoietic Malignancies Cancer Risk Team. How I diagnose and manage individuals at risk for inherited myeloid malignancies. *Blood*. 2016; 128:1800–1813. doi: 10.1182/blood-2016-05-670240

3. Tawana K, Drazer MW, Churpek JE. Universal genetic testing for inherited susceptibility in children and adults with myelodysplastic syndrome and

acute myeloid leukemia: are we there yet? *Leukemia*. 2018; 32:1482–1492. doi: 10.1038/s41375-018-0051-y

4. Peterson LC, Bloomfield CD, Niemeyer CM, et al. Myeloid neoplasms with germline predisposition. In: Swerdlow SH, Campo E, Harris NL, et al., eds. *WHO Classification of Tumors of Haematopoietic and Lymphoid Tissues*. Revised 4th ed. IARC; 2017:121–128.

5. Cerhan JR and Slager SL. Familial predisposition and genetic risk factors for lymphoma. *Blood*. 2015; 126:2265–2273. doi: 10.1182/blood-2015-04-537498

▧ REFERENCES

1. Godley LA and Shimamura A. Genetic predisposition to hematologic malignancies: management and surveillance. *Blood*. 2017;130:424–432. doi: 10.1182/blood-2017-02-735290

2. Churpek JE and Godley LA. Familial acute leukemia and myelodysplastic syndromes In: *UpToDate*, Post, TW ed., UpToDate; 2020.

3. Peterson LC, Bloomfield CD, Niemeyer CM, et al. Myeloid neoplasms with germline predisposition. In: Swerdlow SH, Campo E, Harris NL, et al., eds. *WHO Classification of Tumors of Haematopoietic and Lymphoid Tissues*. Revised 4th ed. IARC; 2017:121–128.

4. The University of Chicago Hematopoietic Malignancies Cancer Risk Team. How I diagnose and manage individuals at risk for inherited myeloid malignancies. *Blood*. 2016;128:1800–1813. doi: 10.1182/blood-2016-05-670240

5. Luo X, Feurstein S, Mohan S, et al. ClinGen myeloid malignancy variant curation expert panel recommendations for germline RUNX1 variants. *Blood Adv*. 2019; 3(20):2962–2979. doi: 10.1182/bloodadvances.2019000644

6. Sood R, Kamikubo Y, Liu P. Role of RUNX1 in hematological malignancies. *Blood*. 2017;129(15):2070–2082. *Blood*. 2018;131(3):373. doi: 10.1182/blood-2017-12-819789

7. Tawana K, Wang J, Renneville A, et al. Disease evolution and outcomes in familial AML with germline CEBPA mutations. *Blood*. 2015;126(10):1214–1223. doi: 10.1182/blood-2015-05-647172

8. Pabst T, Eyholzer M, Haefliger S, Schardt J, Mueller BU. Somatic CEBPA mutations are a frequent second event in families with germline CEBPA mutations and familial acute myeloid leukemia. *J Clin Oncol*. 2008;26(31):5088–5093. doi: 10.1200/JCO.2008.16.5563

9. Savage SA, Bertuch AA. The genetics and clinical manifestations of telomere biology disorders. *Genet Med*. 2010;12(12):753–764. doi: 10.1097/GIM.0b013e3181f415b5

10. Wlodarski MW, Hirabayashi S, Pastor V, et al. Prevalence, clinical characteristics, and prognosis of GATA2-related myelodysplastic syndromes in children and adolescents. *Blood*. 2016;127(11):1387–1518. doi: 10.1182/blood-2015-09-669937

11. Cheah JJC, Hahn CN, Hiwase DK, et al. Myeloid neoplasms with germline DDX41 mutation. *Int J Hematol*. 2017;106(2):163–174. doi: 10.1007/s12185-017-2260-y

12. Berger G, van den Berg E, Sikkema-Raddatz B, et al. Re-emergence of acute myeloid leukemia in donor cells following allogeneic transplantation in a family with a germline DDX41 mutation. *Leukemia*. 2017;31(2):520–522. doi: 10.1038/leu.2016.310

3 Diagnostic Approaches to Hematologic Malignancies

Johnny Nguyen, Rohit Sharma, and Ling Zhang

▨ INTRODUCTION

The current landscape in the classification scheme of hematologic malignancies is a culmination of decades of seminal contributions to the field, including morphology, immunophenotyping, cytogenetics, and the advent of advanced molecular diagnostics. The formal classification of hematologic malignancies has gone through several iterations over the past few decades, from the French-American-British (FAB) Co-Operative Group Classification Systems of 1976 to the updated 4th edition of *WHO Tumours of the Haematopoietic and Lymphoid Tissues*, published in 2017.[1,2] Although morphology remains one of the principal diagnostic tools, the current WHO classification set a precedent by integrating novel genetic information into various diagnostic criteria. With the emergence of next-generation sequencing (NGS) technology, novel genetic mutations and abnormalities are continuously being identified, and their significant roles in disease development and progression are becoming increasingly important in diagnosis and prognosis.[1,3] The updates included in the revision of the 2017 WHO classification better reflect our evolving understanding of the clinical subclassification and prognosis of patient subgroups, discovery of novel mutations, and targeted gene therapy.[4]

▨ MORPHOLOGY

Despite the exponential increase in ancillary studies and molecular diagnostics in the pathologic evaluation of disease, traditional morphologic analysis under conventional bright-field microscopy remains central to the accurate triaging and diagnosing of hematologic disorders. Initial assessment of patient samples relies upon adequate tissue sampling and accurate clinical information. Careful review of Wright-stained peripheral blood smears, Wright-Giemsa–stained bone marrow aspirate smears, or hematoxylin and eosin (H&E) staining of formalin-fixed paraffin-embedded tissue (FFPE) of tissue by experienced hematologists and hematopathologists is an essential step. The resulting morphologic findings usually guide the subsequent laboratory workup and selection of ancillary studies.

The practice of anatomic and clinical pathology mandates maintaining dynamic and broad, but still focused, differential diagnoses when evaluating case material. Unique or unusual cytomorphologic characteristics of neoplastic cells, structures, and infiltrating patterns seen under light microscopy help guide the hematopathologist in diagnosis, for example "flower cells" (Adult T-cell Lymphoma/Leukemia), "faggot cells" (Acute Promyelocytic Leukemia), "hallmark cells" (Anaplastic Large Cell Lymphoma), "cerebriform nuclei" (Sezary Syndrome), or "fried-egg cells" (Hairy Cell Leukemia). These morphologic features may be characteristic but not entirely certain to these particular disease entities. Even within certain disease categories, a spectrum of different morphologic appearances, termed "variants," can be observed in isolation or in combination due to disease heterogeneity. Histological variants may influence clinical management and outcomes and, in such cases, should be documented in pathology reports as well as in clinical notes.

Accurate and reliable histological evaluation requires high-quality preparation of routine hematologic specimens. External factors that mainly adversely affect accurate morphologic diagnosis include poor-quality preparations (e.g., hemodiluted/poorly preserved samples), limited tissue sampling (e.g., fine-needle aspirates), or incomplete ancillary studies. Careful and thorough examination of the entire submitted cytology and tissue specimen is required to avoid "tunnel vision" and identify possible composite lesions.

▧ FLOW CYTOMETRY

Flow cytometry has proven to be an essential diagnostic tool not only for phenotyping hematologic malignancies but also for detecting the presence of minimal residual disease (MRD) and monitoring disease progression.[5,6] It is used to analyze the physical and chemical features of cellular components in an isotonic buffered liquid cellular suspension when passing through one or multiple lasers.[7] The cellular components are labeled with specific antibodies tagged with different fluorochromes. When excited by a laser, the fluorochromes emit light at a specific and narrow wavelength spectrum, which is converted into electrical pulses and then transmitted as "fluorescent intensities" and shown as colored dots on a histogram[7,8] (Figure 3.1). The generation of this "dot plot" allows the quantifiable measurement of tumor-cell characteristics, such as cell size or cell morphology (forward scatter, FSC or FS), granularity or cytoplasmic complexity (side scatter, SSC or SS), and surface and/or cytoplasmic marker expression. In addition to being useful for counting cells or detecting biomarkers, flow cytometry can also be used for cell sorting, protein engineering, and DNA ploidy.[9] Accurate flow cytometric data relies upon proper validation and fine-tuning of important flow cytometer settings, for example, to reduce nonspecific background interference.[10]

It is important to note that flow cytometry is not applicable for the diagnosis of certain hematopoietic neoplasms, such as classical Hodgkin lymphoma, T-cell/histiocyte Rich Large B-cell Lymphoma, Nodular Lymphocyte-Predominant Hodgkin Lymphoma, or Large B-cell Lymphoma with features intermediate between Diffuse Large B-cell

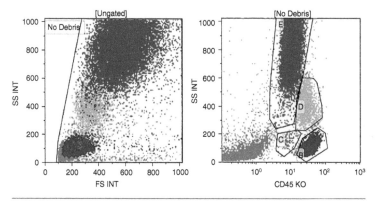

Figure 3.1 Dot blot histogram of flow cytometry.
Forward scatter intensity (FS INT) measures the size of cells, while side scatter intensity (SS INT) measures cellular granularity or internal complexity. CD45 versus SS INT: identifying CD45 negative cells, e.g. erythroid precursors (grey); dim CD45 positive blasts (C, pink); and moderate to bright CD45 positive lymphocytes (B, blue), monocytes (D, green), and a spectrum of maturing granulocytes (E, red) in contrast to cell size.

Lymphoma and classical Hodgkin lymphoma (so-called gray-zone lymphoma). The sensitivity of flow cytometry may be limited due to focal or patchy involvement of tumor cells, extensive necrosis, or tumor-associated fibrosis. The integration of clinical features, morphology, phenotypic studies, and cytogenetic/molecular results is critical to accurate hematopathologic diagnosis in such scenarios. Additionally, caution must be taken when evaluating for clonality in specimens containing a very minute population of neoplastic cells or minimal residual disease (MRD) or in certain nonspecific reactive situations. For instance, florid follicular hyperplasia may produce small subsets of phenotypically identical cells (a monoclonal population of CD10 positive B-cells) which can be mistaken for a lymphoproliferative disorder such as follicular lymphoma.[11] Another example typically seen in the pediatric setting is distinguishing hematogones (non-neoplastic regenerating hematopoietic lymphoid precursors) from abnormal residual leukemic cells in B-lymphoblastic leukemia (B-ALL).[5] Table 3.1 shows commonly used antigens in various flow cytometry parameters and examples of their applications in evaluating hematologic malignancies.

▒ IMMUNOHISTOCHEMICAL STAINING

Immunohistochemical (IHC) staining uses a selected antibody conjugated to peroxidase or other enzyme to bind a specific antigen in tissue specimen(s) or cell clots. After incubating with an enzyme substrate, it results in insoluble particles on the cell surface, cytoplasm, nucleus, or various combinations, which can be visualized by conventional bright-field light microscopy. The quality of IHC results is

Table 3.1 Commonly Used Flow Cytometry Markers in Evaluation of Hematopoietic Neoplasms

Antigen*	Normal Expression	Main Application(s)
CD45	• All B-cells and T-cells • Myeloid precursors • Blasts (dim)	• Mature lymphoid neoplasms • Myeloid malignancies • Acute leukemia, myeloid, T-, B-, or mixed lineages
CD1a	• A subset of thymocytes • Langerhans cells	• Thymoma • T-lymphoblastic leukemia/ lymphoma • Langerhans cell histiocytosis • Negative in ETP-ALL
CD2	• Thymocytes • T/NK-cells • Mast cells	• T/NK-cell lymphoma/ leukemia • Aberrant expression in AML, e.g., microgranular variant APL • Mast cell disorders
CD3	• Thymocytes • T-cells • NK cells (CD3 epsilon, cytoplasmic)	• T-lymphoblastic leukemia/ lymphoma (cytoplasmic) • Mature T-cell lymphoma/ leukemia (surface) • NK cell lymphoma/leukemia (cytoplasmic+/surface–)
CD4	• T-cells • Cortical thymocytes when coexpressing CD8 • Monocytes/histiocytes/ macrophages • PDCs	• T-lymphoblastic lymphoma/ leukemia • AML, CMML, BPDCN
CD5	• Thymocytes • T-cells • Minor B-cell subset	• T-cell lymphoma/Leukemia • CLL/SLL • Mantle cell lymphoma
CD7	• Thymocytes • Mature T-cells • NK cells	• T-cell leukemia/lymphoma • NK/T-cell lymphoma • Aberrant loss of expression is common in MF and among other T-cell malignancies • Aberrant expression in AML
CD8	• Cortical thymocytes when coexpressing CD4 • Mature peripheral T-cells (cytotoxic/ suppressor T cells) • NK cells (30%) • Dendritic cells	• CD8 positive T-cell lymphomas, including MF and PTCL, NOS • A subset of NK cell lymphoma/leukemia

(*continued*)

Table 3.1 Commonly Used Flow Cytometry Markers in Evaluation of Hematopoietic Neoplasms (continued)

Antigen*	Normal Expression	Main Application(s)
CD10	• Immature T-cells and B-cells • Subset of mature T-cells • Germinal center B-cells • Granulocytes	• Diffuse large B-cell lymphoma (germinal center B-cell-like phenotype) • Burkitt lymphoma • Follicular lymphoma • PTCL, follicular T-helper cell type • AILT • B-ALL (Bright; if negative, consider *KMT2A/MLL* gene rearmaments)
CD19	• All B cells, including most normal plasma cells	• B-cell lymphoma/leukemia (Note: May be downregulated post CAR-T immunotherapy) • Aberrantly expressed in myeloid malignancies, e.g., AML with t(8;21)/*RUNX1/RUNX1T1*
CD20	• Mature B-cells (strong) • A subset of precursor/immature B-cells	• Most B-cell lymphomas/leukemias • Dim expression in CLL/SLL • Nodular lymphocyte predominant Hodgkin lymphoma • A subset of plasma cell myeloma
CD23	• Activated B-cells • Follicular dendritic cells	• CLL/SLL • Usually loss of expression in DLBCL
Surface kappa and lambda	• Mature B-cells, polyclonal	• Immunoglobulin light-chain restriction/clonality
Kappa and lambda, cytoplasmic	• Plasma cells, polyclonal	• Monoclonal or light chain restriction in plasma cell neoplasms or lymphoma, e.g., CLL, mantle cell lymphoma, follicular lymphoma, marginal zone lymphoma, lymphoplasmacytic lymphoma, DLBCL
ZAP70	• T-cells, NK cells, precursor B-cells	• CLL/SLL prognostic indicator
CD38	• Plasma cells (bright) • Blast, myeloid, and lymphoid precursors (moderate)	• B-lymphoblastic leukemia/lymphoma • Plasma cell neoplasm • Plasmablastic lymphoma • Primary effusion lymphoma • CLL/SLL prognostic indicator

(continued)

Table 3.1 Commonly Used Flow Cytometry Markers in Evaluation of Hematopoietic Neoplasms (continued)

Antigen*	Normal Expression	Main Application(s)
CD138	• Plasma cells	• Plasma cell neoplasms • Plasmablastic lymphoma • Primary effusion lymphoma carcinoma
CD34	• Myeloblasts • B- and T-cell precursors • Endothelial cells	• AML (e.g., often negative along with HLA-DR in APL) • B- and T-lymphoblastic leukemia/lymphoma • Acute leukemias of ambiguous lineage
TdT	• B- and T-cell precursors	• Thymoma, lymphocyte predominant • B- and T-lymphoblastic leukemia/lymphoma • A subset of AML • A subset of BPDCN (30%) • Acute leukemias of ambiguous lineage
CD117	• Myeloid precursor • Mast cells	• AML • Mast cell disorders • Aberrant expression in T-lymphoblastic leukemia/lymphoma and plasma cell myeloma
HLA-DR	• Stem cell marker • B-cells • Precursor T-cells • Dendritic cells • Monocytes/ Macrophages	• AML (e.g., often negative in APL, see CD34) • Lymphomas
CD13	• Granulocytes, monocytes, and macrophages	• AML • May be aberrantly expressed in B- or T-lymphoblastic leukemia/lymphoma • May be aberrantly expressed in B-cell lymphoma or plasma cell neoplasm
CD14	• Monocytes, histiocytes/macrophages	• AML with monocytic differentiation • CMML

(continued)

Table 3.1 Commonly Used Flow Cytometry Markers in Evaluation of Hematopoietic Neoplasms (continued)

Antigen*	Normal Expression	Main Application(s)
CD33	• Myeloid and monocytic cells	• AML • May be aberrantly expressed in B- or T-lymphoblastic leukemia/lymphoma • May be aberrantly expressed in B-cell lymphoma or plasma cell neoplasm
CD56	• T-cells, activated • NK cells • A subset of large granular lymphocytes	• Mature T-cell lymphoma • T-LGL leukemia • NK cell lymphoma/leukemia • Aberrantly expressed in AML, CMML BPDCN; negative in PDCs
CD64	• Monocytes/Macrophages	• AML • CMML • Extramedullary monocytic sarcoma
CD123	• Normal hematopoietic cells. • PDCs	• BPDCN • AML • B- or T-lymphoblastic leukemia • Hairy cell leukemia • Systemic mastocytosis (negative in normal/reactive mast cells)
Cytoplasmic MPO	• Myeloid precursors	• AML • Acute leukemias of ambiguous lineage

*Only listed markers frequently used and their application.

AILT, angioimmunoblastic T-cell lymphoma; ALL, acute lymphoblastic leukemia/lymphoma; AML, acute myeloid leukemia; APL, acute promyelocytic leukemia; BPDCN, blastic plasmacytoid dendritic cell neoplasm; CLL/SLL, chronic lymphocytic leukemia/small lymphocytic lymphoma; CMML, chronic myelomonocytic leukemia; DLBCL, diffuse large B-cell lymphoma; ETP-ALL, early T-cell precursor acute lymphoblastic leukemia; MF, mycosis fungoides; NOS, not otherwise specified; PDC, plasmacytoid dendritic cell; PTCL, peripheral T-cell lymphoma; T-LGL leukemia, T-cell large granular lymphocytic leukemia.

dependent upon the integrity of the tissue architecture, cell morphology, and antigenicity of target epitopes during specimen processing, including sample harvesting, fixating, and sectioning. In contrast to flow cytometry, IHC studies are performed on tissue with intact or partially retained architecture and interpreted based not only on cell morphology or presence or absence of staining but also on staining pattern and intensity. When interpreting IHC results, one should pay particular attention to the normal counterpart, nonspecific background staining, aberrant, or cross-reactivity.[12] Alternatively, IHCs are also used for those antibodies that are not applicable for flow cytometry or to identify a characteristic localization in neoplastic cells (e.g., membranous and Golgi enhancement of CD30/CD15 in classical Hodgkin lymphoma). Table 3.2 summarizes common markers used in the diagnosis of hematopoietic neoplasms.

Table 3.2 Immunohistochemical Staining Markers Frequently Used in Immunophenotyping

Antigen*	Normal Expression	Application(s)
ALK	• Embryonic neurons, rare in adult CNS	• ALCL, ALK1 positive • ALK positive large B-cell lymphoma
CD30	• Activated B-, T-, and NK cells, monocytes	• ALCL • Other T-cell lymphomas (e.g., PTCL, NOS, MF with increased large cells, a subtype of lymphomatoid papulosis [LyP], ENKTL) • Reed-Sternberg cells in cHL with typical perinuclear dot-like enhancement representing Golgi apparatus • PMBCL • Gray-zone lymphoma (large B-cell lymphoma with features intermediate between DLBCL and cHL) • DLBCL • Plasmablastic lymphoma • Primary effusion lymphoma
CD15	• Granulocytes	• Reed-Sternberg cells in cHL, with perinuclear dot-like enhancement representing the Golgi apparatus • Some AML/granulocytic sarcoma • A small subset of ALL
PAX-5	• B-cells	• B-cell lymphoma/leukemia • Reed-Sternberg cells in cHL (dim expression)
Cyclin D1/BCL-1	• Endothelial cells	• Mantle cell lymphoma • A subset of HCL • A subset of plasma cell myeloma
CD10	• Germinal center B-cells • Immature T- and B-cells • Granulocytes	• DLBCL, GCB type • B- or T-lymphoblastic lymphoma • Burkitt Lymphoma • AILT • PTCL, follicular T-helper cell type
BCL-2	• Inter- and intra-follicular T-cells • Primary follicles and mantle zone B-cells	• Follicular lymphoma (85% of cases) • DLBCL, non-GCB type • Negative in reactive follicular hyperplasia • Negative in Burkitt lymphoma

(*continued*)

Table 3.2 Immunohistochemical Staining Markers Frequently Used in Immunophenotyping (continued)

Antigen*	Normal Expression	Application(s)
BCL-6	• Germinal center B-cells • Follicular T-helper cells	• Follicular lymphoma • DLBCL, GCB or non-GCB type • AILT
MUM1	• B-cells • Plasma cells	• DLBCL, non-GCB type • PMBCL • Plasmablastic lymphoma • Primary effusion lymphoma • Plasma cell neoplasm • ALK positive large B-cell lymphoma • Primary CNS lymphoma
MYC	• None	• Burkitt lymphoma • A subset of DLBCL, including "double expressor" phenotype • High-grade B-cell lymphoma, double or triple hit • High-grade B-cell lymphoma, NOS
Ki-67/ MIB	• Any cells	• Expressed as an estimated percentage to indicate proliferation index of tumor cells (e.g., characteristically high in Burkitt Lymphoma)
Spectrin	• Erythroid precursors • Megakaryocytes	• Percentage and distribution of erythroid precursors • Acute erythroid leukemia • Acute megakaryocytic leukemia
Hemo-globin A	• Erythroid precursors	• Percentage and distribution of erythroid precursors • Acute erythroid leukemia
TCL1	• Non-germinal center B-cells • T-prolymphocytes	• BPDCN • T-prolymphocytic leukemia • Aberrant expression in Burkitt lymphoma/DLBCL
CD43	• Most T-cells • NK cells • Activated B-cells • Granulocytes	• T/NK-cell lymphomas • Myeloid sarcoma • BPDCN • Burkitt lymphoma • Aberrantly expressed in SLL/CLL • A subset of MALToma • Plasma cell neoplasm
Cyto-plasmic MPO	• Myeloid precur-sors	• AML • Myeloid sarcoma • Acute leukemias of ambiguous lineage, T- or B-myeloid

(continued)

Table 3.2 Immunohistochemical Staining Markers Frequently Used in Immunophenotyping (continued)

Antigen*	Normal Expression	Application(s)
Lysozyme	• Mononcyte, histiocyte	• Myeloid Sarcoma
Mast cell tryptase	• Mast cells	• Mast cell disorders
TRAP	• Osteoclasts • Activated macrophages	• HCL

*Only listed markers frequently used and their application.

AILT, angioimmunoblastic T-cell lymphoma; ALCL, anaplastic large cell lymphoma; ALL, acute lymphoblastic leukemia/lymphoma; ATLL, adult T-cell leukemia/lymphoma; BPDCN, blastic plasmacytoid dendritic cell neoplasm; cHL, classical Hodgkin lymphoma; CNS, central nervous system; DLBCL, diffuse large B-cell lymphoma; ENKTL, extranodal NK/T cell lymphoma; GCB, germinal center B-cell; HCL, hairy cell leukemia; MALToma; lymphoma involving the mucosa-associated lymphoid tissue; NOS, not otherwise specified; PMBCL, primary mediastinal large B-cell lymphoma; PTCL, peripheral T-cell lymphoma; TRAP, tartrate-resistant acid phosphatase.

▓ POLYMERASE CHAIN REACTION

Polymerase chain reaction (PCR) was first developed in the early 1980s to amplify selected DNA sequences by using specific primers, a heat-stable DNA-dependent DNA polymerase, and a magnesium-containing buffer. Following it, modified PCRs, including reverse transcriptase PCR (RT-PCR), multiplex PCR, quantitative PCR, quantitative RT-PCR, and allele-specific PCR, have also been developed to detect and monitor hematopoietic disorders that are associated with recurrent cytogenetic translocations (e.g., *PML-RARA, BCR-ABL1, IGH-CCND1, NPM-ALK1*), point mutations (e.g., *JAK2 V617F, BRAF V600E, KITD816V, MYD88 L265P*), or DNA tandem duplication (e.g., *FLT3-ITD*). A common application of PCR in daily practice is to detect antigen T- or B-cell receptor gene rearrangements. Multiplex PCR primers are designed to target highly conserved V-segment regions of T- or B-cell genes to create amplicons that can then be analyzed using the preferred capillary gel electrophoresis method. Running duplicate samples in tandem minimizes false-positive error rates, as monoclonal peaks can be detected in the setting of benign lymphoid hyperplasia secondary to infection, immunodeficiency, or autoimmunity as well as T- or B-cell neoplasms.[13,14] Primer sets, including the Framework 3 (FRIII) and, to a lesser extent, the Framework 2 (FRII) and Framework 1 (FRI) regions of IgH genes and IgK kappa genes, are used for the detection of B-cell lymphomas and TCR beta and gamma genes for T-cell lymphomas.[15,16] Furthermore, ascribing clonality to a specific lineage based solely on PCR gene rearrangement analysis may be misleading, as 5 to 10% of mature and most precursor B-cell neoplasms will exhibit clonal T-cell gene rearrangements, a phenomenon called "lineage infidelity."

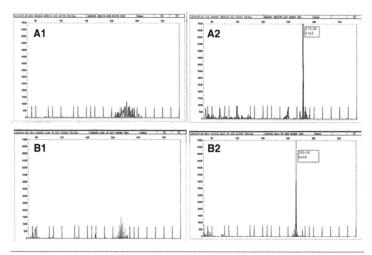

Figure 3.2 Comparison of normal to clonal peak detected by T-cell receptor-gene rearrangement analysis.

Capillary electrophoresis of immunoglobin heavy chain, FR2 (frame region 2) (A 1–2. 1—polyclonal, 2—clonal peak) and T-cell receptor-cell beta gene (B 1–2. 1—polyclonal, 2—clonal peak). Notably, detection of clonality using PCR amplification is suggested when peaks with heights of 2.5 to 3 times the normal background noise are identified.[19]

Lineage infidelity has also been described in T-cell lymphoproliferative disorders.[17] Likewise, it is not uncommon to identify B or T-cell clonal gene rearrangements in some myeloid disorders, such as AML.[18] Thus, caution is needed when interpreting PCR results (Figure 3.2).

When compared with karyotyping, fluorescence in-situ hybridization (FISH), and other tests, PCR analysis increases overall sensitivity. To date, certain PCR assays have gradually been replaced by NGS platforms, due to some inherent limitations of PCR (e.g., detection of gene-specific abnormalities but inability to detect multiple gene alterations simultaneously).

■ CYTOGENETICS

Genetic analysis in hematologic malignancies utilizes both conventional cytogenetic methods (karyotyping and FISH study) and novel approaches, such as comparative genomic hybridization (CGH) (see below). Karyotyping is a test to examine chromosomal abnormalities in a sample of cells. The specimen submitted for cytogenetic study should be freshly harvested and contain sufficient viable cells. The test has been instrumental in detecting recurring genetic abnormalities, numerical and/or structural, in clinical and research settings. The preferred approach is Giemsa-banding (G-banding), which stains various regions within each chromosome analyzed.[20] To analyze the gain or loss of chromosomal materials (and other structural aberrations), the pattern of dark- and light-staining regions in the metaphase stage of cell division is used to characterize abnormal karyotypes.[20] Numerical abnormalities can be manifested with changes affecting complete sets (e.g., triploid or tetraploid) or individual chromosomes (e.g., trisomy or monosomy), while structural abnormalities are often due to chromosomal breakage and further form a new combination from the two broken ends of chromosomes. A disadvantage is that karyotype profiling can only be performed on mitotically active cells and often fails to yield results on cells with low proliferative indexes or no mitotic figures. Neoplasms with highly complex karyotype profiles may not be fully elucidated with conventional karyotyping. Additional cytogenetic evaluation by FISH is necessary when malignancies with cytogenetically identical rearrangements occur, as they may actually have different involved genes at a specific locus. For example, the t(14;18)(q32;q21) can be detected in germinal B-cell type lymphomas with *IgH/BCL-2* gene rearrangement (follicular lymphoma or diffuse large B-cell lymphoma.[21] Occasionally the t(14;18)(q32;q21)/*IgH/BCL-2* gene rearrangement can also be identified in chronic lymphocytic leukemia.[22] Note that some cryptic cytogenetic abnormalities may not be detected using conventional karyotyping (such as in APL).[23]

▮ FLUORESCENCE IN-SITU HYBRIDIZATION

The versatility of sample preparation and sensitivity of probes used in FISH analysis has cemented the methodology in the routine workup of hematologic malignancies (e.g., see DHL section; see PDGFR/FGFR section). The cells used for FISH analysis are typically obtained from the samples submitted for conventional karyotyping, but air-dried bone marrow or blood smears, fresh touch imprint preparations or cytospins, or even frozen or FFPE tissue cassettes are also applicable. FISH studies use fluorescently labeled DNA binding probes that hybridize to metaphase spreads or interphase (non-dividing) nuclei, thus allowing the characterization of cytogenetic changes and detection of some genetic abnormalities not easily shown by conventional karyotyping, such as cryptic chromosomal abnormalities, the origin of marker chromosomes, ring chromosomes, or certain abnormalities hidden in complex cytogenetic aberrations.[24] Dual-color fusion signal probes have been routinely used to identify abnormal fusion signals, although more advanced techniques, such as tri- or four-color FISH, have improved the detection capability to include variant translocations or amplifications. Instead, break-apart probes (adopting the frequent break regions of a gene) are widely used in looking for abnormally separated signals with potential multiple partners (e.g., *c-MYC* translocation to *IgH, IgLK*, or *IgLL; KMT2A/MLL gene* translocation to its multiple partner genes). FISH analysis is more sensitive when compared to conventional karyotyping and allows for more rapid diagnostic turn-around time, particularly when therapeutic management is important, such as identifying *PML-RARA* fusion for t(15;17)(q24;q21) rearrangement in cases of APL.[3] FISH analysis has several drawbacks, including limited available probes, requirement of fluorescence microscopy, and challenges in interpreting FFPE (particularly decalcified trephine core biopsies) or insufficient tumor cells.[24]

COMPARATIVE GENOMIC HYBRIDIZATION

CGH is a particularly useful adjunct molecular study for detecting chromosomal gains, losses, and amplifications.[25] The patient's genomic DNA is labeled with a fluorescent dye, and a reference, normal genomic DNA sample is used for comparison (not necessarily from the same patient). Both normal and patient DNA samples are hybridized to the targets (e.g., oligonucleotides, cDNAs, or genomic fragments) arrayed on a glass slide or other solid platform simultaneously.[19] The differences between the patient's DNA and reference standard correspond to copy number variants/aberrations (CNVs/CNAs). When compared to traditional karyotyping, CGH has two major advantages. First, it can quickly scan an entire genome for imbalances (e.g., aneuploidies, deletions, duplications, and/or amplifications of any locus represented on an array with a higher detection rate). Second, it does not need cell culture to find cells that are undergoing division. The disadvantage of CGH is that it is unable to reveal structural chromosomal abnormalities (e.g., balanced chromosomal translocations, inversions, or mosaicism).[26] The detection of the amplification of such genes as *REL, MYC*, and *BCL-2* has been vital in understanding B-cell lymphomas.[20,21,25,27,28]

SINGLE-NUCLEOTIDE POLYMORPHISM ARRAYS

Single-nucleotide polymorphism (SNP) arrays, in contrast to CGH arrays, are able to detect both CNVs/CNAs and the loss of heterozygosity (LOH) or copy-neutral LOH (CN-LOH), previously termed uniparental disomy (UPD).[29] SNP arrays may be particularly useful when standard cytogenetic and FISH analysis yield negative results, because newer SNP arrays offer the advantage of covering more than 90% of known CNVs by using more than 946,000 probes.[29] Clinically, SNP arrays have been adopted for more accurately assessing DNA ploidy, such as hypodiploidy, in pediatric lymphoblastic leukemia.[30]

NEXT-GENERATION SEQUENCING

Traditional dideoxynucleotide genomic sequencing (Sanger's sequencing), which debuted in 1977, is increasingly being surpassed by NGS platforms, which offer high-resolution, high-throughput data collection.[31] In contrast to Sanger sequencing, NGS allows both the sequencing and detecting of incorporated nucleotides simultaneously in a "massively-parallel" fashion, allowing the previously impractical sequencing of enormous genome sizes to be characterized within hours or days. In NGS, a stepwise reaction occurs in which nucleotides are added, detected simultaneously as they are incorporated into each fragment being sequenced, and washed to remove fluorescent labels or blocking groups (Tables 3.3A and 3.3B). In addition to the DNA

Table 3.3A Common Gene Mutations Identified in Myeloid Neoplasms

Gene	Common/Hotspot Mutations	Protein Class	Associated Disease(s)	Implications Prognostic	Implications Therapeutic
ASXL1	p.G646Wfs* – exon 13	Chromatin/histone modification	MDS, MDS/MPN, AML	Adverse	–
BCOR	–	Transcriptional regulation	MDS, AML	Adverse	–
BCORL1	–	Transcriptional regulation	MDS, AML	–	–
BRAF	p.V600E – exon 15	Signal transduction	LCH	–	BRAF inhibitor (i.e., vemurafenib)
CALR	• 52 bp deletion – p.L367fs*46 – exon 9 (Type 1 mutation) • 5 bp insertion – K385Nfs*47 exon 9 (Type 2 mutation)	Molecular chaperone	MPN, MDS/MPN (e.g., MDS–MPN–RS-T)	Type 1 mutation associated with superior survival compared to Type 2 mutation	–
CBL	–	Signal transduction	MDS, MDS/MPN	Adverse	–
CEBPA	–	Transcriptional regulation	AML	Favorable only when biallelic mutations are present	–
DNMT3A	–	DNA methylation	MDS, MPN, MDS/MPN, AML	Conflicting reports; adverse with concomitant mutation in NPM1 and FLT3-ITD	–

(continued)

Table 3.3A Common Gene Mutations Identified in Myeloid Neoplasms (continued)

Gene	Common/Hotspot Mutations	Protein Class	Associated Disease(s)	Prognostic	Therapeutic
					Implications
ETV6	–	Transcriptional regulation	MDS, AML	Adverse	–
FLT3	6–30 bp internal tandem duplication (ITD) exon 14	Receptor tyrosine kinase	MDS, AML	– Adverse with concomitant *NPM1* and *DNMT3A* mutations – 2017 ELN guidelines*: Mutant allele burden Allelic ratio <0.5 – Favorable; allelic ratio >0.5 – Unfavorable	Type 1 FLT3 inhibitor (i.e., Midostaurin), Type 2 FLT3 inhibitor (i.e., Sorafenib)
	p.D835Y(TKD) –exon 20			Indeterminate	Type 1 FLT3 inhibitor (i.e., Midostaurin)
IDH1	p.R132C – exon 4	DNA methylation	MDS, AML	–	IHD1 inhibitor (i.e., Ivosidenib)
IDH2	p.R140Q – exon 4 p.R712K – exon 4	DNA methylation	MDS, MDS/MPN, AML	Favorable	IDH2 inhibitor (i.e., Enasidenib)
JAK2	p.V617F – exon 14 Exon 12 mutations*	Signal transduction	MPN, MDS/MPN	–	JAK(1/2) inhibitor (i.e., Ruxolitinib)
KIT	p.D816V – exon 17	Receptor tyrosine kinase	AML	Adverse in CBF–AML	–
			SM	–	Multi-kinase/KIT inhibitor (i.e., Midostaurin)

(continued)

Table 3.3A Common Gene Mutations Identified in Myeloid Neoplasms (continued)

Gene	Common/Hotspot Mutations	Protein Class	Associated Disease(s)	Implications	
				Prognostic	Therapeutic
MPL	p.W515L/K – exon 10	Thrombopoietin receptor	MPN	–	–
NPM1	4 bp insertion – exon 12	Nuclear and cytoplasmic protein shuttling	AML	Favorable (in the absence of *FLT3*-ITD)	–
RUNX1	–	Transcriptional regulation	MDS, AML	Adverse	–
SETBP1	–	Transcriptional regulation	MDS, MDS/MPN	Adverse	–
SF3B1	p.K700E – exon 15	RNA splicing	MDS	Favorable	–
SRSF2	–	RNA splicing	MDS	Adverse	–
TP53	–	DNA repair/tumor suppressor	Various myeloid/lymphoid malignancies	Adverse	–
TET2	–	DNA methylation	MDS, MPN, AML	Indeterminate	–

AML, acute myeloid leukemia; bp, base pair; CBF, core binding factor; ITD, Internal tandem duplication; LCH, Langerhans cell histiocytosis; MDS, myelodysplastic syndrome; MDS/MPN, myelodysplastic/myeloproliferative neoplasm; MPN, myeloproliferative neoplasm; SM, systemic mastocytosis; TKD, tyrosine kinase domain.

*ELN, European leukemia net – The mutant allele burden is determined specifically by DNA fragment analysis by measuring the peak height ratio of mutant and wildtype alleles on a fluorescence scale.

Table 3.3B Common Gene Mutations Identified in Lymphoid Neoplasms

Gene	Common/Hotspot Mutations	Protein Class	Associated Disease(s)	Implications Prognostic	Therapeutic
ATM	–	DNA repair	CLL (10%–25%)	Adverse	–
BIRC3	–	Apoptosis regulation	MCL (50%)	–	–
BRAF	p.V600E – exon 15	Signal transduction	CLL (<5%)	Adverse	–
			HCL, MM	–	BRAF inhibitor (i.e., vemurafenib)
CCND3	–	Cyclin dependent kinase regulator	SDRPL	–	–
CXCR4	–	Chemokine receptor	LPL (36%)	Adverse	–
DNMT3A	–	DNA Methylation	AILT	–	–
EZH2	p.Y641 – exon 16	Chromatin/histone modification	FL, DLBCL	–	–
FBXW7	–	Phosphorylation-dependent ubiquitination	T-ALL	Favorable	–
ID3	–	Transcriptional regulation	Burkitt lymphoma	Adverse	–
IgH	–	Antibody mediated immune response	B-cell lymphomas		–
			Plasma cell myeloma	Favorable – Mutation rate >7% when compared to germline *IGHV* sequence & specific D usage of IGHD2 & IGHD3	

(continued)

Table 3.3B Common Gene Mutations Identified in Lymphoid Neoplasms (continued)

Gene	Common/Hotspot Mutations	Protein Class	Associated Disease(s)	Implications Prognostic	Therapeutic
	–	Antibody mediated immune response	CLL	Favorable: Mutation rate >2% when compared to germline IGHV sequence Adverse: Mutation rate <2% when compared to germline IGHV sequence Adverse: Specific V-J usage of *IGHV3-21*	–
			HCL(40%) HCL-v(10%)	Adverse: Specific V-J usage of *IGHV4-34*	
MAP2K1	–	Signal transduction	HCL-v SDRPL	–	–
MYD88	p.L265P – exon 5	NF-kB activation	LPL/WM, CLL, DLBCL (ABC type) (20%), MGUS MALToma (5%) 13%, SMZL	Adverse (DLBCL)	The co-occurrence of *MYD88* L265P mutation and *CD79B* mutation is highly predictive of response to BTK inhibitor, ibrutinib

(continued)

Table 3.3B Common Gene Mutations Identified in Lymphoid Neoplasms (continued)

Gene	Common/Hotspot Mutations	Protein Class	Associated Disease(s)	Implications Prognostic	Therapeutic
NOTCH1	–	Transmembrane receptor protein	T-ALL	Favorable	–
	p.P2514Rfs*4		CLL (8%–15%)	Adverse	
	–		ATLL (30%)	–	
PAX5	–	Transcriptional regulation	DLBCL (4%)	Adverse	–
PRD-M1(BLIMP)	–	Transcriptional regulation	DLBCL (8%)	Adverse	–
SF3B1	p.K700E – exon 15	RNA splicing	CLL	Adverse	–
STAT3	p.Y640F – exon 21 p.D661 – exon 21	Signal transduction	T-LGL leukemia (40%)		–
STAT5B	–	Signal transduction	HSTCL (31%)	–	–
TET2	–	DNA methylation	AILT	–	–
TNFAIP3	–	Ubiquitin-editing enzyme	cHL (44%) PMBCL (36%)	–	–
TP53	–	DNA repair/tumor suppressor	Various myeloid/lymphoid malignancies	Adverse, often associated with complex cytogenetic aberrations	–

AILT, angioimmunoblastic T-cell lymphoma; ALCL, anaplastic large cell lymphoma; ATLL, adult T-cell lymphoma/leukemia; BTK, Bruton's tyrosine kinase; CBF-AML, core binding factor acute myeloid leukemia; cHL, classical Hodgkin lymphoma; CLL/SLL, chronic lymphocytic leukemia/small lymphocytic lymphoma; DLBCL, diffuse large B-cell lymphoma; FL, follicular lymphoma; HCL, hairy cell leukemia; HCL-v, hairy cell leukemia variant; HSTCL, hepato-splenic T-cell lymphoma; IGHV, immunoglobulin heavy chain variable region; LPL/WM, lymphoplasmacytic lymphoma/Waldenström macroglobulinemia; MALToma, lymphoma involving the mucosa-associated lymphoid tissue; MCL, mantle cell lymphoma; MM, multiple myeloma; NOS, not otherwise specified; PMBCL, primary mediastinal large B-cell lymphoma; PTCL, peripheral T-cell lymphoma; SDRPL, splenic diffuse red pulp small B-cell lymphoma; T-ALL, T-cell acute lymphoblastic leukemia/lymphoma; T-LGL leukemia, T-cell large granular lymphocytic leukemia; T-PLL, T-prolymphocytic leukemia.

or RNA sequencing targeted to frequent gene mutations involving myeloid or lymphoid tissue, whole-genomic sequencing (WGS) technology has provided deep insight into the genomic changes in hematopoietic malignances. Using NGS technology, a number of somatic or germline variants, including single nucleotide variants, small insertions (e.g., internal tandem duplication in *FLT3* gene), small deletions, and CNVs, can be identified.[32] Certain structural aberrations, such as chromosomal translocations or inversions, can also be detected. Due to the limitation of inherent short-read lengths produced by NGS methods as compared to Sanger sequencing, the sequenced fragments are compared to a reference genome via computer alignment algorithms to identify abnormalities.[32,33] Gene mutations have been described in nearly every hematologic malignancy and have led to a paradigm shift in the diagnosis, prognosis, and therapeutic implication of our patients (see individual chapters and supplemental tables).

▊ CONCLUSION

An accurate diagnosis and subclassification of hematopoietic malignancies is the initial and important step that guides further clinical treatment decision making. The combination of morphology, immunophenotyping, and cytogenetic analysis is vital to routine pathology practice. Modern technologies including NGS and other advanced molecular methodologies are warranted for new insights into the underlying pathogenesis of malignant hematology, to identify novel prognostic and predictive markers, and to facilitate the development of targeted therapies.

▊ REFERENCES FOR SUPPLEMENTAL READING

1. Papaemmanuil E, Gerstung M, Bullinger L, et al. Genomic classification and prognosis in acute myeloid leukemia. *N Engl J Med.* 2016; 374(23):2209–2221.

2. Swerdlow S, Campo E, Harris NL, et al. *WHO Classification of Tumours of Haematopoietic and Lymphoid Tissues.* Revised 4th ed. IARC Press; 2017.

3. Döhner H, Estey E, Grimwade D, et al. Diagnosis and management of AML in adults: 2017 ELN recommendations from an international expert panel. *Blood.* 2017;129(4):424–447.

4. Iqbal J, Amador C, McKeithan TW, et al. Molecular and genomic landscape of peripheral T-cell lymphoma. In: Querfeld C, Zain J, Rosen ST, eds. *T-Cell and NK-Cell Lymphomas: From Biology to Novel Therapies.* Springer International Publishing; 2019:31–68.

5. Vaqué JP, Martínez N, Batlle-López A, et al. B-cell lymphoma mutations: Improving diagnostics and enabling targeted therapies. *Haematologica.* 2014;99(2):222–231.

▊ REFERENCES

1. Swerdlow S, Campo E, Harris NL, et al. *WHO Classification of Tumours of Haematopoietic and Lymphoid Tissues.* Revised 4th ed. Lyon: IARC Press; 2017.

2. Bennett JM, Catovsky D, Daniel MT, et al. Proposals for the classification of the acute leukaemias. French-American-British (FAB) Co-Operative Group. *Br J Haematol*. Aug 1976;33(4):451–458. doi: 10.1111/j.1365-2141.1976. tb03563.x. PMID: 188440.

3. Jaffe ES, Vardiman JW, Campo E, et al. Cytogenetic analysis and related techniques in hematopathology. *Hematopathology*. 1st ed. St. Louis, MO: Elsevier Saunders; 2011:1058.

4. Arber DA, Orazi A, Hasserjian R, et al. The 2016 revision to the World Health Organization classification of myeloid neoplasms and acute leukemia. *Blood*. 2016;127(20):2391–2405. doi: 10.1182/blood-2016-03-643544.

5. Craig FE, Foon KA. Flow cytometric immunophenotyping for hematologic neoplasms. *Blood*. 2008;111(8):3941–3967. doi: 10.1182/blood-2007-11-120535.

6. Reichard KR, Kroft SH. Flow cytometry in the assessment of hematologic disorders. In: Orazi A, Foucar K, Knowles DM, eds. *Knowles' Neoplastic Hematopathology*. 3rd ed. Wolters Kluwer, 2013:110–145.

7. Macey MG. *Flow Cytometry: Principles and Applications*. Totowa, NJ: Humana Press; 2007.

8. Mach WJ, Thimmesch AR, Orr JA, et al. Flow cytometry and laser scanning cytometry, a comparison of techniques. *J Clin Monit Comput*. Aug 2010;24(4):251–259. doi: 10.1007/s10877-010-9242-4. PMID: 20623376.

9. Darzynkiewicz Z, Halicka H, Zhao H. Analysis of cellular DNA content by flow and laser scanning cytometry. *Adv Exp Med Biol*. 2010;676:137–147. doi: 10.1007/978-1-4419-6199-0_9. PMID: 20687474.

10. Johansson U, Bloxham D, Couzens S, et al. Guidelines on the use of multicolour flow cytometry in the diagnosis of haematological neoplasms. *Br J Haematol*. 2014;165(4):455–488. doi: 10.1111/bjh.12789. PMID: 24620735.

11. Kussick SJ, Kalnoski M, Braziel RM, et al. Prominent clonal B-cell populations identified by flow cytometry in histologically reactive lymphoid proliferations. *Am J Clin Pathol*. Apr 2004;121(4):464–472. doi: 10.1309/4EJ8-T3R2-ERKQ-61WH. PMID: 15080297.

12. Orazi A, Foucar K, Knowles DM, et al. *Knowles' Neoplastic Hematopathology*. 3rd ed. Lippincott Williams & Wilkins (LWW); 2013:91–118.

13. Nihal M, Mikkola D, Wood GS. Detection of clonally restricted immunoglobulin heavy chain gene rearrangements in normal and lesional skin: Analysis of the B cell component of the skin-associated lymphoid tissue and implications for the molecular diagnosis of cutaneous B cell lymphomas. *J Mol Diagn*. 2000;2(1):5–10. doi: 10.1016/S1525-1578(10)60609-5. PMID: 11272902.

14. Elenitoba-Johnson KS, Bohling SD, Mitchell RS, et al. PCR analysis of the immunoglobulin heavy chain gene in polyclonal processes can yield pseudoclonal bands as an artifact of low B cell number. *J Mol Diagn*. 2000;2(2):92–96. doi: 10.1016/S1525-1578(10)60622-8. PMID: 11272894.

15. Trainor KJ, Brisco MJ, Wan JH, et al. Gene rearrangement in B- And T-lymphoproliferative disease detected by the polymerase chain reaction. *Blood*. Jul 1991;78(1):192–196. PMID: 1648975.

16. Hodges E, Krishna MT, Pickard C, et al. Diagnostic role of tests for T cell receptor (TCR) genes. *J Clin Pathol*. Jan 2003;56(1):1–11. doi: 10.1136/jcp.56.1.1. PMID: 12499424.

17. Leonard, DGB. *Molecular Pathology in Clinical Practice*. New York: Springer;2007.

18. Boehm TL, Werle A, Drahovsky D. Immunoglobulin heavy chain and T-cell receptor gamma and beta chain gene rearrangements in acute myeloid leukemias. *Mol Biol Med*. 1987;4(1):51–62. PMID: 3112510.

19. Bejjani BA, Shaffer LG. Application of array-based comparative genomic hybridization to clinical diagnostics. *J Mol Diagn.* Nov 2006;8(5):528–533. doi: 10.2353/jmoldx.2006.060029. PMID: 17065418.

20. Caspersson T, Zech L, Johansson C. Differential binding of alkylating fluorochromes in human chromosomes. *Exp Cell Res.* 1970;60(3):315–319. doi: 10.1016/0014-4827(70)90523-9. PMID: 5422961.

21. Streubel B, Simonitsch-Klupp I, Müllauer L, et al. Variable frequencies of MALT lymphoma-associated genetic aberrations in MALT lymphomas of different sites. *Leukemia.* 2004;18(10):1722–1726. doi: 10.1038/sj.leu.2403501. PMID: 15356642.

22. Braekeleer MD, Tous C, Guéganic N, et al. Immunoglobulin gene translocations in chronic lymphocytic leukemia: A report of 35 patients and review of the literature. *Mol Clin Oncol.* May 2016;4(5):682–694. doi: 10.3892/mco.2016.793. PMID: 27123263.

23. O'Keefe CL, Tiu R, Gondek LP, et al. High-resolution genomic arrays facilitate detection of novel cryptic chromosomal lesions in myelodysplastic syndromes. *Exp Hematol.* 2007;35(2):240–251. doi: 10.1016/j.exphem.2006.09.016. PMID: 17258073.

24. Bridge JA. Advantages and limitations of cytogenetic, molecular cytogenetic, and molecular diagnostic testing in mesenchymal neoplasms. *J Orthop Sci.* 2008;13(3):273–282. doi: 10.1007/s00776-007-1215-1. PMID: 18528664.

25. Kallioniemi A, Kallioniemi OP, Sudar D, et al. Comparative genomic hybridization for molecular cytogenetic analysis of solid tumors. *Science.* 1992;258(5083):818–821. doi: 10.1126/science.1359641. PMID: 1359641.

26. Bi W, Borgan C, Pursley AN, et al. Comparison of chromosome analysis and chromosomal microarray analysis: What is the value of chromosome analysis in today's genomic array era? *Am J Med Genet.* 2013;15(6):450–457. doi: 10.1038/gim.2012.152. PMID: 23238528.

27. Hsi ED. *Hematopathology.* Philadelphia, PA: Churchill Livingstone Elsevier; 2007:1058.

28. Palanisamy N, Abou-Elella AA, Chaganti SR, et al. Similar patterns of genomic alterations characterize primary mediastinal large-B-cell lymphoma and diffuse large-B-cell lymphoma. *Genes Chromosom Cancer.* 2002;33(2):114–122. doi: 10.1002/gcc.10016. PMID: 11793437.

29. Song J, Shao H. SNP array in hematopoietic neoplasms: A review. *Microarrays.* 2016;5:1. doi: 10.3390/microarrays5010001.

30. Okamoto R, Ogawa S, Nowak D, et al. Genomic profiling of adult acute lymphoblastic leukemia by single nucleotide polymorphism oligonucleotide microarray and comparison to pediatric acute lymphoblastic leukemia. *Haematologica.* 2010;95(9):1481–1488. doi: 10.3324/haematol.2009.011114. PMID: 20435627.

31. Sanger F, Nicklen S, Coulson AR. DNA sequencing with chain-terminating inhibitors. *Proc Nat Acad Sci.* 1977;74(12):5463–5467. doi: 10.1073/pnas.74.12.5463. PMID: 271968.

32. Merker JD, Valouev A, Gotlib J. Next-generation sequencing in hematologic malignancies: What will be the dividends? *Therap Adv Hematol.* 2012;3(6):333–339. doi: 10.1177/2040620712458948. PMID: 23606936.

33. Mardis ER. Next-generation sequencing platforms. *Annu Rev Anal Chem (Palo Alto Calif).* 2013;6:287–303. doi: 10.1146/annurev-anchem-062012-092628.

4   Minimal Residual Disease Assays

Pukhraz Basra and Silvia Tse Bunting

INTRODUCTION

Measurable/minimal residual disease (MRD) has been defined as the detection of leukemic cells at levels below morphologic detection, post-chemotherapy. MRD testing aids in determining the patients' response to treatment, the effectiveness of therapy, and the presence of potential risk of relapse. MRD monitoring has become part of routine clinical practice in the management of patients with acute myeloid leukemia (AML), acute lymphoblastic leukemia (ALL), multiple myeloma (MM), chronic lymphocytic leukemia, and chronic myeloid leukemia (CML). The presence of MRD at the end of induction has been shown to be an independent prognostic indicator.[1–3] Increasing evidence now indicates that the ability to identify residual disease below the morphology threshold is an important tool for refining the approach to risk classification. An ideal MRD test should be able to discriminate between the minute populations of neoplastic cells and cells that are regenerative or normal.

METHODS

There are three different methods being developed for MRD detections with various sensitivity and efficiency: multiparameter flow cytometry (MFC), polymerase chain reaction (PCR), and next-generation sequencing (NGS). Table 4.1 highlights major differences between the three methods.

MRD TESTING IN ACUTE MYELOID LEUKEMIA

Assessment of post-treatment remission is traditionally based primarily on morphology, with AML relapse conventionally defined as more than 5% blasts in the bone marrow not attributable to other causes. Reportedly, more than 50% of adult patients with AML relapse after attaining morphologically defined complete remission (CR) with induction chemotherapy. Methods for MRD detection denote the presence of leukemia cells down to white-blood-cell levels ranging from $1:10^3$ to $1:10^6$, compared with 1:20 in morphology-based assessments. Each methodology differs in the proportion of patients to whom it can be applied and in its sensitivity to detect MRD. It is expected that the integration of baseline factors, such as clinical, pathologic characteristics including genetic features at diagnosis, and assessment of MRD will improve

Table 4.1 Differences in Methods for MRD Detections

	Methods	Sensitivity	Pros	Cons
MFC	MFC uses disease-specific panels of fluorochrome-labeled monoclonal antibodies to identify aberrantly expressed antigens located on the neoplastic cells.	Variable and lab-dependent; usually for B-ALL: 0.01%; AML: 0.1%	Quick turnaround time (could be hours); wide availability; Ability to differentiate between normal regenerative changes and residual leukemia	High demand for technical processing and professional interpretation
PCR	PCR is used to amplify targets of known genetic abnormalities; quantitative assays can also be used to monitor treatment response.	Variable depending on each assay and individual lab; some with a sensitivity of 0.001%.	Relatively robust and reliable technology.	Limited to cases with known abnormalities and availability of the tests.
NGS	NGS allows parallel and repeated sequencing of millions of small DNA fragments and can be used to evaluate a few genes or an entire genome.	Variable depending on individual lab; some could achieve 0.001%	Ability to assay large numbers of mutated genes could help trace the evolution of malignant clones	Technical demand and professional proficiency

ALL, acute lymphoblastic leukemia; AML, acute myeloid leukemia; MFC, multiparameter flow cytometry; NGS, next-generation sequencing; PCR, polymerase chain reaction.

risk assessment. However, no well-adopted guidelines or recommendations are available on how and when to apply MRD assessments and how to translate the results to clinical practice in adult patients.

It is now well established that MRD detected by MFC is an independent prognostic factor for relapse, relapse-free survival, and overall survival in patients with AML.[1] A working group for the European

Leukemia Network established a cutoff of 0.1%. It is strongly recommended to submit the first bone marrow pull for MRD analysis, at least for follow-up bone marrow samples intended for MFC MRD, preferably using the same volume across time points and patients. The evaluation of the use of peripheral blood is ongoing. Early study by flow cytometry showed that it cannot be recommended due to lack of correlation with bone marrow.[5] However, a recent study showed that a qPCR in peripheral blood is an informative tool for disease surveillance in patients with childhood AML (Juul-Dam KL, et al., *Br J Haematol*. 2020). The present concept for MRD assessment during treatment is to use MRD for risk analysis at an early time point prior to consolidation therapy. Not much is known about the optimal time intervals for clinically relevant sequential measurements of MRD during post-therapy follow-up (Feller N, et al., *Leukemia*. 2004). Due to the significance of MRD and the challenges of AML MRD detection, it might be prudent to utilize multiple testing modalities to ensure true MRD negativity.

1. **MFC:** For the detection of MRD via MFC, two separate approaches have been used: (a) the leukemia-associated immunophenotype (LAIP) approach, which defines LAIPs at diagnosis and tracks them in subsequent samples; and (b) the different-from-normal (DfN) approach, which is based on the identification of aberrant differentiation/maturation profiles at follow-up. The DfN approach can be applied if information from diagnosis is not available and also to detect new aberrancies, together with disappearance of diagnosis aberrancies, referred to in earlier literature as "immunophenotype shifts." These may emerge from leukemia evolution or clonal selection. However, in some instances, a distinct population, differing from the initial one, can be seen. It may represent a shift of the initial clone/population or the emergence of a chemotherapy-resistant subpopulation. Whether this will lead to relapse is impossible to determine, but in such instances, closer surveillance of the patient is suggested.[4]

2. **PCR:** This approach is usually of high sensitivity and therefore currently considered the gold standard. In general, it is suggested that a MRD platform should be able to detect leukemic cells to a level of 0.1% (1 in 1,000 mutated cells). It is recommended to use real-time qPCR platforms for MRD assessment because of their established high sensitivity.[1] However, its applicability is limited to the ~40% of AML patients who harbor one or more suitable abnormalities. For molecular MRD, these abnormalities are limited to acute promyelocytic leukemia (APL), AML with inv (16) (*CBFB-MYH11*), AML with t(8;21) (AML1-ETO), and AML with *NPM1*-mutated. In APL, the most important MRD end point is the achievement of PCR negativity for *PML-RARA* at the end of consolidation treatment, which is associated with a low risk of relapse and high chance of long-term

survival. Despite the prognostic value of MRD in *CBFB-MYH11* AML in terms of relapse rate, no effect was noted on overall survival in multivariate analysis, probably because of the relatively high response rates of inv (16) AML to salvage treatment. The presence of measurable NPM1 transcripts in PB after at least two cycles of cytotoxic chemotherapy is associated with a high risk of relapse (>80%).

3. **NGS:** In light of the challenges of the MFC method and the limitations of the PCR-based method, the NGS-based approach might provide a good alternative in AML MRD detection. This theory is supported by a recent study by Jongen-Lavrencic, et al. (*NEJM* 2018); notably, patients who were both NGS and MFC negative had the best outcomes.

▓ MRD TESTING WITH ACUTE LYMPHOBLASTIC LEUKEMIA

1. **MFC:** It has been a long-standing tradition to use MFC to assess MRD in pediatric ALL patients due to the effort of Children's Oncology Group. This effort has significantly improved the survival of pediatric ALL patients. The most challenging aspect of MRD detection in B lymphoblastic leukemia is differentiating leukemic blasts from post-induction regeneration of normal immature lymphoid cells (hematogones), which express some common ALL-associated antigens. In addition, the bone marrow sample hypocellularity and, in some patients, phenotypic shift can create diagnostic challenges. For T-cell acute lymphoblastic leukemia (T-ALL), the markers of immaturity disappear during induction therapy; thus, an expansive antibody panel is needed to identify aberrant phenotypes. The currently accepted MRD level of sensitivity for B-ALL is 0.01%, while the sensitivity level for T-ALL is 0.1% (Roshal M, et al., *Cytometry B Clin Cytom.* 2010).

2. **PCR:** As discussed in the AML section, the PCR method requires a known sequence variation, thus limiting the use of the technology. The sensitivity varies, depending on individual tests.

3. **NGS:** The quantitation of MRD for B-ALL can be determined by NGS for rearranged IgH (VDJ), IgH (DJ), IgK, and IgL receptor-gene sequences. ClonoSeq® (Adaptive Biotechnologies, Seattle, WA) is an FDA-cleared test for evaluating for MRD for B-ALL. Extracted genomic DNA quality is assessed, and rearranged immune receptors are amplified with a multiplex PCR. Sequencing libraries are prepared from barcoded amplified DNA samples, which are then sequenced by synthesis with NGS. The study requires diagnostic samples to be used as an ID for MRD tracking. The ClonoSeq® Assay provides robust quantitative measurements of MRD frequencies from 10^{-4} to 10^{-6}. The sensitivity is correlated with the amount of input material (i.e., genomic DNA). Currently, no FDA-cleared MRD

assay exists for T-ALL, but the quantitation of MRD for T-ALL can be determined by NGS for T-cell receptor-gene sequences.

▣ MRD TESTING WITH MULTIPLE MYELOMA

Multiple myeloma often recurs due to residual malignant cells, drug resistance, and/or persistence of resistant dormant subclones. Molecular analyses remain pivotal for defining high-risk myeloma and are used in updated patient stratifications, while MRD testing is likely to be incorporated into standard follow-up for myeloma. Recent studies have confirmed the prognostic impact of MRD status as an independent variable for outcome. A bone marrow biopsy performed after completion of therapy is essential to assess response status. Heterogeneous bone marrow infiltration and peripheral blood dilution can be major hurdles to the evaluation of MRD, making an adequate bone marrow sample imperative to disease evaluation.

1. **MFC:** CD45 (in conjunction with light scatter characteristics), CD38, and CD138 are the best markers for the discrimination of plasma cells. In addition, the expression of CD19, CD56, CD117, CD20, CD28, CD27, and CD81, together with cytoplasmic immunoglobulin light-chain restriction, allows a clear discrimination between normal/reactive versus monoclonal plasma cells (Feller N, et al., *Leukemia*. 2004). MFC often underestimates the number of plasma cells due to their survival during the process. However, conventional-flow MRD approaches can discriminate aberrantly expressed cell surface markers in approximately 90% of patients (with a sensitivity of detecting 10^{-4} atypical PC in normal bone marrow) (Rawstrom AC, *Haematologica*. 2008). A recently published study showed that the sensitivity could reach 10^{-5} in high performance analysis (Soh KT, *Curr Protoc Cytom*. 2019).

2. **PCR:** MRD analysis by PCR detects persistent malignant plasma cells through the amplification of a tumor-specific molecular marker. The *IGH* rearrangement is used as a marker of clonality in various B-cell malignancies. PCR remains one of the most sensitive approaches to detect residual malignant plasma cells, reaching a sensitivity of 10^{-5} (van der Velden VH, et al., *Leukemia*. 2007). Unfortunately, it requires time-consuming labor and is not widely available because of its dependence on patient-specific primers and probes for quantitative PCR.

3. **NGS:** ClonoSeq® (Adaptive Biotechnologies, Seattle, WA) is an FDA-cleared test for evaluating for MRD in patients with multiple myeloma. Please see NGS section for MRD for B-Acute Lymphoblastic Leukemia.

4. **Imaging Studies:** For the evaluation of extramedullary disease, imaging studies should be used in combination with MFC and molecular studies. Studies have reported that PET/CT-negative

patients had better progression-free and overall survival rates compared to those of PET/CT-positive patients (Zamagni E, et al., *Clin Cancer Res*. 2015).

5. **Cell-Free DNA:** Recent studies have identified circulating DNA fragments carrying tumor-specific sequence alterations in the blood of patients with solid tumors; various studies have also found that myeloma-specific alterations (VDJ rearrangements or somatic genomic alterations) can also be identified and tracked in cell-free DNA circulating in blood (Mithraprabhu S, *Leukemia*. 2017).

▒ REFERENCES FOR SUPPLEMENTAL READING

1. Schuurhuis GJ, Heuser M, Freeman S, et al. Minimal/measurable residual disease in AML: a consensus document from the European LeukemiaNet MRD working party. *Blood*. 2018;131:1275–1291.

2. Della Starza I, Chiaretti S, De Propris MS, et al. Minimal residual disease in acute lymphoblastic leukemia: technical and clinical advances. *Front Oncol*. 2019;9:726.

3. Caers J, Garderet L, Kortüm KM, et al. European myeloma network recommendations on tools for the diagnosis and monitoring of multiple myeloma: what to use and when. *Haematologica*. 2018;103(11):1772–1784.

4. Ravandi F, Walter RB, Freeman SD. Evaluating measurable residual disease in acute myeloid leukemia. *Blood Adv*. 2018;2(11):1356–1366.

5. Loken MR, Chu SC, Fritschle W, et al. Normalization of bone marrow aspirates for hemodilution in flow cytometric analyses. *Cytometry B Clin Cytom*. 2009;76(1):27–36.

5 Polycythemia Vera

Misty Dawn Shields
and Kenneth S. Zuckerman

INTRODUCTION

Polycythemia vera (PV) is a chronic myeloproliferative neoplasm (MPN), most closely related to essential thrombocythemia (ET) and primary myelofibrosis (MF). PV is characterized by an elevated red cell mass (RCM), and is associated with mutation of the *JAK2* kinase in almost all cases. PV is predominantly diagnosed in patients ages 60 years and older, and no gender preference has been identified. PV is associated with decreased survival due to cardiovascular complications, most importantly thrombosis, as well as fibrotic progression to post-PV MF or leukemic transformation to acute myeloid leukemia (AML). Treatment of PV is focused on preventing thrombosis and bleeding complications and reducing vasomotor and constitutional symptoms, but it is not known to reduce the risk of progression to post-PV MF or transformation to AML and does not appear to prolong survival. Current risk stratification helps identify patients at higher risk of potential morbidity and mortality from PV and define criteria for risk-adapted treatment (including low-dose aspirin, phlebotomy, and cytoreductive agents). There is no clearly defined role for transplantation, unless in progression to post-PV MF or AML.

DIAGNOSIS

2016 WHO CLASSIFICATION

Requires All Three Major Criteria *OR* First Two Major Criteria + One Minor Criterion

Major Criteria

1. Hgb greater than 16.5 g/dL (male), Hgb greater than 16 g/dL (female) *OR* HCT greater than 49% (male), HCT greater than 48% (female)
2. Bone marrow (BM) trilineage myeloproliferation with pleomorphic megakaryocytes
3. Presence of *JAK2* mutation

Minor Criterion

1. Subnormal serum erythropoietin (EPO) level

Initial laboratory evaluation should include a CBC with differential, lactate dehydrogenase (LDH), serum EPO level, and molecular testing for *JAK2* V617F exon 14 mutation (~95% of WHO-defined PV). If negative, and the patient has features consistent with the diagnosis of PV, testing for a *JAK2* exon 12 or 13 mutation (present in 2% to 4% of cases) should be ordered. Bone marrow aspiration and biopsy (BM Asp/Bx) are necessary in most cases to differentiate PV with thrombocytosis, from ET; to help diagnose rare cases of *JAK2* unmutated PV; and to obtain a baseline measurement (or absence) of reticulin fibrosis (BM Asp/Bx features are summarized in Table 5.1). Although data show that BM Asp/Bx is not necessary to confirm a diagnosis of PV if the patient has Hgb >18%/HCT >60% or red blood cell mass >125% of expected, it remains a useful diagnostic test for baseline level of fibrosis. A focused physical exam should assess for a palpable spleen (~40%), although other signs, such as conjunctival plethora or ruddy cyanosis, may be found. History of constitutional symptoms, such as fatigue and pruritus; splenomegaly (early satiety and/or left upper quadrant abdominal pain); thrombosis (both arterial and venous as well as unusual sites, such as portal vein and splanchnic vein); bleeding episodes; and microvascular symptoms, such as headaches, lightheadedness, visual disturbances, atypical chest pain, erythromelalgia, and paresthesias, should be obtained. Family history should be evaluated for relatives with increased red blood cell counts, prior phlebotomies, or histories of any MPN or myeloid malignancy.

The differential diagnosis of physiologic and non-physiologic erythrocytosis includes (A) low EPO states, such as hypertransfusions

Table 5.1 Comparison of BM Aspirate/Biopsy Diagnostic Features Between PV and ET

PV Bone Marrow	ET Bone Marrow
Hypercellular	Normocellular to sometimes mildly hypercellular
Panmyelosis	Increased number of megakaryocytes, but no erythroid hyperplasia and no/modest granulocytic hyperplasia, with no significant left-shift of granulocytic or erythroid differentiation
Loose clusters of mature megakaryocytes of different sizes with polymorphous appearance	Marked proliferation of megakaryocytes with predominance of giant forms with abundant mature cytoplasm, deeply lobated or hyperlobated forms ("staghorn" nuclei), located diffusely or in small loose clusters
Lack of detectable iron by Prussian blue staining	Stainable iron is present in 40% to 70% at diagnosis

with pRBCs ("blood doping"), familial erythrocytosis caused by EPO receptor mutations, and PV; (B) hypoxia-driven erythrocytosis with normal-elevated EPO states, such as residence in a high altitude, severe chronic hypoxemic lung disease, obesity-hypoventilation or sleep apnea (possible, rarely proven), hemoglobinopathies with high oxygen affinity, chronic tobacco use, or end-stage renal disease; (C) non-physiologic with elevated EPO states and malignancy, such as renal cell, hepatocellular, ovarian, or parathyroid carcinomas, exogenous EPO or androgenic steroid administrations, or Von Hippel-Lindau (VHL) gene inactivating mutations.

▓ KEY DIAGNOSTIC DILEMMA

PV often presents with concomitant thrombocytosis, which can make it difficult to distinguish PV from ET, as the *JAK2* V617F mutation can also be seen in 50% to 60% of ET patients. This situation has been especially difficult in patients with "masked PV," whose Hgb/HCT levels do not meet diagnostic criteria; however, inclusion of BM characteristics can almost always can help distinguish these two diagnoses, most notably the cellularity of the bone marrow (Table 5.1).

▓ PROGNOSIS

PV is a chronic MPN that is incurable with current therapies other than hematopoietic stem cell transplantation, which is rarely indicated in the absence of post-PV MF or transformation to AML. Median overall survival (OS) of 14.1 years has been reported for all PV patients. In a study of more than 1,500 patients with PV, risk factors associated with decreased OS included older age, leukocytosis, venous thrombosis, and abnormal karyotype. Mayo Clinic Prognostic Scoring System risk score (summarized in Table 5.2) yields a median overall survival of 28, 19, and 11 years for low risk, intermediate risk, and high risk, respectively. Notably, reduced OS in PV is associated with cardiovascular complications and progression to post-PV MF and AML. The 10-year risk for transformation to post-PV MF is ~10%, and leukemic transformation to 3% to 5%. However, the risk of thrombosis exceeds 20% in the first 5 to 10 years, and in patients with marked thrombocytosis (platelets >1,000×10^9/dL), acquired von Willebrand-like syndrome can increase the risk of bleeding. Pre-existing risk factors (such as

Table 5.2 Mayo Clinic Prognostic Scoring System for PV

Age >67	5 points	*Low risk*	*0 points*
Age 56–67 years	2 points	*Intermediate risk*	*1–2 points*
Leukocytes >15,000	1 point	*High risk*	*≥3 points*
Prior thrombosis	1 point		

cardiovascular disease, HTN, diabetes, and tobacco use) are associated with an increased risk of thrombosis or other cardiovascular complications. Failure to maintain HCT below 45% and having elevated total WBC count (variably defined as >9,000, >11,000, or >15,000/µl, or above the normal range) also are increased risk factors for thrombosis.

▧ TREATMENT

The primary treatment goal is to reduce the risk of thrombosis without increasing the bleeding risk and to ameliorate symptoms. Unfortunately, current treatments have not been shown to prolong survival or alter the natural history of PV, other than reducing the risk of thrombosis or its potential risk of fibrotic or leukemic transformation. Therefore, the current treatment approach is to tailor therapy to a patient's risk stratification (Table 5.3). Low-dose aspirin therapy with phlebotomy (goal HCT <45) is recommended for all patients with PV, regardless of risk group or gender. Pruritus sometimes can be managed with low-dose aspirin, selective serotonin reuptake inhibitors (SSRIs), phototherapy, and/or antihistamines. Risk-adapted therapies include cytoreductive agents, such as hydroxyurea, interferon-α, and ruxolitinib, and less frequently busulfan. The RESPONSE trial studied the role of ruxolitinib (JAK1/2 kinase inhibitor) in phlebotomy-dependent, hydroxyurea-intolerant or -unresponsive PV patients with splenomegaly, randomized 1:1 to ruxolitinib versus standard of care (SOC; including hydroxyurea, IFN-α, anagrelide, immunomodulators, and pipobroman) with primary endpoints of HCT control and 35% reduction in splenic volume by week 32, that was achieved in 21% ruxolitinib versus 1% SOC (HCT control 60% [73% durable at 5 years] versus 19%). Of note, ruxolitinib was associated with higher rates of herpes zoster infections (6%) versus SOC (0%). Additionally, the RESPONSE-2 trial tested a similar patient population as above without splenomegaly, with a primary endpoint of HCT control achieved in 62% of patients versus 19% with SOC. Symptoms most improved with ruxolitinib (i.e., >90% change in symptom score) include pruritus, sweating, and symptomatic splenomegaly. Recurrent thrombosis is twice as likely in PV compared to non-MPN. Vitamin K antagonists have been the cornerstone for lifelong anticoagulation with splanchnic vein thrombosis (SVT) and long-term anticoagulation in cerebral venous thrombosis (CVT) in PV. The role of direct oral anticoagulants in high-risk MPN as well as recurrent thrombosis has not been well established, and use should be on an individualized basis.

▧ GENOMICS AND PERSONALIZED MEDICINE

The role of personalized medicine for PV is yet to be elucidated into translational practice; however, recent advances have shown promising data for diagnosis, prognostication, and treatment

Table 5.3 Risk Stratification of PV and Risk-Adapted Therapy

Risk Category	Therapy
Low risk without extreme thrombocytosis (≥1 or 1.5 million)	Low-dose aspirin + phlebotomy
Low risk with extreme thrombocytosis (≥1 or 1.5 million)	Low-dose aspirin (if ristocetin cofactor activity >30% and no history of significant bleeding) + phlebotomy
High risk	Low-dose aspirin once or twice daily + phlebotomy + hydroxyurea or pegylated interferon
High-risk refractory or intolerant to hydroxyurea	Low-dose aspirin once or twice daily + phlebotomy + ruxolitinib or pegylated interferon (age <65) or busulfan (≥65)
Treatment specifics	
Low-dose aspirin	81 mg daily (USA)/100 mg daily (outside USA)
Phlebotomy	Goal HCT <45%
Hydroxyurea	Start 500 mg daily and titrate to maximum 2000–2500 mg daily, with goal of normalization of blood counts
Interferon-α (pegylated)	Initial dose of 45 mcg weekly, titrated to usual maintenance dose of 90–180 mcg weekly
Ruxolitinib	Usual starting dose of 10–15 mg twice daily, titrated as needed for reduction of phlebotomy requirements, platelet count, and improvement of splenomegaly symptoms and side effects
Busulfan	Start at 2–4 mg/day, withhold when platelets <200 k/mcL or absolute neutrophil count <1500/mcL, and restart at half dose
Thrombosis (SVT, CVT, VTE, Arterial)	Vitamin K antagonist, typically long-term versus lifelong, could consider DOAC on individualized basis

planning. Risk-stratification models with mutations of splicesome genes (*SRSF2*) as well as *ASXL1 and IDH2* mutations, in addition to International Prognostic Scoring System (IPSS), may demonstrate independent predictive impact on overall survival, per Mutation-Enhanced International Prognostic Scoring Systems for

PV (MIPSS-PV) risk models. Recent preclinical studies suggest that hypoxia-inducible factor–regulated (HIF-regulated) target genes (IL1RAP, F3, SELP, VEGFA, SLC2A1) play a key role in pro-thrombo-inflammatory state of JAK2 V617F–mutated PV. Interestingly, CHIT1 (chitotriosidase), an enzyme found in macrophage activation, inflammation-induced remodeling, fibrosis, and pathologic erythropoiesis in PV, may have a diagnostic role as a circulating biomarker, as serum levels are significantly higher in PV or post-PV MF than in ET, post-ET MF, or primary MF.

POTENTIAL PRACTICE-CHANGING CLINICAL TRIALS

Several recent clinical trials investigating novel long-acting pegylated interferon, histone deacetylase (HDAC) inhibitors, MDM2 inhibitors, and JAK1/2 inhibitors have shown promising results in PV.

PROUD-PV and its extension study CONTINUATION-PV were Phase III randomized, controlled, open-label studies comparing novel monopegylated interferon alfa-2b (ropeginterferon alfa-2b) with hydroxyurea, for complete HCT response with normalization of spleen size, initially over 12 months (21% versus 28%) and then rolled over to 36 months to assess long-term response (53% versus 38%, $p = .04$), suggestive as a valuable durable long-term treatment option in PV without splenomegaly.

Phase I study of the MDM2 inhibitor idasanutlin with or without interferon alfa-2a in PV was safe (no dose-limiting toxicities) with promising ORR after six cycles of 58% alone, and 50% in combination, with median duration of response 16.8 months. Global Phase II trials are ongoing.

REFERENCES FOR SUPPLEMENTAL READING

1. Vannucchi A. How I treat polycythemia vera. *Blood.* 2014;124(22): 3212–3220.
2. Vannucchi A, Kiladjian J, Verstovsek S. Ruxolitinib versus standard therapy for the treatment of polycythemia vera. *N Eng J Med.* 2015; 372(5):426–435.
3. Tefferi A, Vannucchi M, Barbui, T. Polycythemia vera treatment algorithm 2018. *Blood Can J.* 2018;8:3.
4. Yacoub A, Mascarenhas J, Hoffman R. Pegylated interferon alfa-2a for polycythemia versa or essential thrombocythemia resistant or intolerant to hydroxyurea. *Blood.* 2019;134(18):1498–1509.
5. Tefferi A, Guglielmelli P, Vannucchi A. Mutation-enhanced international prognostic systems for essential thrombocythaemia and polycythaemia vera. *Br J Haematol.* 2020 Apr;189(2):291–302. doi: 10.1111/bjh.16380

6 Essential Thrombocythemia

Nikesh N. Shah and Kenneth S. Zuckerman

■ INTRODUCTION

Essential thrombocythemia (ET) is a *BCR-ABL1*-negative clonal myeloproliferative disorder associated with chronic thrombocytosis. Approximately 90% of patients have a somatically acquired mutually exclusive "driver" mutation in *JAK2, CALR*, or *MPL* that results in the upregulation of the *JAK-STAT* pathway. It is diagnosed by excluding causes of reactive thrombocytosis and other chronic myeloproliferative disorders, such as chronic myeloid leukemia (CML), polycythemia vera (PV), and primary myelofibrosis (PMF). The Surveillance, Epidemiology, and End Results (SEER) data have shown the incidence of ET in the United States to be 1.0 to 2.5 per 100,000 cases per year, with a median onset age between 50 and 60 years. However, as many as 20% may be younger than 40 years of age. Childhood ET is rare and appears to be relatively benign. When ET is diagnosed in childhood, ruling out whether the disorder is acquired or familial is reasonable. Interestingly, there is a female preponderance, with a ratio of 2:1. Up to 50% of patients present incidentally after a complete blood count (CBC) is obtained for other workup, while others can present with disease-related symptoms or complications, such as vasomotor symptoms, visual changes, dizziness, headache, thrombosis, bleeding, or first-trimester fetal loss. ET is also characterized by an increased risk of thrombosis and transformation to acute myeloid leukemia (AML) and post-ET myelofibrosis (MF).

■ DIAGNOSIS

Initial prospective studies to establish diagnostic criteria were undertaken by the Polycythemia Vera Study Group (PVSG) and World Health Organization (WHO). Revised WHO criteria for the diagnosis of ET require all four major criteria or the first three major criteria and one minor criterion.

WHO 2016 DIAGNOSTIC CRITERIA

Major Criteria

- Sustained platelet count ≥450 × 10^9/L
- Bone marrow biopsy showing megakaryocyte proliferation with increased number of large and mature megakaryocytes, with

hyperlobulated nuclei and no significant increase or left shift of neutrophil granulopoiesis or erythropoiesis and a very rarely minor (grade 1) increase in reticulin fibers
- Not meeting WHO criteria for *BCR-ABL1*-positive CML, PV, PMF, myelodysplastic syndrome (MDS), or other myeloid neoplasm
- Demonstration of *JAK2, CALR*, or *MPL* mutation

Minor Criterion
- Presence of a clonal marker (*ASXL1, EZH2, TET2, IDH1/IDH2, SRSF2*, or *SR3B1* mutation) or absence of evidence for reactive thrombocytosis

Most patients are asymptomatic at presentation, but some may experience constitutional symptoms, such as weight loss; fatigue; vasomotor symptoms, such as headache, lightheadedness, erythromelalgia, or livedo reticularis; acroparesthesia; or thrombotic or hemorrhagic episodes. Splenomegaly is rarely present on physical examination. Initial laboratory evaluation includes CBC with differential, comprehensive metabolic panel (CMP), serum ferritin, and serum erythropoietin. Diagnostic workup should also include mutation analysis for *JAK2, CALR, and MPL* mutations (Table 6.1). Bone marrow aspiration and biopsy are important for diagnosis and help differentiate "true" ET from prefibrotic/early PMF by the lack of reticulin fibrosis at onset, along with isolated megakaryocytic hyperplasia and differences in morphologic abnormalities. Bone marrow in ET patients typically shows randomly distributed or loosely clustered large to giant megakaryocytes with deeply folded staghorn nuclei surrounded by mature cytoplasm.

▨ PROGNOSIS

In 2012, the International Prognostic Score for ET (IPSET) for overall survival was derived from the evaluation of 867 patients diagnosed with ET, according to the 2008 WHO criteria. Based on prognostic factors of age (≥60 years), leukocytosis (≥11,000/mcl), and history of thrombosis, patients were divided into low- (0–1), intermediate- (2), and high-risk (3–4) groups. Ten-year thrombosis-free survival rates in the low-, intermediate-, and high-risk groups were 89%, 84%, and 69%, respectively (Figure 6.1). IPSET does not predict risk of evolution to post-ET MF or AML. In 2020, the Mutation-Enhanced International Prognostic Systems for Essential Thrombocythemia (MIPSS-ET), which incorporates molecular aberrations, has been proposed as an updated model to prognosticate survival. Patients are divided into low- (0–1), intermediate- (2–5), and high-risk (≥5) groups based on presence of male sex (1 point), age ≥60 years (4 points), presence of adverse mutations (*SRSF2, SF3B1, U2AF1, TP53;* 2 points), and leukocyte count ≥11,000/mcl (1 point). This method has not yet been prospectively validated. Both IPSET and MIPSS-ET stratify patients by survival, and the IPSET-thrombosis score was developed to assess

Table 6.1 Frequencies of Acquired Mutations in Essential Thrombocythemia

Gene	Mutations/Exons Involved	Genomic Location	Frequency in ET	Prognostic Impact
JAK2	Exon 14; V617F	9p24	60%	Increased thrombotic risk
CALR	Exon 9 type 1: 52-bp deletion type 2: 5-bp insertion	19p13.2	25%–30%	
MPL	Exon 10 S505N, W515K/L/A	1p34	3%–5%	
JAK2, CALR, and MPL negative			10%	
SRSF2	Inactivating mutations	17q25.1	2%	Adverse risk
SF3B1	Inactivating mutations	2q33.1	3%–5%	Adverse risk
U2AF1	Inactivating mutations	21q22.3	1%	Adverse risk
TP53	Inactivating mutations	17p13.1	2%	Adverse risk

ET: essential thrombocythemia.

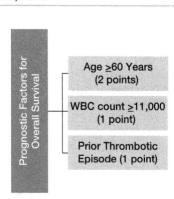

Figure 6.1 Factors associated with overall survival (IPSET score).

factors associated with increased risk of venous thromboembolism (VTE) (Figure 6.2). Based on this score, three thrombosis risk groups were identified—low, intermediate, and high (Table 6.2). A revised

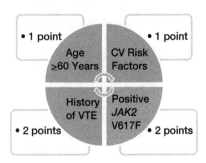

Cardiovascular (CV) Risk Factors:
Diabetes, Hypertension, Smoking

Figure 6.2 Factors associated with increased risk of thrombosis (IPSET score).

Table 6.2 Thrombotic Events Based on Revised IPSET Score		
Risk Groups	**Risk Factors**	**Thrombosis Risk/Year**
Very low risk	1. No VTE history 2. Age ≤60 years 3. *JAK2*-unmutated	• If CV risk factors: 1.05% • If no CV risk factors: 0.44%
Low risk	1. No VTE history 2. Age ≤60 years 3. *JAK2*-mutated	• If CV risk factors: 2.57% • If no CV risk factors: 1.59%
Intermediate risk	1. No VTE history 2. Age >60 years 3. *JAK2*-unmutated	• If CV risk factors: 1.64% • If no CV risk factors: 1.44%
High risk	1. VTE history at any age **OR** 2. Age >60 years and *JAK2*-mutated	• If CV risk factors: 4.17% • If no CV risk factors: 2.36%
CV, cardiovascular; VTE, venous thromboembolism.		

IPSET-thrombosis model was proposed and has been independently validated. The revised model has four risk groups: very low (no VTE history, age ≤60 years, *JAK2* unmutated), low (no VTE history, age ≤60 years, *JAK2*-mutated), intermediate (no VTE history, age > 60 years, *JAK2*-unmutated), and high (VTE history or age > 60 years with *JAK2* mutation). Though not incorporated into the original or revised IPSET-thrombosis models, leukocytosis is associated with an increase in thrombotic risk by 60%, as shown in a large meta-analysis of more than 30,000 patients with ET and PV. Genetic mutations are playing a larger role in prognostication in ET. Patients with *JAK2*V617F mutation tend to have higher hemoglobin, while those with *CALR* mutation tend to have higher platelet counts. As discussed above, *JAK2*V617F mutation is independently associated with increased thrombosis risk in comparison with *CALR* mutation. Cumulative thrombosis risk of *JAK2*V617F versus *CALR* has been shown to be 12% versus 3% (at 5 years), 22% versus 5% (at 10 years), and 33% versus 12% (at 15 years), respectively. *TP53* mutations have shown increased risk of leukemic transformation, whereas spliceosome mutations (*SF3B1* and *U2AF1*) are associated with lower rate of MF-free survival. A retrospective review of 133 patients showed decreased overall survival, leukemia-free survival, and MF-free survival, in patients with adverse-risk mutations (*SRSF2, SF3B1, U2AF1, TP53*).

▨ TREATMENT

Unfortunately, current therapies do not appear to alter the natural history of ET and do not prevent progression to post-ET MF or AML. Goals of treatment are symptom management and reduction of thrombosis and hemorrhage risk (Figure 6.3). Treatment can help minimize complications and control symptoms. National Comprehensive Cancer Network (NCCN) guidelines have incorporated the revised IPSET score into treatment recommendations, while European LeukemiaNet (ELN)

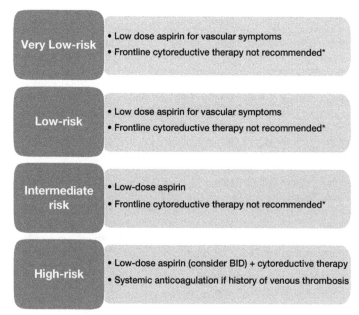

Very Low-risk
• Low dose aspirin for vascular symptoms
• Frontline cytoreductive therapy not recommended*

Low-risk
• Low dose aspirin for vascular symptoms
• Frontline cytoreductive therapy not recommended*

Intermediate risk
• Low-dose aspirin
• Frontline cytoreductive therapy not recommended*

High-risk
• Low-dose aspirin (consider BID) + cytoreductive therapy
• Systemic anticoagulation if history of venous thrombosis

* Consider initiating cytoreductive therapy for symptomatic progression (new thrombosis, major bleeding, splenomegaly, or intractable disease-related symptoms).

Figure 6.3 Current treatment recommendations for essential thrombocythemia.

still relies on the 2012 IPSET score. Both guidelines recommend aspirin for reduction of cardiovascular (CV) risk and cytoreductive therapy for high-risk patients. High-risk patients should be considered for twice-daily aspirin to effectively suppress thromboxane A2 synthesis, although this recommendation has not yet been updated in the guidelines. Systemic anticoagulation is also recommended for high-risk patients with history of venous thrombosis.

ASPIRIN
Aspirin should be used with caution in patients with thrombocytosis >1 million/mcl due to increased bleeding risk via acquired von Willebrand's disease (aVWD). Thus, such patients should be screened, and aspirin should be avoided in patients with ristocetin cofactor activity <30% due to increased risk of hemorrhage. Low-dose aspirin (≤100 mg/day) is only recommended if the ristocetin cofactor activity is ≥30%. The optimal dosing of aspirin in ET is not known, and patients who are high risk or who remain symptomatic with microvascular complications despite once-daily dosing can be considered for twice-daily low-dose aspirin. Anticoagulation can be continued with low-dose once-daily aspirin in patients who have a history of VTE and patients who are at risk for arterial thrombosis.

HYDROXYUREA
The cytoreductive agent Hydroxyurea (HU) is an antineoplastic drug that blocks deoxynucleotide synthesis by inhibiting the enzyme ribonucleotide reductase and can control symptoms associated with thrombocytosis and hepatosplenomegaly. HU is the preferred cytoreductive agent for most patients. The recommended initial dose is 15 mg/kg per day, and the dosage should be adjusted to limit neutropenia and anemia while maintaining a platelet count ≤600 × 10^9/L (Tefferi et al. *Blood Cancer J.* 2018). HU reduces the risk of thrombosis from 24% to less than 4% in high-risk patients with median follow-up of 27 months (maximum of 42 months). Side effects include nausea, vomiting, diarrhea or constipation, oral and skin ulceration, hyperpigmentation of the skin and nails, and mood changes. Rare complications include fever, abnormal liver function tests, and secondary hematologic malignancies. HU is relatively contraindicated in pregnancy, women of childbearing age, or during breast feeding; interferon should be used in these situations. HU can also induce megaloblastic features due to inhibition of vitamin B12 and folic-acid synthesis.

PEGYLATED INTERFERON-α
Pegylated interferon-α (IFN-α) is the treatment of choice in pregnancy, women of childbearing age, or patients failing treatment with HU. The starting dose is 45-mcg subcutaneously (SQ) once a week, titrated monthly to a goal dose of 90-, 135-, or 180-mcg SQ once a week to minimize toxicity (based on response and tolerance). Based

on response, IFN-α may be discontinued gradually, decreasing the dose by 45 mcg/week every 6 months and to 45 mcg every other week for final taper. The phase 2 MPD-RC 111 study evaluated IFN-α in 65 ET patients resistant or intolerant to HU. The ORR was 69%, with 43% CR and 26% PR. Patients with *CALR* mutation showed higher CR rates (56% vs. 28% in *CALR*-unmutated patients). The phase 3 MPN-RC 112 study randomized 168 patients with high-risk ET and PV to IFN-α versus HU. Outcomes were similar, with ORR at 12 months 69.8% with HU and 78% with IFN-α. IFN-α was associated with more grade 3–4 toxicities (51.3% vs. 30.8%). Common toxicities included headache, fatigue, weakness, nausea, depression, or, less often, transaminitis.

ANAGRELIDE

Anagrelide is an oral imidazoquinoline derivative, which inhibits platelet aggregation via the platelet anti-cyclic adenosine monophosphate (cAMP) phosphodiesterase activity and inhibits platelet production by interfering with megakaryocyte proliferation and maturation. It should be considered a treatment option only after failure of other options, such as pegylated-interferon and busulfan, due to increased incidence of arterial thrombosis, bleeding complications, and fibrotic progression. Side effects are related to vasodilator and inotropic effects, such as headache, fluid retention, tachycardia/palpitations, and diarrhea. Less common complications include anemia, heart failure, and acquired idiopathic cardiomyopathy. In the United Kingdom Medical Research Council Primary Thrombocythemia 1 Study, 809 patients were randomly assigned based on PVSG criteria to hydroxyurea versus anagrelide (with aspirin in both groups). After median follow-up of 39 months, patients in the anagrelide group experienced increased risk of arterial thrombosis (mostly transient ischemic attacks), hemorrhage, and a slightly higher rate of transformation to MF but lower risk of venous thrombosis. There was no difference in progression to AML or death. Anagrelide was compared to HU in the WHO-classified ET study (ANAHYDRET). 259 untreated high-risk patients with ET were enrolled, and anagrelide was non-inferior to HU with regard to thrombosis, bleeding, or rate of discontinuation after follow-up of 730 patient-years. Only 28% of patients were on aspirin in both groups.

BUSULFAN

Busulfan is an alkylating agent also used in ET, typically after progression or intolerance on HU. Busulfan can achieve sustained complete hematologic response in more than 80% of patients (Alvarez-Larran, et al., *Ann Hematol.* 2014). The starting dose is 2 to 4 mg daily orally, and treatment is held when platelets drop below 400 to 600 $\times$ 10^9/L. Once the platelet count increases, treatment can be resumed at a lower dose. The primary adverse effect is myelosuppression. Some studies have shown an increased risk of leukemic transformation, although this has not been consistently observed.

OTHER TREATMENT OPTIONS

Ruxolitinib is a *JAK* inhibitor approved for use in PV and MF that has been shown to have some activity in ET. The recommended starting dose is 15 to 20 mg twice daily for control of constitutional symptoms. The MAJIC-ET study randomized 58 patients with ET intolerance or resistance to hydroxycarbamide/hydroxyurea to ruxolitinib versus best available therapy. Response rates and toxicities were similar between both groups, with CR at 1 year 46.6% in the ruxolitinib group and 44.2% in the best available therapy group. It can cause dose-related myelosuppression. In post-ET MF, supportive care for management of cytopenias is important and is briefly described as follows:

- *JAK* inhibitors: Ruxolitinib and fedratinib are FDA-approved for treatment of post-ET MF. Additional *JAK* inhibitors aimed at reducing symptom burden include momelotinib (SIMPLIFY-2 trial) and pacritinib (PERSIST trial).

- Lenalidomide: The recommended starting dose is 10 mg daily for 21 of 28 days or thalidomide (starting dose 50 mg daily) plus prednisone for first 3 months (dose schedule of 30 mg daily for first month, then 15 mg daily for second month, then 15 mg every other day for third month).

- Splenectomy: This is reserved for patients with symptomatic splenomegaly who are unresponsive or intolerant to myelosuppressive agents or *JAK* inhibitors.

- Allogeneic hematopoietic stem cell transplantation: Myeloablative or nonmyeloablative chemotherapy can be an option in intermediate-two or high-risk patients (based on the Dynamic International Prognostic Scoring System [DIPSS] score).

POTENTIAL PRACTICE-CHANGING CLINICAL TRIALS

- RESET-272 is an ongoing phase 2 trial of ruxolitinib versus anagrelide in patients with ET resistance or intolerance to hydroxyurea (NCT03123588).

- NCT04262141 is an early-phase trial in ET or PV patients that is studying IMG-7289, lysine-specific demethylase 1 (LSD1) inhibitor, which has previously shown activity in MF.

- Aspirin Regimens in Essential Thrombocythemia (ARES) is a randomized phase 2 trial evaluating aspirin dosing in ET and the effect on platelet thromboxane production (EudraCT 2016-002885-30).

Ongoing studies in post-ET MF include the following:

- ESSENTIAL is a study including selinexor in MF refractory or intolerant to *JAK* inhibitors (NCT03627403).

- FREEDOM is a trial evaluating long-term efficacy and safety of fedratinib in intermediate- and high-risk MF patients previously treated with ruxolitinib (NCT03755518).

- MOMENTUM is a phase 3 trial randomizing patients to momelo-tinib versus danazol for anemic MF patients (NCT04173494).
- NCT03222609 is a phase 2 study evaluating tolerability and efficacy of navitoclax +/− ruxolitinib.

▦ REFERENCES FOR SUPPLEMENTAL READING

1. Barbui T, Vannucchi AM, Buxhofer-Ausch V, et al. Practice-relevant revision of IPSET-thrombosis based on 1019 patients with WHO-defined essential thrombocythemia. *Blood Cancer J.* 2015;5(11):e369.

2. Carobbio A, Ferrari A, Masciulli A, et al. Leukocytosis and thrombosis in essential thrombocythemia and polycythemia vera: a systematic review and meta-analysis. *Blood Adv.* 2019;3(11):1729–1737. doi: 10.1182/bloodadvances.2019000211

3. Harrison CN, Mead AJ, Panchal A, et al. Ruxolitinib vs best available therapy for ET intolerant or resistant to hydroxycarbamide. *Blood.* 2017;130(17):1889–1897. doi: 10.1182/blood-2017-05-785790

4. Tefferi A, Guglielmelli P, Lasho TL, et al. Mutation-enhanced international prognostic systems for essential thrombocythaemia and polycythaemia vera. *Br J Haematol.* 2020; doi: 10.1111/bjh.16380 [Epub ahead of print]

5. Tefferi A, Vannucchi AM, Barbui T. Essential thrombocythemia treatment algorithm 2018. *Blood Cancer J.* 2018;8(1):2. doi: 10.1038/s41408-017-0041-8

6. Yacoub A, Mascarenhas J, Kosiorek H, et al. Pegylated interferon alfa-2a for polycythemia vera or essential thrombocythemia resistant or intolerant to hydroxyurea. *Blood.* 2019;134(18):1498–1509. doi: 10.1182/blood.2019000428

7 Primary Myelofibrosis

Carmelo J. Blanquicett and Andrew Kuykendall

▓ INTRODUCTION

Primary myelofibrosis (PMF) is a chronic myeloproliferative neoplasm (MPN) characterized by constitutional symptoms, progressive cytopenias, hepatosplenomegaly, extramedullary hematopoiesis, and a propensity to transform into acute myeloid leukemia (AML). Myelofibrosis (MF) can occur de novo (PMF) or after a previous diagnosis of polycythemia vera (PV) or essential thrombocythemia (ET) (PPV-MF or PET-MF, respectively). The median age at diagnosis is between 60 and 65 years old. It is the least common of the *BCR-ABL1*-negative MPNs but the most symptomatic, with patients frequently experiencing fatigue, constitutional symptoms, and bone pain. The course of the disease is extremely variable, with some patients progressing quickly to AML, while others can be monitored without treatment for decades. Allogeneic hematopoietic cell transplant (AHCT) carries curative potential but is reserved for fit patients with higher-risk disease. Otherwise, treatment is palliative and focused on improving constitutional symptoms, splenomegaly, and cytopenias.

▓ DIAGNOSIS

Overt PMF should be distinguished from pre-fibrotic PMF, PPV-MF, or PET-MF. 2016 World Health Organization (WHO) Diagnosis Criteria for overt PMF must meet all three major criteria and at least one minor criterion:

Major Criteria

- Megakaryocyte proliferation and atypia on bone marrow biopsy accompanied by reticulin and/or collagen fibrosis grade 2 or 3
- Not meeting WHO criteria for chronic myeloid leukemia (CML), PV, ET, myelodysplastic syndromes (MDS), or other myeloid neoplasm
- Presence of clonal marker (*JAK2 V617F, JAK2* exon 12, *CALR* exon 9, *MPL* exon 10 mutations) OR absence of reactive bone marrow fibrosis

Minor Criteria

- Leukoerythroblastosis
- Leukocytes $\geq 11 \times 10^9$/L
- Increased serum lactate dehydrogenase (LDH)

- Anemia
- Palpable splenomegaly

Initial evaluation should include a complete blood count (CBC) with differential, complete metabolic panel (CMP), LDH, uric acid, bone marrow biopsy with cytogenetics, and molecular testing for *BCR-ABL1*, *JAK2*V617F, *JAK2* exon 12, *MPL*, and/or *CALR* mutations; however, triple negative disease (absence of a driving mutation in *JAK2*, *MPL*, or *CALR*) can be seen in up to 10% of individuals. Efforts to obtain a bone marrow aspirate are often met with a "dry tap," whereby an aspirate is unable to be obtained. Tear drop cells (dacrocytes) and leukoerythroblastic findings (i.e., nucleated red blood cells, immature myeloid cells) are seen on peripheral blood analysis. A focused physical exam should specifically assess for hepatosplenomegaly and signs and symptoms of anemia and thrombocytopenia.

■ KEY MANAGEMENT DILEMMA

Most patients will require therapy for MF-related symptoms. Due to the heterogeneity of the disease and the lack of disease-modifying therapies, treatment should be individualized. Patients with symptomatic splenomegaly and/or significant constitutional symptoms are likely to benefit from a *JAK2* inhibitor, such as ruxolitinib or fedratinib. In the absence of symptomatic splenomegaly and/or constitutional symptoms, *JAK2* inhibitors are unlikely to provide clinical benefit and may worsen hematologic parameters. Patients with severe anemia may benefit from erythropoietin-stimulating agents (ESAs), danazol, or immunomodulating drugs (e.g., lenalidomide, pomalidomide, or thalidomide). In most cases, clinical trials are a preferred option.

■ PROGNOSIS

Numerous prognostic scoring systems in MF have been developed over the last decade. Historical prognostic systems rely solely upon clinical data with inputs that include anemia, advanced age, constitutional symptoms, leukocytosis, and the presence of peripheral blasts. Contemporary prognostic scoring systems have increasingly relied upon molecular information. Select prognostic scoring systems have been summarized below to include clinically driven (DIPSS), genomically driven (GIPSS), and hybrid (MIPSS70-plus v2.0; see http://www.mipss70score.it/) models. MIPSS70-plus v2.0 represents the most comprehensive model to date; incorporates multiple tiers of cytogenetic data, gender-adjusted hemoglobin levels, and high-risk mutations, resulting in a five-tiered model with very low–, low-, intermediate-, high-, and very high–risk designations. MYSEC-PM is a prognostic model specifically developed to predict survival in secondary MF (i.e., post-ET MF and post-PV MF) and outperforms

PMF risk models (DIPSS, GIPSS, MIPSS70-plus v2.0) in this group of patients.6

Regardless of the model used, high-risk patients have a median life expectancy in the 1- to 2-year range, while low-risk patients have median expected survival of ≥10 years, highlighting the heterogenous nature of this disease (Table 7.1).

▓ TREATMENT

Treatment of MF is largely palliative in nature. AHCT offers the only curative option, but the vast majority of patients do not receive AHCT due to disease- or patient-related factors. The benefit of AHCT is limited to high-, intermediate-2-, and highly selected intermediate-1 risk patients due to the significant morbidity and mortality associated with this treatment.

Apart from AHCT, treatment typically aims at improving constitutional symptoms (e.g., fever, chills, night sweats, anorexia with weight loss) and symptomatic splenomegaly or improving cytopenias. For the former, *JAK2* inhibition has shown great benefit, while treatment options for the latter situation are varied and have exhibited less consistent benefit.

Numerous *JAK2* inhibitors have been evaluated in clinical trials with ruxolitinib and fedratinib, both currently approved for the treatment of intermediate- and high-risk MF. Ruxolitinib, a *JAK1/2* inhibitor, was approved in 2011 after demonstrating remarkable spleen-size reduction and symptom benefit versus placebo (COMFORT-I) and best available therapy (COMFORT-II). Fedratinib, a selective *JAK2* inhibitor with concomitant *FLT3* inhibition, was approved in 2019 after demonstrating significant spleen-size reduction compared to placebo (JAKARTA). Approval for fedratinib was considerably delayed due to a clinical hold over concerns with encephalopathy. Ultimately, fedratinib was approved, albeit with a black-box warning describing the potential for encephalopathy, including Wernicke's. Momelotinib and pacritinib are *JAK2* inhibitors that have demonstrated activity in MF and are currently in the late stages of clinical development, with potential advantages in patients who have concurrent anemia or thrombocytopenia, respectively (Table 7.2).

For patients whose primary clinical manifestations of MF are attributed to cytopenias, *JAK2* inhibitors offer little therapeutic benefit. In these patients, ESAs, androgens, and immune-modulators, such as lenalidamide and thalidomide, can be used. These agents have largely been evaluated retrospectively or in the context of small phase 2 studies lacking comparator arms. Responses rates range from 20% to 30% and are not durable (Table 7.3). Luspatercept, an erythroid maturation agent, is currently being studied in MF-related anemia, with encouraging results demonstrated in combination with ruxolitinib in transfusion-dependent patients (ASH 2019).

Table 7.1 Select Prognostic Scoring Systems and Associated Survival Data Based on the Corresponding Scoring System

	DIPSS (2010)	GIPSS	MIPSS 70+ Version 2.0
Clinical	• Hemoglobin <10 g/dl (2 points) • Age ≥65 years (1 point) • Constitutional symptoms (1 point) • Leucocytes >25 × 10⁹/L (1 point) • Circulating Blasts ≥1% (1 point)	• N/A	• Moderate anemia, Hgb 8–10 g/dl (1 point) • Severe anemia, Hgb <8 g/dl (2 points) • Constitutional symptoms (2 points) • Circulating blasts ≥2% (1 point)
Genetic	• N/A	• VHR karyotype (2 points) • Unfavorable karyotype (1 point) • Type 1/like CALR absent (1 point) • ASXL1 mutation (1 point) • SRSF2 mutation (1 point) • U2AF1Q157 mutation (1 point)	• VHR karyotype (4 points) • Unfavorable karyotype (3 points) • ≥2 HMR mutated genes (3 points) • 1 HMR mutation (2 points) • CALR type 1/like mutation absent (2 points)
Associated Survival Data (Median Survival)	• Low risk: 0 points (not reached) • Intermediate-1 risk: 1–2 points (14 years) • Intermediate-2 risk: 2 points (4 years) • High risk: 3–5 points (2 years)	• Low risk: 0 points (26.4 years) • Intermediate-1 risk: 1 point (8 years) • Intermediate-2 risk: 2 points (4.2 years) • High risk: ≥3 points (2 years)	• Very low risk: 0 points (not reached) • Low risk: 1–2 points (16.4 years) • Intermediate risk: 3–4 points (7.7 years) • High risk: 5–8 points (4.1 years) • Very high risk: ≥9 points (1.8 years)

Table 7.2 Overview of Treatment Options

	ESAs	Androgens (e.g., Danazol)	Hydroxyurea	IFN	Lenolidamide +/- prednisone	Low-Dose Thalidomide +/- Prednisone	Ruxolitinib	Fedratinib
Constitutional Symptoms	No effect	No effect	+	+/-	+	No effect	++	++
Splenomegaly	-	No effect	++	++	+	+	++	++
Anemia	+	+	-	-	+	++	-	-
Thrombocytopenia	-	+	-	-	+/-	++	-	-
Overall Survival	No effect	No effect	No effect	No effect	No effect	No effect	Modest increase—noted after 3 years	Unavailable (insufficient follow-up data)
Side Effects		Liver toxicity	- Leg/mouth ulcerations - Nail changes - Alopecia * No RCTs showing increased leukemogenic potential	- Flulike symptoms - Bone marrow suppression - Depression	- Thrombocytopenia - Fatigue - Mild neutropenia - Rash	- Constipation - Paresthesias - Mild neutropenia - Rash	- Marrow suppression (dose-related) - "Cytokine rebound" reaction - Opportunistic infections (i.e., varicella reactivation) - Increase in non-melanoma skin cancers	- Anemia - Thrombocytopenia - Fatigue - GI symptoms (nausea, diarrhea) - Transaminitis - Encephalopathy, including Wernicke's

A variety of treatment options exist for MF, though the benefit profile of each differs.
The above trial summarizes standard treatments while noting their beneficial (+) as well as deleterious (–) effects on common MF symptoms. Side effect profiles for these therapies vary as well.

ESA, erythropoietic-stimulating agents; GI, gastrointestinal; IFN, interferon; RCT, randomized controlled trial.

Table 7.3 Newer PMF Treatment Options, Respective Targets, and Late-Phase Clinical Trials Evaluating These Agents

Agent(s)/ Regimen	Targets	Clinical Trial Phase	Primary Endpoint
Ruxolitinib	*JAK1-/ JAK2-* inhibitor	III (COMFORT-I)	Reduction by at least 35% in the spleen volume at 24 weeks
		III (COMFORT II)	Percentage of patients with at least 35% reduction in spleen volume at 24 and 48 weeks
Pacritinib	*JAK2/ IRAK-1/ FLT3-* inhibitor	III (PERSIST-2)	Rates of patients achieving 35% or more spleen volume reduction and 50% or more reduction in total symptom score (TSS) at week 24
		III (PERSIST-1)	Spleen volume reduction of 35% or more from baseline at week 24
		II (PAC203)	Spleen volume reduction at 24 weeks
		III (PACIFICA)	Change in spleen volume at 24 weeks
Fedratinib	*JAK2-/ FLT3-* inhibitor	II (ARD11936)	Percentage reduction in spleen volume at 12 weeks
		III (JAKARTA)	Spleen response (≥35% reduction in spleen volume from baseline) at week 24 and confirmed 4 weeks later
Momelotinib	*JAK1-/ JAK2-/ ACVR1-* inhibitor	III (SIMPLIFY 2)	Reduction by at least 35% in spleen volume at 24 weeks compared with baseline in previously ruxolitinib-treated patients (endpoint not met)
		III* (MOMENTUM)	Total symptom score response rate at week 24
		III (SIMPLIFY 1)	Reduction by at least 35% in spleen volume at 24 weeks compared with baseline (momelotinib shown to be non-inferior to ruxolitinib for spleen response but inferior for symptom response in the secondary endpoint analysis: 28% vs 42%)

*In progress

Source: Adapted from Brewersdorf et al. *Cancer Manag Res.* 2019;11:10777–10790.

■ POTENTIAL PRACTICE-CHANGING CLINICAL TRIALS

Despite the successes of *JAK2* inhibition, current treatments lack the ability to modify the underlying disease. Current research is aimed at developing novel agents in addition to synergistic combinations. While two *JAK2* inhibitors have received FDA-approval, two additional *JAK2* inhibitors are in late-phase clinical trials. Momelotinib is a *JAK1/2* inhibitor that has shown encouraging effects on anemia and transfusion dependency. Despite setbacks in two previous phase 3 clinical trials (SIMPLIFY-1 and SIMPLIFY-2), it is currently being investigated in a phase 3 randomized controlled trial (MOMENTUM) versus danazol. Pacritinib, a *JAK2/FLT3/IRAK1* inhibitor, is also being investigated in a phase 3 study focusing on MF patients with severe thrombocytopenia, a group for whom current treatment options are extremely limited. Beyond *JAK2* inhibitors, novel agents being explored include the erythroid maturation agent luspatercept, a modified activin receptor type IIB (ActRIIB) fusion protein antagonist that has demonstrated activity in improving anemia in transfusion-dependent patients receiving ruxolitinib. Combination treatments are also actively being investigated. CPI-0610, a selective and potent bromodomain and extra-terminal domain (BET) inhibitor, demonstrated efficacy in terms of spleen volume reduction and symptom control when used in combination with ruxolitinib in the phase II MANIFEST trial. Recombinant human pentraxin-2 (PRM-151) has been shown to reduce bone marrow fibrosis and improve spleen size and symptoms, leading to its current and ongoing evaluation in a phase 2 trial. Imetelstat, a 13-mer oligonucleotide targeting human telomerase ribonucleic acid (RNA), was associated with impressive overall survival in a cohort of relapsed/refractory MF patients who had otherwise been shown to have a dismal prognosis. Without a control arm, these results have been challenging to contextualize. Nevertheless, this represents an encouraging trend in that the focus has been placed on potential disease modification rather than on improvements in spleen volume and symptom burden.

■ REFERENCES FOR SUPPLEMENTAL READING

1. Verstovsek S, Mesa RA, Gotlib J, et al. A double-blind, placebo-controlled trial of ruxolitinib for myelofibrosis. *N Engl J Med.* 2012;366(9):799–807.

2. Tefferi A, Pardanani A. Myeloproliferative neoplasms: a contemporary review. *JAMA Oncol.* 2015;1(1):97–105.

3. Cervantes F. How I treat myelofibrosis. *Blood, J Am Soc Hematol.* 2014;124(17):2635–2642.

4. Cervantes F, Dupriez B, Pereira A, et al. New prognostic scoring system for primary myelofibrosis based on a study of the International Working Group for Myelofibrosis Research and Treatment. *Blood, J Am Soc Hematol.* 2009;113(13):2895–2901.

5. Passamonti F, Cervantes F, Vannucchi AM, et al. A dynamic prognostic model to predict survival in primary myelofibrosis: a study by the IWG-MRT (International Working Group for Myeloproliferative Neoplasms Research and Treatment). *Blood, J Am Soc Hematol.* 2010;115(9):1703–1708.

6. Passamonti F, Giorgino T, Mora B, et al. A clinical-molecular prognostic model to predict survival in patients with post polycythemia vera and post essential thrombocythemia myelofibrosis. *Leukemia.* 2017;31(12):2726–2731. doi: 10.1038/leu.2017.169

7. Mesa RA, Gotlib J, Gupta V, et al. Effect of ruxolitinib therapy on myelo-fibrosis-related symptoms and other patient-reported outcomes in COMFORT-I: a randomized, double-blind, placebo-controlled trial. *J Clin Oncol.* 2013;31(10):1285.

8. Harrison CN, Vannucchi AM, Kiladjian JJ, et al. Long-term findings from COMFORT-II, a phase 3 study of ruxolitinib vs best available therapy for myelofibrosis. *Leukemia.* 2016;30(8):1701–1707. doi: 10.1038/leu.2016.148

9. Mascarenhas J, Hoffman R, Talpaz M, et al. Results of the PERSIST-2 phase 3 study of pacritinib (PAC) versus best available therapy (BAT), including ruxolitinib (RUX), in patients (pts) with myelofibrosis (MF) and platelet counts < 100,000/μl. *Blood.* 2016;128(LBA-5).

10. Mesa RA, Vannucchi AM, Mead A, et al. Pacritinib versus best available therapy for the treatment of myelofibrosis irrespective of baseline cyto-penias (PERSIST-1): an international, randomised, phase 3 trial. *Lancet Haematol.* 2017;4(5):e225–e236.

11. Gerds AT, Savona MR, Scott BL, et al. Results of PAC203: a randomized phase 2 dose-finding study and determination of the recommended dose of pacritinib. *Blood.* 2019;134(Suppl 1):667.

12. Harrison CN, Gerds AT, Kiladjian JJ, et al. Pacifica: a randomized, con-trolled phase 3 study of pacritinib vs. physician's choice in patients with primary myelofibrosis, post polycythemia vera myelofibrosis, or post essential thrombocytopenia myelofibrosis with severe thrombocytopenia (platelet count < 50,000/mL). *Blood.* 2019;134(Suppl 1):4175.

13. Pardanani A, Tefferi A, Jamieson C, et al. A phase 2 randomized dose-ranging study of the JAK2-selective inhibitor fedratinib (SAR302503) in patients with myelofibrosis. *Blood Can J.* 2015;5(8):e335–e335.

14. Harrison CN, Schaap N, Vannucchi AM, et al. Janus kinase-2 inhibitor fed-ratinib in patients with myelofibrosis previously treated with ruxolitinib (JAKARTA-2): a single-arm, open-label, non-randomised, phase 2, multi-centre study. *Lancet Haematol,* 2017;4(7):e317–e324.

15. Harrison CN, Vannucchi AM, Platzbecker U, et al. Momelotinib versus best available therapy in patients with myelofibrosis previously treated with ruxolitinib (SIMPLIFY 2): a randomised, open-label, phase 3 trial. *Lancet Haematol.* 2018;5(2):e73–e81.

8   Chronic Myelogenous Leukemia

Chetasi Talati, Dasom Caroline Lee,
and Javier Pinilla-Ibarz

▓ INTRODUCTION

Chronic myelogenous leukemia (CML) is a hematologic disorder accounting for 15% to 20% of adult leukemias with median age of onset of 67 years. However, there is also a significant smaller group that comprises adolescents and young adults (AYA) who are diagnosed between the ages of 15 and 29 years. Ionizing radiation is a known risk factor to the development of the disease. The majority of CML cases are molecularly defined by the presence of the Philadelphia chromosome (Ph), which is a reciprocal translocation resulting from the fusion of the breakpoint cluster region (*BCR*) gene on 22q11.2 and the Abelson murine leukemia (*ABL1*) gene on 9q34.1. Thus, t(9;22)(q34.1;q11.2) results in a *BCR-ABL1* fusion product with abnormal tyrosine kinase activity, which plays a central role in the abnormal cell proliferation.

CML is differentiated into three phases:

1. Chronic: 85% of patients are in this stage at diagnosis.
2. Accelerated: Leukocyte counts are challenging to control with treatment as neutrophil differentiation becomes impaired.
3. Blast phase: Lymphoid or myeloid blasts proliferate, uncontrollably resembling acute leukemia.

If chronic phase CML (CP-CML) is left untreated, it will eventually progress to accelerated phase (AP-CML) or blast phase (BP-CML) in 3 to 5 years. Early recognition and targeted treatment with novel tyrosine kinase inhibitors (TKIs) are crucial to improving patient outcomes and disease-specific survival.

▓ DIAGNOSIS

Accepted diagnostic criteria for CP-, AP-, and BP-CML are described below based on World Health Organization (WHO) 2016 classification. For BP-CML, Modified MD Anderson Cancer Center criteria and International Bone Marrow Transplant Registry (IBMTR) criteria are also widely accepted and described below:

WHO 2016 CRITERIA:

1. **CP-CML:** Not meeting the criteria of AP-CML and BP-CML

2. **AP-CML:** ≥1 of the hematologic/cytogenetic criteria or response to TKI criteria

   A. **Hematologic/Cytogenetic Criteria:**
   - Persistent or increased white blood count (WBC) (>10 × 10^9/L) unresponsive to therapy
   - Persistent or increasing splenomegaly unresponsive to therapy
   - Persistent thrombocytosis (>1000 × 10^9/L) unresponsive to therapy
   - Persistent thrombocytopenia (<100 × 10^9/L) unrelated to therapy
   - 20% or more basophils in the peripheral blood
   - 10%–19% blasts in the peripheral blood and/or bone marrow
   - Additional clonal chromosomal abnormalities in Ph+ cells at diagnosis that include "major route" abnormalities (second Ph, trisomy 8, isochromosome 17q, trisomy 19), complex karyotype, or abnormalities of 3q26.2
   - Any new clonal chromosomal abnormality in Ph+ cells that occurs during therapy

   B. **"Provisional" Response-to-TKI Criteria:**
   - Hematologic resistance to the first TKI (or failure to achieve a complete hematologic response to the first TKI) **OR**
   - Any hematologic, cytogenetic, or molecular indications of resistance to two sequential TKIs **OR**
   - Occurrence of two or more mutations in *BCR-ABL1* during TKI therapy

3. **BP-CML:**

   A. **WHO 2016 Criteria:**
   - ≥20% blasts in the blood or bone marrow **OR**
   - Extramedullary infiltrates of leukemic blasts

   B. **Modified MD Anderson Cancer Center Criteria (Used by Clinical Trials):**
   - Peripheral blood myeloblasts ≥15% and <30%
   - Peripheral blood myeloblasts and promyelocytes combined ≥30%
   - Peripheral blood or bone marrow basophils ≥20%
   - Platelet count ≤ 100 × 109/L unrelated to therapy
   - Additional clonal cytogenetic abnormalities in Ph+ cells

   C. **IBMTR Criteria:**
   - ≥30% myeloblasts in the blood **AND/OR** bone marrow
   - Extramedullary infiltrates of leukemic blasts

Symptoms can include generalized fatigue, abdominal pain and discomfort (left upper quadrant), weight loss, and early satiety from symptomatic splenomegaly and bleeding/bruising episodes. The physical exam should include assessing spleen size by palpation. Laboratory testing should include complete blood count (CBC) and comprehensive metabolic panel (CMP). A complete hematologic evaluation, including bone marrow biopsy and aspiration, flow cytometry, cytogenetic analysis, and molecular ancillary studies (i.e., fluorescence in situ hybridization [FISH] analysis for t(9;22) (q34.1;q11.2) *BCR-ABL1*), should be performed at the time of diagnosis to establish the specific phase of CML. Quantitative real-time polymerase chain reaction (qRT-PCR) for *BCR-ABL1* fusion transcripts should also be obtained at time of diagnosis and subsequently every 3 months to monitor treatment response (Tables 8.1 and 8.2). Patients with negative qRT-PCR for *BCR-ABL1* transcript in the setting of a positive cytogenetic or FISH result should be investigated for alternative splicing variants (i.e., p190 or p230), for which a specific polymerase chain reaction (PCR) can be ordered. The majority of CML cases involve the major BCR (M-BCR), which creates the fusion protein p210; however, involvement of the μ-BCR breakpoint region creates the larger fusion protein p230, which is associated with greater neutrophilic maturation and possibly thrombocytosis. Involvement of the minor-BCR, or m-BCR (p190), is more

Table 8.1 Response Criteria Definitions

Type of Response	Definition
CHR	• Platelets <450 × 10⁹/L AND • White cells <10 × 10⁹/L AND • No circulating immature myeloid cells AND • <5% basophils on differential AND • No palpable splenomegaly
PCyR	1%–35% Ph+ cells*
CCyR	No Ph+ cells*; fewer than 1 out of 200 nuclei *BCR-ABL1*–positive by FISH
MMR	*BCR-ABL*^{IS} ≤0.10%
MR$^{4.0}$	*BCR-ABL*^{IS} <0.01%
MR$^{4.5}$	*BCR-ABL*^{IS} <0.0032%
Molecularly Undetectable Leukemia	*BCR-ABL* transcripts nonquantifiable and nondetectable

CCyR, complete cytogenetic response; CHR, complete hematologic response; MMR, major molecular response; PCyR, partial cytogenetic response.

*At least 20 metaphases analyzed on conventional cytogenetics of bone marrow aspirate

Table 8.2 Response Expectations for First-Line Therapy/Second-Line After Intolerance

Time (Months)	Optimal Response	Treatment Failure
3	$BCR\text{-}ABL^{IS}$ ≤10% and/or PCyR	No CHR or Ph+ cells >95% by karyotyping
6	$BCR\text{-}ABL^{IS}$ <1% and/or CCyR	$BCR\text{-}ABL^{IS}$ >10% or Ph+ cells >35% by karyotyping
12	$BCR\text{-}ABL^{IS}$ ≤0.1% (MMR)	$BCR\text{-}ABL^{IS}$ >1% or CCyR not achieved
At any time	$BCR\text{-}ABL^{IS}$ ≤0.1% (MMR)	Loss of CHR, loss of CCyR, confirmed loss of MMR*, $BCR\text{-}ABL1$ kinase domain mutation, additional cytogenetic abnormality in Ph+ cells

CCyR, complete cytogenetic response; CHR, complete hematologic response; MMR, major molecular response.

*Confirmed loss of MMR = two consecutive results showing $BCR\text{-}ABL1$ greater than 0.1%, of which one is ≥1%.

frequently encountered in Ph-positive B-ALL (see $BCR\text{-}ABL1$ + B-ALL section) but also can be rarely found in patients with CP-CML (typically with monocytosis).

▓ KEY DIAGNOSTIC DILEMMA

The differential diagnosis for CML includes a leukemoid reaction, chronic myelomonocytic leukemia (CMML), chronic neutrophilic leukemia (CNL), and atypical CML. CMML usually has characteristics of both myeloproliferative neoplasm (MPN) and myelodysplastic syndromes (MDS) with persistent monocytosis of greater than 1,000 cells/mcL with anemia and/or thrombocytopenia. Atypical CML features leukocytosis and splenomegaly but lacks the Ph chromosome and thus is categorized with MDS/MPN (see MDS/MPN section). CNL commonly harbors the colony-stimulating factor 3 receptor ($CSF3R$) T618I mutation along with SET binding protein 1 ($SETBP1$) and is associated with a poor prognosis (see Chapter 6). BP-CML can be difficult to differentiate from acute myeloid leukemia (AML), but the presence of basophilia, splenomegaly, clinical history of prior CML, and $BCR\text{-}ABL1$ positivity are useful features for diagnosing BP-CML.

▓ PROGNOSIS

Risk stratification can be accomplished using the Sokal, Hasford, or European Treatment and Outcome Study (EUTOS) scores (*Int J Hematol.* 2014;100(4):379–385; online calculator for all three scores available at http://bloodref.com/myeloid/cml/sokal-hasford).

■ TREATMENT
INITIAL TREATMENT—WITHOUT CONFIRMATION

- Hydroxyurea is used for cytoreduction with an elevated WBC (>50 × 10⁹/L) while confirmation of the Ph is being obtained.
- Allopurinol can be used to minimize complications associated with tumor lysis (see Chapter 52).

FRONTLINE TREATMENT IN CP-CML

- Low risk (Sokal): Imatinib 400 mg daily, nilotinib 300 mg BID, dasatinib 100 mg daily, or bosutinib 400 mg PO daily (*J Clin Oncol.* 2010;28:424–430; *J Clin Oncol.* 2014;32:415–423; *Blood.* 2012;119:1123–1129; *Lancet Oncol.* 2011;12:841–851; *J Clin Oncol.* 2018;36(3):231–237)
- Intermediate or high risk (Sokal): Nilotinib 300 mg BID, dasatinib 100 mg daily, or bosutinib 400 mg PO daily (*Blood.* 2012;119:1123–1129; *Lancet Oncol.* 2011;12:841–851; *J Clin Oncol.* 2018;36(3):231–237)

The ENESTnd study comparing nilotinib to standard-dose imatinib showed a cumulative rate of major molecular response (MMR) at 5 years of 77% with nilotinib and 60% with imatinib and an $MR^{4.5}$ of 54% and 31%, respectively. Rate of transformation to accelerated or blast phase was also significantly lower (2.1%–3.2% vs 6.7%, respectively). The DASISION study comparing dasatinib to standard-dose imatinib had cumulative MMR rates at 5 years of 76% with dasatinib and 64% with imatinib and an $MR^{4.5}$ of 42% and 33%, respectively. Rate of transformation to accelerated or blast phase was lower (2.5% vs 5.8%). Certain mutations have shown better response rates to nilotinib (V299L, F317L/V/I/C), whereas some respond better to dasatinib (E255K/V, F359V/C/I). The BFORE trial comparing bosutinib 400 mg PO daily to standard-dose imatinib resulted in MMR rate at 12 months (primary endpoint) of 47.2% compared to 36.9%, respectively (p = .02). Rate of disease progression to accelerated/blast phase was 1.6% with bosutinib and 2.5% with imatinib.

FRONTLINE TREATMENT IN AP-CML AND BP-CML

The goal is to control and bring the disease back to chronic phase and to proceed to hematopoietic stem cell transplant (HSCT). Imatinib and dasatinib have been FDA-approved for all phases of CML, including blast crisis. Nilotinib and bosutinib are only FDA-approved for chronic and accelerated phases but are not to be used in blast phase. Ponatinib has been approved for T315I in all phases and in its absence when no other TKIs are indicated. If previous therapy includes interferon (IFN) or hydroxyurea only, imatinib, nilotinib, bosutinib, or dasatinib can be initiated with plans to proceed with HSCT. If the patient progressed on prior treatment with a TKI, a mutation profile should be performed to guide subsequent therapy. Ponatinib or dasatinib can be used along with chemotherapy in patients without T315I mutation. If T315I mutation is identified, ponatinib is the only active TKI available. If TKIs fail and the patient is in myeloid blast crisis, anthracycline- and cytarabine-based induction regimens can be used. For a lymphoid blast crisis, use of hyperfractionated cyclophosphamide, vincristine, Adriamycin, and dexamethasone (Hyper-CVAD in cycles 1, 3, 5, and 7; methotrexate, solumedrol, cytarabine as part of cycles 2, 4, 6, and 8) in conjunction with a TKI (typically dasatinib or ponatinib) is recommended. Patients in blast crisis should receive allogeneic stem cell transplant during first remission to improve outcomes when feasible.

PATIENTS WITH RESISTANCE OR INTOLERANCE TO TKI

Omacetaxine mepesuccinate is a protein synthesis inhibitor that has a role in the treatment of advanced phase CML in patients with docu-mented intolerance to prior therapy with two or more TKIs. Two phase 2 trials (CML-202 and CML-203) assessed 51 patients with AP-CML and 44 patients with BP-CML, with primary endpoint being maintenance or attainment of major hematologic response (MHR). MHR was noted in 37% of AP-CML and 9% of BP-CML patients (Khoury et al., *Leuk Lymphoma*; 56(1):120–127).

WHEN TO PROCEED WITH ALLOGENEIC STEM CELL TRANSPLANT

The advent of TKI therapy with excellent response rates and low side-effect profiles compared to HSCT has reduced its necessity in chronic phase. HSCT should only be considered after failure of one or two TKIs and in case of hematologic intolerance. HSCT remains controversial in patients with T315I mutations in chronic phase. For patients in AP- or BP-CML, HSCT should be considered after disease control (blast <5%). The 5-year overall survival (OS) for transplant is 40% in AP-CML and 10% in BP-CML.

▓ MONITORING RESPONSE TO TKI THERAPY

Current guidelines recommend monitoring for *BCR-ABL1* transcript levels via peripheral blood qRT-PCR at diagnosis and every 3 months while receiving TKI therapy. This should be continued for a total of 2 years after complete cytogenetic response (CCyR) has been achieved. After 2 years, qRT-PCR should be done every 3 to 6 months. If increase in the transcript level is observed (at least 1-log increase), qRT-PCR should be repeated in 1 to 3 months. Bone marrow cytogenetics are needed at the time of diagnosis and to assess for cytogenetic response at 3 months. If at the 3-month evaluation, PCyR or *BCR-ABL1* less than 10% has been achieved, one can continue the same dose of TKI. If this criterion is not met, switching to alternate TKI or dose escalation of imatinib is suggested after consideration of adher-ence and drug interactions. At 12 months, if CCyR is not achieved, the recommendation is to switch to an alternate TKI. A bone marrow biopsy should be performed whenever CCyR or MMR is not achieved in 1 year to confirm that the disease has not progressed. If there is disease progression to accelerated or blast phase from chronic phase, *BCR-ABL* kinase domain mutation analysis should be performed. During CP-CML, when there are any signs of hematologic or cytogenetic relapse, mutation analysis is recommended. Furthermore, lack of PCyR or presence of *BCR-ABL1* transcript level greater than 10% at 3 and 6 months mandates *BCR-ABL* kinase domain mutation analysis. At 12 months, if CCyR or MMR is not achieved, mutational analysis should be performed.

▧ TREATMENT-FREE REMISSION

Treatment-free remission (TFR) can be achieved in carefully selected patients with CP-CML who have reached and maintained deep molecular response ($\geq$MR$^{4.0}$; *BCR-ABL* $\leq$ 0.01% *BCR-ABL* IS) for $\geq$2 or more years. The most important major change in the field is the potential for TKI discontinuation in patients with deep molecular remission, as initial studies have shown safety (i.e., response can be recaptured) and durability of remission following discontinuation (30%–50% TFR; *Lancet Haematol.* 2015;2(12):e528–e535; *J Clin Oncol.* 2014;32(5):424–430). Feasibility of discontinuation of TKI has been evaluated in several clinical trials; based on such studies, National Cancer Centers Network (NCCN) has devised eligibility criteria for TKI discontinuation:

1. Adult patients (age $\geq$18) with CP-CML who have prior quantifiable *BCR-ABL1* transcript and have been treated with any approved TKI therapy for at least 3 years
2. Patients who also have achieved and maintained deep molecular response for $\geq$2 years, as demonstrated by at least four tests that are performed at least 3 months apart

Patients who maintain MMR (MR^3; *BCR-ABL1* $\leq$ 0.1% IS) after TKI discontinuation should be closely followed with monthly molecular monitoring for one year, every 2 months for the second year, and every 3 months thereafter. They should have easy access to qPCR test with sensitivity of detection of at least MR$^{4.5}$ (*BCR-ABL-ABL1* $\leq$ 0.0032% IS) and ability to provide results within 2 weeks. Such close follow-up after TKI discontinuation is critical, because approximately 40% to 60% of patients who discontinue TKI therapy experience molecular relapse within 12 months. They should also be monitored for TKI withdrawal syndrome, which presents as diffuse musculoskeletal pain or pruritis. If loss of MMR is detected, TKI therapy should be resumed within 4 weeks with monthly molecular monitoring until MMR is achieved. For those who achieve MMR after resumption of TKI therapy, molecular monitoring every 3 months indefinitely is recommended. For those who fail to achieve MMR, *BCR-ABL1* kinase domain mutation testing is recommended with monthly molecular monitoring for 6 months.

▣ POTENTIAL PRACTICE-CHANGING CLINICAL TRIALS

Asciminib, a fourth-generation TKI that targets native and mutated *BCR-ABL1,* including the T315I mutation, demonstrated a substantial and durable MMR by 12 months in 48% of evaluable patients and MMR by 12 months in 28% of patients with T315I mutation in a phase I clinical trial of patients heavily pretreated with CML (*N Engl J Med.* 2019 Dec 12;381(24):2315–2326). Another phase I clinical trial that assesses asciminib in combination with nilotinib in CML is currently being investigated (NCT02081378). PETALs (NCT02201459), DASAPEG (NCT01725204), and PINNACLE (NCT02001818) are ongoing trials studying the effects of combining IFN with TKIs, such as nilotinib or dasatinib. Because complete molecular remission (CMR) may be curative, *BCR-ABL* independent factors eradicating MRD are being studied. Ruxolitinib is an oral agent that targets the *JAK-STAT* pathway and disrupts a protective niche for leukemic stem cells, leading to increased TKI-induced apoptosis. A phase I clinical trial demonstrated that ruxolitinib in combination with nilotinib was well tolerated and resulted in a promising molecular response (40% of undetectable *BCR-ABL* transcripts by 6 months), which warrants further investigation (*Leuk Res.* 2018 Nov;74:89–96). Another clinical trial that investigates maintenance of TFR after treatment with ruxolitinib plus TKI therapy in CP-CML in patients who failed TKI discontinuation is also being conducted (NCT03610971).

▣ REFERENCES FOR SUPPLEMENTAL READING

1. Baccarani M, Deininger MW, Rosti G, et al. European LeukemiaNet recommendations for the management of chronic myeloid leukemia. *Blood.* 2013;122(6):872–874.

2. Cortes J, Kantarjian H. How I treat newly diagnosed CP-CML. *Blood.* 2012;120(7):1390–1397.

3. Druker BJ, Guilhot F, O'Brien SG, et al. Five-year follow-up of patients receiving imatinib for chronic myeloid leukemia. *N Engl J Med.* 2006;355(23):2408–2417.

4. Hugues T, Deininger M, Hocchaus A, et al. Monitoring CML patients responding to treatment with tyrosine kinase inhibitors: review and recommendations for harmonizing current methodology for detecting BCR-ABL transcripts and kinase domain mutations and for expressing results. *Blood.* 2006;108:28–37.

5. Ross D, Hughes T. How I determine if and when to recommend stopping tyrosine kinase inhibitor treatment for chronic myeloid leukemia. *Br J Haematol.* 2014;166(1):3–11.

6. Hughes TP, Mauro MJ, Cortes JE, et al. Asciminib in chronic myeloid leukemia after ABL kinase inhibitor failure. *N Engl J Med.* 2019 Dec 12;381(24):2315–2326.

7. Sweet K, Hazlehurst L, Sahakian E, et al. A phase I clinical trial of ruxolitinib in combination with nilotinib in chronic myeloid leukemia patients with molecular evidence of disease. *Leuk Res.* 2018 Nov;74:89–96.

9   Chronic Neutrophilic Leukemia

Yenny Alejandra Moreno Vanegas, Arun Kadamkulam Syriac,

and Utkarsh Acharya

▨ INTRODUCTION

Chronic neutrophilic leukemia (CNL) is a rare *BCR/ABL*-negative myeloproliferative disorder. It is characterized by a sustained mature neutrophilia without dysgranulopoiesis. Clinical presentation includes hepatosplenomegaly, myeloid marrow hyperplasia due to granulocyte proliferation, and absence of the *BCR/ABL* fusion gene. The diagnosis of CNL has been historically challenging and has ultimately relied on the exclusion of alternate reactive and myeloproliferative disorders, including chronic myelogenous leukemia (CML) and chronic myelomonocytic leukemia (CMML). The discovery of the oncogenic driver mutation *CSF3R* has helped provide a biomarker for this difficult diagnosis. Given the diagnostic challenges and paucity of reported cases, limited epidemiologic data exist. Nevertheless, recent literature indicates that CNL affects mostly elderly patients, with a median age of diagnosis of 66.5 years in the largest series of 40 patients. There is a slight male preponderance (56% to 58% of the cases). The clinical course includes chronic and an accelerated or blast phase with the possibility of progression to myelodysplastic syndrome (20%) and acute myeloid leukemia (AML). This condition has limited management options and a generally unfavorable prognosis, with survival rates of less than 2 years.

▨ DIAGNOSIS

Most patients exhibit no overt symptoms, and the diagnosis of CNL is incidentally entertained because of a protracted and unexplained leukocytosis. However, symptomatic patients most commonly report fatigue with rare accompanying symptoms, including weight loss, bone pain, pruritus, hepatosplenomegaly, gout, and bleeding diathesis due to platelet dysfunction, thrombocytopenia, and/or neoplastic cells infiltrating vascular walls. Patients with bleeding symptoms out of proportion to their platelet counts should be evaluated for acquired von Willebrand's disease and other platelet/coagulation disorders. As noted in Table 9.1, accurate diagnosis of CNL relies on a thorough clinical history, complete blood count (CBC), abdominal imaging, and bone marrow examination. A diagnosis of CNL is contingent upon the exclusion of alternate myeloproliferative disorders, including CML and CMML. In 2016, the World Health Organization (WHO) classification was updated to include *CSF3R*-T618I and other activating mutations in *CSF3R* as diagnostic markers.

Table 9.1 Distinguishing Features Between aCML and CNL

Characteristics	aCML	CNL
Peripheral Leukocytosis	>13 × 109/L	>25 × 10⁹/L
• Neutrophils	Left shift	>80% of leukocytes
• Basophils	Minimally increased	Not increased
• Monocytes	Variable, <1 × 109/L	<1 × 109/L
• Immature Granulocytes	>10%	<10%
• Myeloblasts	<20%	<1%
• Granulocytic Dysplasia	Present	Absent
Bone Marrow		
• Myeloid Hyperplasia	Present	Present
• Myeloblasts	<20%	<5%
• Neutrophilic Maturation Pattern	Dysplasia	Normal
Clinical		
• Infectious or Inflammatory Process	Absent	Absent
• Median Age	60–80 years	60–80 years
• Median Survival	25 months	23.5 months
• Hepatosplenomegaly	Present	Present
• Mucocutaneous Bleeding	Present	Present
BCR/ABL Fusion Gene, PDGFRA, PDGFRB, FGFR1 Rearrangements	Absent	Absent
Evidence of Alternate MPN (PV, ET, MF)	Absent	Absent
Mutation in CSF3R	Up to one third SETBP and/or ETNK1 mutation positive, and rarely CSF3R, 10%	Usually present (60%–100% of cases)

aCML, atypical chronic myelogenous leukemia; CNL, chronic neutrophilic leukemia; ET, essential thrombocythemia; MF, myelofibrosis; MPN, myeloproliferative neoplasms; PV, polycythemia vera.

2016 WHO CLASSIFICATION OF CNL

1. Peripheral blood white blood cells (WBC) ≥25 × 10^9/L
   - Segmented neutrophils plus band forming ≥80% of WBCs
   - Neutrophil precursors (promyelocytes, myelocytes, and metamyelocytes) <10% of WBC
   - Myeloblasts rarely observed
   - Monocyte count <1 × 10^9/L
   - No dysgranulopoiesis

2. Hypercellular bone marrow
   - Neutrophil granulocytes increased in percentage and number
   - Normal neutrophilic maturation
   - Myeloblasts <5% of nucleated cells

3. Not meeting WHO criteria for *BCR-ABL1+* CML, polycythemia vera (PV), essential thrombocythemia (ET), or primary myelofibrosis (PMF)

4. No rearrangement of *PDGFRA, PDGFRB, FGFR1,* or *PCM1-JAK2*

5. Presence of *CSF3R*-T618I, other activating *CSF3R* mutation, or, in the absence of a *CSF3R* mutation, persistent neutrophilia (at least 3 months); splenomegaly; and no identifiable cause of reactive neutrophilia, including the absence of a plasma cell neoplasm or, if present, demonstration of clonality of myeloid cells by cytogenetic or molecular studies

KEY DIAGNOSTIC DILEMMA

The diagnosis of atypical CML (aCML) can be confused with CNL, as they both can present in the same manner and have similar laboratory findings. After close evaluation, there are several key features that can distinguish the two leukemias (Table 9.1). For instance, in CNL, the peripheral leukocytosis counts are generally greater than 25 × 10^9/L, with a median leukocyte count of 39 × 10^9/L, as opposed to aCML, with counts greater than 13 × 10^9/L. Importantly, CNL is characterized by the presence of more mature granulopoietic forms (>80% are at the band and segmented stage of neutrophil development), with minimal to no circulating blasts. The absence of monocytosis, eosinophilia, and basophilia is another key finding. Peripheral smear and bone marrow aspirate may show immature granulocytes (>10% in the peripheral blood), and granulocytic dysplasia is another important diagnostic difference between aCML and CNL.

2016 WHO CLASSIFICATION OF ACML

1. Peripheral blood (PB) leukocytosis due to increased numbers of neutrophils and their precursors (promyelocytes, myelocytes, metamyelocytes) comprising ≥10% of leukocytes

2. Dysgranulopoiesis, which may include abnormal chromatin clumping

3. No or minimal absolute basophilia; basophils usually <2% of leukocytes

4. No or minimal absolute monocytosis; monocytes <10% of leukocytes

5. Hypercellular bone marrow (BM) with granulocytic proliferation and granulocytic dysplasia, with or without dysplasia in the erythroid and megakaryocytic lineages

6. Less than 20% blasts in the blood and BM

7. No evidence of *PDGFRA*, *PDGFRB*, or *FGFR1* rearrangement or *PCM1-JAK2*

8. Not meeting WHO criteria for *BCR-ABL1+* CML, PMF, PV, or ET*

*Cases of myeloproliferative neoplasms (MPN), particularly those in accelerated phase and/or in post-PV or post-ET myelofibrosis, if neutrophilic, may simulate aCML. A previous history of MPN, the presence of MPN features in the BM, and/or MPN-associated mutations (in *JAK2*, *CALR*, or *MPL*) tend to exclude a diagnosis of aCML. Conversely, a diagnosis of aCML is supported by the presence of *SETBP1* and/or *ETNK1* mutations. The presence of a *CSF3R* mutation is uncommon in aCML and, if detected, should prompt a careful morphologic review to exclude an alternative diagnosis of CNL or other myeloid neoplasms.

■ DIAGNOSTIC ADVANCES

Cytogenetic analysis is typically normal in CNL patients. However, various aberrations, including del(11q), del(20q), add (21), and del(12p), have been reported in myeloid disorders, but none is specific to CNL. Considerable advances in molecular profiling have led to the identification of *CSF3R*, which encodes the receptor for colony-stimulating factor 3, a cytokine responsible for the differentiation and proliferation of myeloid cell lines. These observations gave rise to possible therapeutic targets. Mutations in *CSF3R* have been associated with severe congenital neutropenia and are reported in 60% to 100% of WHO-defined CNL cases from previously reported cohorts. Two major mutations include *CSF3R*-T618I and *CSF3R*-T615A. These point mutations have been shown to produce constitutive activation of tyrosine kinases that will cause activation of the JAK-STAT pathway and the SRC tyrosine kinase pathway. These mutations, in addition to truncation of the *CSF3R* protein, have also been described in approximately 25% of CNL patients. Other concomitant mutations that have been evaluated in other myeloid malignancies can also be observed in CNL. The most common of these mutations include *SETBP1*, *ASXL1*, and *SRSF2*. Both *SETBP1* and *ASXL1* mutations in CNL have been associated with a poor prognosis, and *SETBP1* has been anecdotally implicated in resistance to ruxolitinib.

▨ PROGNOSIS

CNL falls within a heterogeneous spectrum of myeloproliferative disorders, and prognostic data are limited, given the scarcity of published manuscripts. Although not specifically defined (as in CML), CNL has a chronic phase, an accelerated phase, and a blast phase. Disease acceleration often manifests with progressive neutrophilia with resistance to therapy. Median overall survival is reportedly 23.5 months, according to existing literature. The most common disease complications include transformation to AML, which may occur in approximately 20% of cases and at a median of 21 months from initial diagnosis. The most common causes of mortality include intracranial hemorrhage because of evolving thrombocytopenia, leukemic transformation, and iatrogenic-related complications from therapy (e.g., infections). Poor prognosis factors of CNL are not clear. On multivariable analysis, only the presence of *ASXL1* mutations and thrombocytopenia at diagnosis were independently predictive of shortened survival. Other studies have shown that both *SETBP1* and *ASXL1* mutations may be associated with poor prognosis in CNL and CMML. The presence of *SETBP1* mutation can be associated with progression of blast-phase transformation. Interestingly, the presence of *CSF3R* variants has not been shown to affect survival based on historical data. However, newer studies have shown that *CSF3R*-T618I mutated individuals exhibit adverse clinical features and reduced life expectancy when compared to other variants.

▨ TREATMENT

Optimal management strategies to address CNL have yet to be perfected, and the decision to treat should be based on patient performance status, symptoms, and clinician/patient preferences. Currently, there is no standard of care, and none of the therapeutic agents has shown benefits of survival, other than for a small fraction of patients who undergo stem cell transplant. Hydroxyurea is the most commonly utilized cytoreductive agent to control leukocytosis and reduce spleen size; however, most patients exhibit unintended cytopenias or become refractory to therapy with continued use. Other therapies include interferon-alpha or its pegylated form, hypomethylating agents, ruxolitinib, thalidomide, cladribine, and imatinib. None of these treatments has induced remission. Alternatively, splenic debulking to control abdominal symptoms was previously incorporated into treatment but is no longer recommended due to the ensuing and severe leukocytosis observed after the procedure. For patients with transformed acute leukemia, standard "7 + 3" induction is recommended; however, remission is seldom achieved as in most transformed/secondary acute leukemias. Allogeneic hematopoietic stem cell transplant (HSCT) has also been reported via case reports but is accompanied by high mortality and failure rates. As such, no standardized practice exists to date for the treatment of such patients.

■ POTENTIAL PRACTICE-CHANGING CLINICAL TRIALS

Identification of the *CSF3R*-T618I mutation has been a target of interest when exploring novel therapeutic strategies for this challenging condition. Based on anecdotal evidence exhibiting the cytoreductive and hematologic efficacy of ruxolitinib in a CNL patient harboring *CSF3R*-T618I mutation, the general applicability of JAK inhibition in this disease group has generated notable interest. Accordingly, a phase 2 study (NCT02092324) examined the efficacy of ruxolitinib in 44 patients with aCML and CNL with data reported in December 2019. The results from this trial demonstrated an overall response rate of 35% in the entire cohort, with response rates favoring treated patients with CNL and/or those harboring *CSF3R*-T618I mutation. This is the first trial to formally explore the efficacy of JAK/STAT inhibition in patients with CNL and may invoke a paradigm shift in treatment of this rare condition. Further research pertaining to the diagnostic, therapeutic, and prognostic significance of molecular profiling in this disease is ongoing.

■ REFERENCES FOR SUPPLEMENTAL READING

1. Bain BJ, Brunning RD, Vardiman J, et al. Chronic neutrophilic leukaemia. In: Swerdlow S, Campo E, Harris NL, eds. *WHO Classification of Tumours of Haematopoietic and Lymphoid Tissue*. Geneva, Switzerland: World Health Organization; 2008:38–39.

2. Barbui T, Thiele J, Gisslinger H, et al. The 2016 WHO classification and diagnostic criteria for myeloproliferative neoplasms: document summary and indepth discussion. *Blood Can J*. 2018;8:15.

3. Elliott MA, Hanson CA, Dewald GW, et al. WHO-defined chronic neutrophilic leukemia: a long-term analysis of 12 cases and a critical review of the literature. *Leukemia*. 2005;19:313–317.

4. Maxson JE, Gotlib J, Pollyea DA, et al. Oncogenic *CSF3R* mutations in chronic neutrophilic leukemia and atypical CML. *N Engl J Med*. 2013;368:1781–1790.

5. Szuber N, Tefferi, A. Chronic neutrophilic leukemia: new science and new diagnostic criteria. *Blood Can J*. 2018;8:19.

6. Vardiman JW, Bennett JM, Bain BJ, et al. Atypical chronic myeloid leukaemia, BCR-ABL1 negative. In: Swerdlow SH, Campo E, Lee Harris N, et al., eds. *WHO Classification of Tumors of Haematopoietic and Lymphoid Tissues*. Lyon, France: IARC Press; 2008:80–81.

7. Szuber N, Finke CM, Lasho TL, et al. *CSF3R*-mutated chronic neutrophilic leukemia: long-term outcome in 19 consecutive patients and risk model for survival. *Blood Can J*. 2018;8(2):21.

8. Szuber N, Elliott M, Tefferi A. Chronic neutrophilic leukemia: 2020 update on diagnosis, molecular genetics, prognosis, and management. *Am J Hematol*. 2020 Feb;95(2):212–224.

9. Dao KT, Gotlib J, Deininger MM, et al. Efficacy of ruxolitinib in patients with chronic neutrophilic leukemia and atypical chronic myeloid leukemia. *J Clin Oncol*. 2020;38(10):1006–1018. doi: 10.1200/JCO.19.00895

10 Systemic Mastocytosis

Kristen Gonter-Aubin and Andrew Kuykendall

▨ INTRODUCTION

Systemic mastocytosis (SM) is a clonal disorder leading to expansion of the mast cell population and accumulation of mast cells in tissues. A rare disease diagnosed in both children and adults, it is estimated to affect about 1 in 10,000 people. Children commonly present with isolated cutaneous involvement, while adults more commonly show evidence of systemic infiltration. Symptoms are largely due to activation of the allergic response, tissue invasion, and subsequent mast cell granule release. The diagnosis is based primarily on evidence of proliferation of abnormal mast cells with concomitant elevated tryptase and the presence of a somatic mutation in *KIT*. Treatment aims to improve disease-related symptoms and decrease mast cell burden. The emergence of targeted therapies has begun to shift the long-standing treatment paradigm.

▨ DIAGNOSIS

2016 World Health Organization (WHO) Diagnostic Criteria require 1 major criterion + 1 minor criterion **OR** 3 minor criteria.

Major Criterion

1. Presence in bone marrow or other noncutaneous tissue of multifocal dense aggregates containing ≥15 mast cells in aggregates

Minor Criteria

1. Mast cells with atypical morphology or spindled shaped, comprising more than 25% of the total mast cells in the bone marrow or noncutaneous tissue, *OR* more than 25% of total mast cells in bone marrow aspirate either immature or atypical
2. *KIT D816V* mutation detected in bone marrow, blood, or other extracutaneous organs (~90% of SM patients)
3. Bone marrow or other noncutaneous mast cells abnormally expressing CD2 and/or CD25 surface markers
4. Serum tryptase level persistently >20 ng/mL (patient must be in baseline state, and this criterion is only valid if there is no concurrent clonal myeloid disorder)

DIAGNOSTIC PEARLS

- Cytopenias, cytoses, or elevated lactate dehydrogenase (LDH) may suggest a concomitant associated hematologic neoplasm (AHN) and should prompt further investigation.
- Sanger sequencing and next-generation sequencing often lack the sensitivity needed to capture *KIT* mutations, which may lead to false negatives. Highly sensitive polymerase chain reaction (PCR) assays are required and can be performed on peripheral blood samples.
- In the setting of an AHN, particularly acute myeloid leukemia (AML), SM can often be overlooked in the pathologic evaluation of a bone marrow specimen due to poor staining.

▓ KEY DIAGNOSTIC DILEMMA

A significant subset of SM patients (~40%) exhibit evidence of AHN. These patients are categorized by the 2016 WHO classification as having SM with an associated hematologic neoplasm (SM-AHN). This was referred to as SM with an associated clonal hematologic non-mast cell lineage disease (SM-AHNMD) in WHO 2008. In 90% of patients, the associated hematologic disease is myeloid in origin, with chronic myelomonocytic leukemia (CMML) being a common partner. Associated lymphoproliferative diseases have also been reported but are much less common. SM-AHN patients are more likely to be older, male, and more symptomatic than patients with SM. The associated hematologic disorder is often aggressive, requires therapy, and should be notated in the diagnostic section of the pathology report. *KIT*-targeting agents (i.e., midostaurin, avapritinib) have shown benefit for patients with SM-AHN, though progression to AML is still observed, suggesting that the AHN often drives prognosis (Tables 10.1 and 10.2).

▓ PROGNOSIS

The prognosis for patients with SM is variable. Patients with indolent systemic mastocytosis (ISM) likely have a prognosis similar to the age-adjusted population, while those with mast cell leukemia have nearly 100% expected mortality at 2 years. Between those two extremes, advanced SM has a 5-year overall survival (OS) rate of approximately 30% to 35%, while SM-AHN has a 5-year OS rate of approximately 20%. The international prognostic scoring system for mastocytosis (IPSM) is a simple, validated prognostic tool. In those with non-advanced mastocytosis, age ≥60 and an alkaline phosphatase level ≥100 U/L were prognostic of inferior OS and progression-free survival (PFS). Patients with no risk factors (low risk) had a 10-year OS of 98.1%, while those with one or two risk factors had 10-year OS of 87.1% and 52.1%, respectively. In those with

Table 10.1 "B" and "C" Findings Stratify SM by Symptoms

"B" Findings: Organ involvement without organ dysfunction	"C" Findings: Organ involvement with organ dysfunction
1. Bone marrow biopsy >30% mast cell infiltration and/or total tryptase >20 ng/mL	1. Bone marrow destruction manifested by ≥1 cytopenia with no apparent non–mast cell hematologic malignancy
2. Signs of dysplasia or myeloproliferation in non–mast cell lineages (not meeting criteria for AHNMD)	2. Skeletal involvement with large osteolytic lesions or pathologic fractures
3. Hepatomegaly without impairment of liver function, palpable splenomegaly without hypersplenism, and/or lymphadenopathy on palpation or imaging	3. Palpable hepatomegaly with evidence of liver dysfunction, portal HTN, or ascites
	4. Malabsorption with weight loss due to GI infiltration

AHNMD, associated clonal hematologic non–mast cell disease; GI, gastrointestinal; HTN, hypertension.

advanced mastocytosis, age >60, tryptase level 125 ng/mL or higher, leukocyte count 16×10^9/L or higher, hemoglobin ≤11 g/dL, platelet count ≤100 × 10^9/L, and skin involvement were prognostic of inferior OS and PFS. OS of those with ASM and ≤1 risk factor was comparable to those with non-advanced mastocytosis and one to two risk factors. Those with ASM and two to five risk factors had significantly worse OS.

▇ TREATMENT

Treatment is based on utilization of a wide variety of agents to try to mitigate symptoms from mast cell activation or to reduce mast cell burden. In ISM or smoldering systemic mastocytosis (SSM), treatment is typically targeted at avoidance of triggers, symptom-directed treatment, and treatment of concomitant osteoporosis/osteopenia. The ongoing PIONEER study is evaluating avapritinib in patients with ISM/SSM. For patients with ASM and SM-AHN, treatment is aimed at improving organ damage inflicted by mast cell proliferation while reducing the mast cell burden. Increasingly, *KIT*-targeting agents , such as midostaurin, are being used in this setting, though treatment of the AHN often takes precedence. Cladribine can lead to rapid cytoreduction, but cytopenias and opportunistic infections are common (Table 10.3).

Table 10.2 WHO Classification of Mastocytosis

CM	1. UP (also known as MPCM)
	2. Diffuse cutaneous mastocytosis (almost exclusively seen in children)
	3. Solitary mastocytoma of skin
Solid Mast Cell Tumors	1. Mast cell sarcoma
	2. Extracutaneous mastocytoma
	*No evidence of SM, a localized destructive growth pattern, and high-grade cytology are common.

Subtypes of SM

1. ISM
   a. Meets criteria for SM
   b. No "C" findings
   c. No evidence of AHN

SSM	**Isolated bone marrow mastocytosis**
• ISM, but with 2 or more "B" findings	• ISM plus bone marrow involvement, no skin involvement
• Generally high burden of MC	• Generally low burden of MC

2. SM-AHN	Distinct entity per WHO classification Meets criteria for SM and criteria for AHN
3. ASM	• Meets criteria for SM • 1 or more "C" findings • No evidence of mast cell leukemia
4. MCL	• Meets criteria for SM ≥10% immature mast cells in peripheral blood and/or ≥20% immature/atypical mast cells on bone marrow aspirate • Rare variant: aleukemic MCL, <10% circulating mast cells, and no skin lesions – Extremely poor prognosis

AHN, associated hematologic neoplasm; ASM, aggressive systemic masto-cytosis; CM, cutaneous mastocytosis; ISM, indolent systemic mastocytosis; MCL, mast cell leukemia; MPCM, maculopapular cutaneous mastocytosis; SM, systemic mastocytosis; SM-AHN, systemic mastocytosis with associated hematologic neoplasm; SSM, smoldering systemic mastocytosis; UP, urticara pigmentosa.

Mastocytosis can be divided into CM, SM, and solid mast cell tumors. Within these categories, the disease is further stratified based on organ involvement and organ dysfunction. These classifications differ prognostically and serve to guide therapeutic approach. Often, patients with "C" findings require cytotoxic therapy.

▩ POTENTIAL PRACTICE-CHANGING CLINICAL TRIALS

Phase 1 and 2 trials with Avapritinib/BLU-285, a small molecule kinase inhibitor that selectively inhibits activation-loop mutants of *KIT,* has shown promising results across all subtypes of SM. A phase 1 dose

Table 10.3 Treatments for SM		
Symptomatic	**Cytoreductive**	
Antihistamines	**Interferon alpha 2b**	
– H1 antagonists to prevent pruritus and flushing – H2 antagonists to control abdominal symptoms – Dual H1 and serotonin-receptor antagonist, cyproheptadine, can potentially treat both	– 1 million units 3×/week – with gradual dose escalation – maximum = 5 million units/day; can be given with prednisone – ORR (~50%) – May relieve bone pain and bony lesions	
Leukotriene antagonists	**Cladribine** (2-CdA) 5 mg/m² daily for 5 days Q4-8 wk	
– Can be used in conjunction with antihistamines	– ORR ~70% – Possibly more effective in ISM	
Mast cell stabilizers	**Glucocorticoids** (e.g., prednisone 1 mg/kg)	
– Helps with GI symptoms	– May provide temporary benefit	
Aspirin	**Tyrosine kinase inhibitors**	Imatinibᵃ
– Can help control flushing and/or angioedema		– Useful in those **without** *KIT* D816V mutation
Epinephrine		Dasatanib
– To be used for anaphylactic events		– Active in vitro, disappointing in vivo
Omalizumab		Midostaurin
– Anti-IgE humanized monoclonal ab – Case reports suggest prevention of recurrent anaphylaxis		– Active against mutated mastocytosis

ᵃ*KIT* D816V mutation induces resistance to imatinib. Patients should be screened prior to therapy.

GI, gastrointestinal; ISM, indolent systemic mastocytosis; ORR; objective response rate.

escalation/expansion trial (NCT02561988) in 69 (39 evaluable) ASM patients noted overall response rates and complete response (CR)/partial hematologic recovery (CRh) rates of 77% and 23%, respectively, with 93% of evaluable patients having a ≥50% reduction in both bone marrow mast cells and serum tryptase level. Data from the phase 2 trial (NCT03580655) in ASM are pending. A randomized phase 2 trial (NCT03731260) in patients with ISM/SSM noted rapid reduction of ≥50% in serum tryptase levels and mast cell burden in patients treated at all dose levels. A 30% improvement in mastocytosis-related symptoms and quality of life was seen with avapritinib compared to placebo, independent of dose. No grade 3 adverse events were reported. Ripretinib/DCC-2618, a *KIT* and *PDGFRA* switch control inhibitor, is currently being studied in patients with advanced malignancies, including ASM, SM-AHN, and MCL (NCT02571036). This agent has the potential to inhibit exon 17 *KIT* mutations that are resistant to conventional kinase inhibitors.

■ REFERENCES FOR SUPPLEMENTAL READING

1. Theoharides TC, Valent P, Akin C. Mast cells, mastocytosis, and related disorders. *N Engl J Med.* 2015;373:163–172.

2. Valent P, Akin C, Metcalfe DD. Mastocytosis: 2016 updated WHO classification and novel emerging treatment concepts. *Blood.* 2017;129(11):1420–1427. doi: 10.1182/blood-2016-09-7318933

3. Reiter A. George T, Gotlib J. New developments in diagnosis, prognostication and treatment of advanced systemic mastocytosis. *Blood.* doi: 10.1182/blood.2019000932 [Published online ahead of print February 27, 2020]

4. Lim KH, Tefferi A, Lasho TL, et al. Systemic mastocytosis in 342 consecutive adults: survival studies and prognostic factors. *Blood.* 2009;113:5727–5736.

5. Wang SA, Hutchinson L, Tang G, et al. Systemic mastocytosis with associated clonal hematological non-mast cell lineage disease (SM-AHNMD): clinical significance and comparison of chromosomal abnormalities in SM and AHNMD components. *Am J Hematol.* 2013;88:219–224.

6. Sperr WR, Kundi M, Alvarez-Twose I, et al. International prognostic scoring system for mastocytosis (IPSM): a retrospective cohort study. *Lancet Haematol.* 2019;6(12):e638–e649. doi: 10.1016/S2352-3026(19)30166-8e

11 PDGFRA/PDGFRB/FGFR1 Myeloid Neoplasms

Joseph Clara and Eric Padron

■ INTRODUCTION

Myeloid and lymphoid neoplasms with eosinophilia and abnormalities of platelet-derived growth factor receptor alpha (*PDGFRA*), platelet-derived growth factor receptor beta (*PDGFRB*), and fibroblast growth factor receptor 1 (*FGFR1*) comprise a group of rare hematologic neoplasms associated with eosinophilia, which result from the formation of a fusion gene that encodes an aberrant, constitutively activated tyrosine kinase. They are considered to be very rare (<1/100,000), but their exact incidences are unknown. The most prevalent fusion gene among them, *FIP1L1-PDGFRA*, is estimated to be present in around 10% of idiopathic hypereosinophilia cases in developed countries. There is a marked male predominance (M:F ratio of ~17:1) in neoplasms related to *PDGFRA* fusion, with a median age of onset in the 40s, and a more moderate male predominance in disease related to *PDGFRB* (M:F ratio of 2:1) and *FGFR1* (M:F ratio of 1.5:1), with a median age of onset of 40 and 32 years, respectively. While these entities are grouped together based on genetic/molecular similarities, they exhibit variable clinical manifestations and are also distinguished by their respective sensitivities to the tyrosine kinase inhibitor imatinib. The most common presentations of disease associated with *PDGFRA*, *PDGFRB*, and *FGFR1* fusions are chronic eosinophilic leukemia (CEL), chronic myelomonocytic leukemia (CMML), and myeloproliferative neoplasm (MPN) or T-lymphoblastic lymphoma, respectively, although a spectrum of hematologic manifestations can be seen in each group. Eosinophil-mediated organ damage is most likely to occur in neoplasms involving *PDGFRA* and may involve the skin, spleen, gastrointestinal (GI) tract, lungs, and heart. Lymph node involvement and systemic systems, such as fever, weight loss, night sweats, and fatigue, are more common in *FGFR1* disease. *PDGFRA*- and *PDGFRB*-associated neoplasms demonstrate an almost invariable and dramatic response to imatinib, while *FGFR1*-associated disease is not sensitive to imatinib and has no clinically recognized targeted treatment. However, encouraging preliminary results have been reported from a phase II trial with the *FGFR* inhibitor pemigatinib (see below). The understanding of the unique cytogenetic and molecular abnormalities of these entities along with the advent of targeted tyrosine kinase inhibitors has led to major improvements in outcomes for a large proportion of patients with these illnesses, with the exception of those with *FGFR1* abnormalities.

▦ DIAGNOSIS

2008 World Health Organization (WHO) Diagnostic Criteria of Myeloid and Lymphoid Neoplasms With Eosinophilia and Abnormalities of *PDGFRA, PDGFRB,* or *FGFR1*

- Diagnostic criteria of an MPN (or acute myeloid leukemia [AML] or lymphoblastic leukemia/lymphoma) with eosinophilia associated with *FIP1L1-PDGFRA*:
  - An MPN (or AML or lymphoblastic leukemia/lymphoma) with prominent eosinophilia
  - Presence of an *FIP1L1-PDGFRA* fusion gene (interstitial deletion del(4)(q12q12))
- Diagnostic criteria of MPN associated with *ETV6-PDGFRB* fusion gene or other rearrangement of *PDGFRB*:
  - An MPN, often with prominent eosinophilia and sometimes with neutrophilia or monocytosis
  - Presence of t(5;12)(q31~q33;p12) or a variant translocation or demonstration of an *ETV6-PDGFRB* fusion gene rearrangement of *PDGFRB*
- Diagnostic criteria of MPN or acute leukemia associated with *FGFR1* rearrangement:
  - An MPN with prominent eosinophilia and sometimes with neutrophilia/monocytosis or acute leukemia (i.e., AML or precursor T-cell/B-cell lymphoblastic leukemia/lymphoma [often with peripheral blood or bone marrow eosinophilia])
  - Presence of t(8;13)(p11;q12) or a variant translocation leading to *FGFR1* rearrangement demonstrated in myeloid cells, lymphoblasts, or both

2016 WHO Updates to Myeloid and Lymphoid Neoplasms Associated With Eosinophilia and Rearrangements of *PDGFRA, PDGFRB,* or *FGFR1* or With *PCM1-JAK2* (*Blood.* 2016; 127(20):2391–2405)

- Criteria remain the same, but it is now recognized that a subset of cases do not have eosinophilia.
- New provisional entity: myeloid neoplasm with t(8;9)(p22;q24.1); *PCM1-JAK2*
  - Eosinophilia, left-shifted erythroid predominance, lymphoid aggregates, and usually evidence of myelofibrosis (possibly imitating primary myelofibrosis [PMF]) may rarely present as the precursor lymphoid neoplasms B- or T-acute lymphoblastic leukemia (ALL) and may respond to *JAK* inhibitors
- *ETV6-JAK2* and *BCR-JAK2* mutated neoplasms are best classified under the new provisional entity, *BCR-ABL1*-like B-ALL

Evaluation includes complete blood count (CBC) with differential; peripheral blood smear; blood chemistries; serum tryptase, serum IgE, and vitamin $B_{12;}$ bone marrow biopsy with cytogenetic analysis; immunophenotyping; molecular analysis for *FIP1L1-PDGFRA;* and assessment for end-organ damage based on signs and symptoms, including serum troponin, electrocardiogram, echocardiogram, pulmonary function tests/bronchoscopy, biopsy of affected tissues, and computerized tomography (CT) scan of chest/abdomen/pelvis. The *FIP1L1-PDGFRA* fusion gene results from a cryptic del(4)(q12) and is the most common cytogenetic abnormality in neoplasms with *PDGFRA* rearrangement. This 800-kb deletion is undetectable by karyotype, and molecular testing is often required with real-time polymerase chain reaction (RT-PCR), nested RT-PCR, or fluorescence in situ hybridization (FISH) analysis. A markedly elevated serum vitamin B_{12} (>2,000 pg/mL) or tryptase level (>11.5 ng/mL) may be used as a surrogate marker for *FIP1L1-PDGFRA*-positive disease when testing for the gene fusion is unavailable. Cytogenetics should be carried out to screen for abnormalities involving *PDGFRB* and *FGFR1* as well as other variants of *PDGFRA*. The most common partner fusion gene associated with *PDGFRB* is *ETV6*, which results from t(5;12)(q31-33;p12), and the most common partner fusion gene associated with *FGFR1* is *ZNF198*, resulting from t(8;13)(p11;q12). *PDGFRB* and *FGFR1* abnormalities detected on cytogenetic testing should be confirmed by RT-PCR or FISH studies. Rarely, *PDGFRB* rearrangements are cytogenetically occult but can be detected by RT-PCR or ribonucleic acid (RNA)-sequencing analysis.

▓ KEY DIAGNOSTIC DILEMMA

T- and B-cell lymphoblastic leukemia/lymphoma may present with eosinophilia (see B-cell ALL and T-cell ALL; Chapters 18 and 20), which may be primary/clonal or secondary, and assessment for *PDGFR* and *FGFR1* rearrangements should be carried out (Figure 11.1).

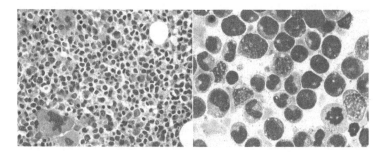

Figure 11.1 Bone marrow core biopsy and aspirate typical of a representative patient with lymphoblastic leukemia/lymphoma with eosinophilia and *FGFR1* rearrangement showing marked hypercellularity with infiltration by lymphoblasts, a significant myeloid preponderance, and increase in eosinophils.

▣ PROGNOSIS

There is substantial variability in the natural history among these three entities based on their respective responsiveness, or lack there of, to imatinib. CEL and hypereosinophilic syndrome (HES) historically have poor prognoses, but neoplasms with *PDGFRA/B* rearrangements are exquisitely sensitive to imatinib, with almost all patients exhibiting rapid and sustained hematologic and molecular responses. In addition, primary and acquired resistance to imatinib is extremely rare in this group of patients. In contrast, myeloid and lymphoid neoplasms with *FGFR1* abnormalities are usually not responsive to imatinib, and patients typically undergo an aggressive course terminating in AML within 1 to 2 years despite treatment with aggressive chemotherapy and stem cell transplantation. There are currently no validated prognostic models or scoring systems for this rare group of diseases.

▣ TREATMENT

The efficacy of treatment with imatinib is well established in patients with neoplasms associated with rearrangements of *PDGFRA/B,* and thus it is currently the standard of care. Hematologic and molecular remissions are rapidly attainable in most cases of *PDGFRA/B.* Ongoing treatment appears necessary, as relapse is common after discontinuation of imatinib, and remission is able to be reestablished with the resumption of treatment. FISH and/or molecular studies may be used to monitor response to imatinib in cases involving *PDGFRA/B.* The optimal dose of imatinib to achieve and sustain a molecular remission has not been established, but doses ranging from 100-mg weekly to 400-mg daily have proven effective. Left ventricular dysfunction and cardiogenic shock have been reported after initiation of imatinib, and prophylactic systemic corticosteroids are recommended during the first 7 to 10 days of treatment initiation in patients with evidence of cardiac involvement and/or elevated serum troponin levels. There have been isolated reports of acquired resistance to imatinib, and treatment options in these cases would be an increased dose of imatinib, an alternative tyrosine kinase inhibitor, or allogeneic hematopoietic cell transplantation (HCT). Bone marrow transplantation has been successful in *FIP1L1-PDGFRA*-positive HES/CEL and remains the only curative option, but it should be reserved for aggressive cases that are resistant to tyrosine kinase inhibitors. In *FGFR1* disease, there has been a paucity of data until recently regarding the use of small molecule inhibitors, and induction with AML or ALL regimens (e.g., Hyper-CVAD) followed by allogeneic stem cell transplantation has been recommended for amenable patients. The oral *FGFR1, -2,* and *-3* inhibitor pemigatinib has demonstrated encouraging responses, and treatment with an *FGFR1* inhibitor on a clinical trial should be considered for patients with *FGFR1*-rearranged disease.

PATIENTS WITH *FIP1L1-PDGFRA* FUSION GENE

- Imatinib 100-mg daily is the FDA-recommended starting dose. Increased doses up to 300 to 400 mg/day may be necessary in some patients who fail to demonstrate sufficient responses. Maintenance dosing of 100 to 200 mg weekly may be sufficient to sustain a molecular remission (*Br J Haematol.* 2008;141(2):200–204. doi: 10.1111/j.1365-2141.2008.07033.x; *Haematologica.* 2007 Sep;92(9):1173–1179. doi: 10.3324/haematol.11420; *Medicine.* 2013;92:e1Ye9. doi: 10.1097/MD.0b013e3182a71eba).

PATIENTS WITH *PDGFRB-* AND *PDGFRA*-VARIANT FUSION GENES

- Imatinib 400-mg daily. In patients with *PDGFRB*-associated disease, 10-year overall survival (OS) rate of 90%, and 6-year progression free survival (PFS) 88% (*Blood.* 2014;123(23):3574–3577. doi.org/10.1182/blood-2014-02-555607).

PATIENTS WITH *FGFR1* FUSION GENES

- Intensive chemotherapy with such regimens as Hyper-CVAD followed by early allogeneic stem cell transplantation.
- FGFR1 inhibitor (e.g., pemigatinib clinical trial). Preliminary phase II data of pemigatinib, overall response 85%, complete cytogenetic response in 46% (*Blood.* 2018;132(Supplement 1):690. doi: https://doi.org/10.1182/blood-2018-99-110388).

▓ POTENTIAL PRACTICE-CHANGING TRIALS

Given the rarity of this group of hematologic neoplasms combined with established definitive treatment for a large proportion of cases, there are few active trials focused on them. Updated results from the ongoing phase II trial of pemigatinib are expected to be informative for the management of *FGFR1*-rearranged disease (NCT03011372). Other targeted treatments, including ponatinib and PKC412 (midostaurin), have demonstrated activity in a few isolated cases of *FGFR1*-associated disease (*Leukemia.* 2016 Apr;30(4):947–950; *Proc Natl Acad Sci USA.* 2004 Oct;101(40):14479–14484). Another trial is investigating the use of the FGFR1-4 inhibitor futibatinib and includes patients with myeloid or lymphoid neoplasms with *FGFR1* rearrangements (NCT04189445). Other recurrent genetic abnormalities have been identified in myeloid and lymphoid neoplasms with eosinophilia and may soon be included in this category. These include rearranged *JAK2* (*PCM1-JAK2* fusion) and *FLT3* (*ETV6-FLT3* fusion). There are two reports of hematologic remission and cytogenetic response in two patients with CEL and *PCM1-JAK2* fusion treated with the *JAK1/2* inhibitor ruxolitinib, but remissions can be variable, with some lasting for a limited duration (*Blood.* 2012;120(7):1529–1531;

J Clin Oncol. 2013;31:e269–e271; *Ann Hematol*. 2015;94:233–238. https://doi.org/10.1007/s00277-014-2221-y). Clinical trials are currently investigating the use of ruxolitinib in *JAK2*-rearranged or -mutated eosinophilic neoplasms (NCT03801434 and NCT00044304).

▨ REFERENCES FOR SUPPLEMENTAL READING

1. Gotlib J. Tyrosine kinase inhibitors and therapeutic antibodies in advanced eosinophilic disorders and systemic mastocytosis. *Curr Hematol Malig Rep*. 2015;10:351–361. doi: 10.1007/s11899-015-0280-3

2. Shomali W, Gotlib J. World Health Organization–defined eosinophilic disorders: 2019 update on diagnosis, risk stratification, and management. *Am J Hematol*. 2019;94(10):1149–1167. doi: 10.1002/ajh.25617

3. Baer C, Muehlbacher V, Kern W. Molecular genetic characterization of myeloid/lymphoid neoplasms associated with eosinophilia and rearrangement of *PDGFRA, PDGFRB, FGFR1* or *PCM1-JAK2. Haematologica*. 2018;103(8):e348–e350. doi: 10.3324/haematol.2017.187302

4. Kilon AD. How I treat hypereosinophilic syndromes. *Blood*. 2015;126(9):1069–1077. doi: 10.1182/blood-2014-11-551614

5. Vega F, Medeiros LJ, Bueso-Ramos CE, et al. Hematolymphoid neoplasms associated with rearrangements of *PDGFRA, PDGFRB*, and *FGFR1*. *Am J Clin Pathol*. 2015;144:377–392. doi: 10.1309/AJCPMORR5Z2IKCEM

12 Myelodysplastic Syndromes

Anthony M. Hunter, David A. Sallman,

and Rami Komrokji

■ INTRODUCTION

The myelodysplastic syndromes (MDS) are a heterogeneous group of clonal myeloid disorders characterized by cytopenias, bone marrow (BM) dysplasia, ineffective hematopoiesis, and increased risk for transformation to acute myeloid leukemia (AML). The incidence is 4.8 per 100,000 people per year, and the median age at diagnosis is 70 to 75 years of age. The disease is rare in people younger than 40 years old but increases to a maximum of 55.8 per 100,000 among patients in their 80s and older.

■ DIAGNOSIS

Peripheral blood cytopenias and related complications are the predominant presenting feature of MDS, with 90% of patients presenting with anemia. A pathologic diagnosis of MDS requires persistent peripheral blood cytopenias with one or more of the following criteria established: (a) morphologic dysplasia in ≥10% of cells in at least one hematopoietic cell lineage, (b) increased BM myeloblasts (≥5% but <20%), or (c) presence of an MDS-defining cytogenetic abnormality. Every patient should be evaluated with a complete blood count with differential, reticulocyte count, and peripheral smear. BM aspiration and biopsy with iron staining and cytogenetic studies by standard G-banding chromosomal analysis or, if not obtainable, fluorescence in situ hybridization (FISH) is required. Molecular profiling via next-generation sequencing (NGS) should be incorporated into routine clinical care due to its impact on diagnosis, prognosis, treatment, and eligibility for clinical trial enrollment. Erythropoietin (EPO), red blood cell folate, and vitamin B12 levels should be checked along with iron studies and thyroid-stimulating hormone to evaluate the anemia. The history should assess the duration, severity, and acceleration of cytopenias and should also investigate prior infections, transfusion history, bleeding problems, and prior exposure to chemotherapy or toxic chemicals.

Patients with MDS are classified by WHO based on number of dysplastic lineages, cytogenetic abnormalities, presence of BM ring sideroblasts (RS), and percentage of BM blasts (Table 12.1). In the WHO

Table 12.1 2016 WHO Classification[1]

WHO Category	Peripheral Blood	BM
MDS with SLD (MDS-SLD)	Cytopenia (1–2 lines) <1% blasts	Dysplasia (1 line) <5% blasts RS <15%/<5%[†]
MDS with MLD (MDS-MLD)	Cytopenia (1–3 lines) <1% blasts	Dysplasia (2–3 lines) <5% blasts RS <15%/<5%[†]
MDS with RS (MDS-RS)[*]	Cytopenia (1–3 lines) <1% blasts	Dysplasia (1–3 lines) <5% blasts RS ≥15%/≥5%[†]
MDS with excess blasts (MDS-EB-1 & MDS-EB-2)	Cytopenia (0–3 lines) MDS-EB-1: 2–4% blasts MDS-EB-2: 5–19% blasts	Dysplasia (1–3 lines) MDS-EB-1: 5–9% blasts MDS-EB-2: 10–19% blasts or Auer rods present
MDS with isolated del(5q)[**]	Cytopenia (1–2 lines) <1% blasts	Dysplasia (1–3 lines) <5% blasts
MDS unclassifiable (MDS-U)[***]	Cytopenia (1–3 lines) 1% or <1% blasts	Dysplasia (0–3 lines) <5% blasts

Cytopenias are defined as hemoglobin <10 g/dL, platelet count <100 × 10^9/L, and absolute neutrophil count <1.8 × 10^9/L. To be classified as dysplasia, >10% of any cell lineage must be dysplastic. PB monocytes must be <1 × 10^9/L (suggests diagnosis of chronic myelomonocytic leukemia, CMML).

[†]If *SF3B1* mutation is present.

[*]Subclassified as MDS-RS with single or multi-lineage dysplasia (MDS-RS-SLD or MDS-RS-MLD) based on presence of 1 or 2–3 dysplastic lineages, respectively. Pancytopenia with RS is classified as MDS-RS-MLD.

[**]Del(5q) alone or with 1 additional abnormality, except –7 or del(7q).

[***]1% peripheral blasts needs to be confirmed on 2 separate occasions. MDS-U diagnosis is also made with SLD and pancytopenia or presence of an MDS-defining cytogenetic abnormality in the absence of dysplasia (adapted from *Blood*. 2016; 127:2391–2405).

BM, bone marrow; CMML, chronic myelomonocytic leukemia; MDS, myelodysplastic syndromes; MLD, multilineage dysplasia; SLD, single lineage dysplasia; RS, ring sideroblasts; WHO, World Health Organization.

2016 update, mutation of *SF3B1* is diagnostic of MDS-RS if there is at least 5% BM RS (*Blood*. 2011;118:6239–6246).

Additional testing, including assessment for a paroxysmal nocturnal hemoglobinuria (PNH) clone (see Chapter 11), may be considered in specific patients. If the presenting features include gastrointestinal disorders and neuropathy, copper and ceruloplasmin levels should be checked to rule out copper deficiency, which may mimic MDS.

■ PROGNOSIS

The most widely used prognostic systems include the International Prognostic Scoring System (IPSS) and the Revised IPSS (IPSS-R, Table 12.2). Although the IPSS has historically been used for clinical trials and treatment recommendations in MDS, the IPSS-R further refines prognostication with additional stratification based on severity of cytopenias and cytogenetic categories. Therapeutic recommendations have traditionally been based on separating patients into lower-risk ([LR] i.e., low and intermediate-1 [int-1] by IPSS) and higher-risk ([HR] i.e., int-2 and high by IPSS) categories. This distinction has been more challenging with the IPSS-R due to the presence of five categories (with intermediate patients included in both LR and HR trials), but a score of ≤3.5 has been proposed to define LR disease.

Table 12.2 IPSS-R

Score Value						
Prognostic variable	0	0.5	1	1.5	2	3	4
Cytogenetic*	Very good	–	Good	–	Intermediate	Poor	Very poor
Marrow blasts (%)	≤2	–	>2–<5	–	5–10	>10	–
Hemoglobin	≥10	–	8–<10	<8	–	–	–
Platelets	≥100	50–<100	<50	–	–	–	–
ANC	≥0.8	<0.8	–	–	–	–	–

IPSS-R risk category (% of population)	**Overall score**	**Median survival (year) in the absence of therapy**	**25% AML progression (year) in the absence of therapy**
Very low (19)	≤1.5	8.8	Not reached
Low (38)	>1.5–≤3.0	5.3	10.8
Intermediate (20)	>3.0–≤4.5	3	3.2
High (13)	>4.5–≤6.0	1.6	1.4
Very high (10)	>6.0	0.8	0.7

*Very good: –Y, del(11q); Good: normal karyotype, del(5q), del(12p), del(20q) double deletion including del(5q); Intermediate: del(7q), +8, +19, i(17q) and any other single or double independent clones; poor: –7, inv(3)/t(3q)/del(3q), double including –7/del(7q), complex (3 abnormalities); very poor: complex (>3 abnormalities).

AML, acute myeloid leukemia; ANC, absolute neutrophil count; IPSS-R, Revised International Prognostic Scoring System.

In addition to defined scoring systems, NGS has revolutionized prognostication, with ~90% of patients having detectable mutations. Mutations of *ASXL1, EZH2, ETV6, RUNX1,* and *TP53* were identified to predict for inferior overall survival (OS), independent of IPSS.[2] In contrast, only mutations in *SF3B1* predict for improved OS. The largest cohort reported to date (*n* = 2,173) identified improved OS in patients with *SF3B1* mutations, while mutations in *TP53, CBL, EZH2, RUNX1, U2AF1,* and *ASXL1* predicted for inferior OS (*Blood.* 2015;126(23):907). *TP53* mutations are perhaps the strongest predictor of inferior outcomes in patients with MDS, found in the majority of patients with complex karyotype and up to 20% of patients with isolated del(5q) (*Leukemia.* 2016;30:666–673; *BJH.* 2013;160:660–672). *TP53* mutations predict for inferior outcomes with lenalidomide (Len) in del(5q) patients, shorter duration of response to hypomethylating agent (HMA), and inferior outcomes with allogeneic hematopoietic cell transplantation (allo-HCT). Studies incorporating somatic mutations into prognostic models are ongoing, with the likely creation of a computational molecular model in the coming years based on work by the International Working Group.

■ TREATMENT

Managing MDS is complicated by advanced age of patients, presence of non-hematologic comorbidities, and comparative inability to tolerate intensive therapies. Moreover, AML arising from MDS is associated with lower response rate (RR) to treatment than is de novo AML, though CPX-351 (liposomal combination of daunorubicin/cytarabine) has demonstrated improved OS (see Chapter 15). Treatment selection is based on risk stratification, presenting symptoms, and patient-specific factors, such as age, performance status, comorbidities, and preference. In patients with LR-MDS (see Prognosis), the primary goal of treatment is to improve cytopenias and ameliorate symptoms, while with HR disease, the goal is to alter the natural history of the disease by prolonging OS and delaying transformation to AML. Asymptomatic LR and potentially HR patients should be monitored with active surveillance. Supportive care is an important component for all MDS patients (Table 12.3). The only curative therapy available is allo-HCT, which should be considered in all appropriate patients with HR disease as well as LR patients refractory to treatment.

FRONTLINE TREATMENT: LOWER-RISK PATIENTS WITH ISOLATED DEL(5Q)

- Len 10 mg PO 21/28 days or continuous with transfusion independence (TI) in 67% of patients and 50% to 60% cytogenetic response.[3] Len should be initiated at the 10 mg dose, based on potentially higher efficacy, although dose reductions are frequently required.

Table 12.3 Supportive Care Therapy Options in the Treatment of MDS Patients

Supportive Care	
Category	Practical Notes
Hematopoietic cytokines (G-CSF, GM-CSF, ESAs)	Consider for refractory, symptomatic cytopenias in LR patients.
	Lower EPO levels (<500 mU/mL, particularly <200 mU/mL) and lower transfusion requirement (<2/mo) are predictive of ESA response.
Thrombocytopenia	Give transfusions for severe thrombocytopenia (<10 × 10^9/L) or bleeding.
	While not FDA-approved, the TPO-receptor agonists romiplostim and eltrombopag have activity in LR-MDS.
Anemia	Standard of care for symptomatic anemia in MDS is leuko-reduced and irradiated red blood cell transfusion.
	EPO <500: rHu EPO (epoetin alpha 40–60,000 U SC/wk or darbepoetin alpha 150–500 mcg q2-3 wk); response should be seen in 6–8 weeks. If no response to EPO alone, consider addition of G-CSF, given synergism (especially in patients with >15% RS).
Iron overload management (deferoxamine–IM/SC deferasirox-PO)	Monitor serum ferritin levels and organ dysfunction. Target ferritin of <1,000 ng/mL in LR patients who are expected to have >20 transfusions, ongoing transfusions, and/or ferritin >2,500 ng/mL.

EPO, erythropoietin; ESA, erythropoiesis stimulating agent; G-CSF, granulocyte colony-stimulating factor; GM-CSF, granulocyte-monocyte colony-stimulating factor; LR, lower risk; LR-MDS, lower-risk myelodysplastic syndromes; MDS, myelodysplastic syndromes; RS, ring sideroblasts; TPO, thrombopoietin.

FRONTLINE TREATMENT: LOWER-RISK PATIENTS WITHOUT ISOLATED DEL(5Q)

- Erythropoiesis stimulating agents (ESA): Responses observed in 20% to 40% of patients. Patients with low EPO levels (<500 mU/mL, particularly if <200 mU/mL) and low transfusion burden (<2 U/month) have RR up to 50% to 70% with ESAs, compared to <10% with high EPO and transfusion burden (*Br J Haematol.* 2003;120(6):1037–1046).
- Although Len is not FDA-approved, approximately 25% to 35% of non-del(5q) LR-MDS patients develop TI when treated with

it, with improved RR seen in combination with ESA (*J Clin Oncol.* 2016;34:2988–2996; *Leukemia. 2016*;30:897–905. *Blood.* 2019;134:842).

- HMA therapy (azacitidine [AZA] or decitabine [DAC]) has shown RR similar to those in HR patients (10%–20% CR, 30%–40% HI). At least 4–6 cycles should be given prior to considering treatment failure. AZA in LR-MDS is often given on a 5-day schedule (*J Clin Oncol.* 2009:1850–1856), and 3-day regimens of AZA and DAC have been explored (*Blood.* 2017;130(13):1514–1522).

- ATG with or without cyclosporine is most effective in younger (<60 years) patients, HLA-DR15+, hypoplastic MDS, normal cytogenetics, shorter duration of transfusion dependence, and patients with a PNH clone present; trilineage responses can occur (*J Clin Oncol.* 2008;26:2505–2511).

FRONTLINE TREATMENT: HIGHER-RISK PATIENTS, TRANSPLANT INELIGIBLE

- The only proven disease-modifying therapy in HR-MDS, AZA 75 mg/m^2 × 7 days is the standard of care based on the AZA-001 phase 3 trial demonstrating an improvement in median OS (24.5 months vs. 15 months with conventional care).[4] Of note, outcomes in "real-world" cohorts have demonstrated less optimistic outcomes, with median OS of 14–17 months (*Leukemia.* 2015;29(9):1875–1881).

- While no clear OS benefit has been demonstrated, DAC remains an option, with similar RR observed.

- Intensive chemotherapy can be considered, but with lower RR and often short durations of remission.

FRONTLINE TREATMENT: HIGHER-RISK PATIENTS, TRANSPLANT ELIGIBLE

- Allo-HCT is the only curative treatment for MDS and should be considered in all patients with limited comorbidities at time of diagnosis (*Blood.* 2004;104(2):579–585). While the impact of therapy prior to allo-HCT remains inconclusive, high disease burden at time of transplant is predictive of inferior outcomes, and HMAs are frequently used as a bridge to transplant (*Blood.* 2014;123(15):2333–2342; *Biol Blood Marrow Transplant.* 2012;18(8):1211–1218).

- Low-dose HMA maintenance therapy post-transplant can be tolerated, but no clear benefit has been documented (*Blood.* 2018;132(Supplement 1):971).

- Long-term survival after allo-HCT in patients with *TP53* mutations is rare, and thus only highly selected patients should be considered, and clinical trials are preferred (*J Clin Oncol.* 2014;32:2691–2698).

RELAPSE/REFRACTORY PATIENTS

- If LR-MDS, other available therapies (noted above), clinical trials, or allo-HCT may be considered.
- Outcomes after HMA failure are dismal, and thus clinical trial is preferred.

▨ POTENTIAL PRACTICE-CHANGING CLINICAL TRIALS

Therapeutic agents with disease-modifying capacity in MDS are lacking, and appropriate candidates should be considered for enrollment into clinical trials. Luspatercept, a recombinant fusion protein that binds TGF-β superfamily ligands, demonstrated TI in 38% of patients in a phase 3 trial of transfusion-dependent, LR-MDS with RS and is pending FDA review, with expected approval.[5] The Bcl-2 inhibitor venetoclax has shown promising efficacy in combination with HMA, leading to FDA approval in AML, with multiple studies in HR-MDS ongoing. Advancements in NGS are leading to the development of targeted therapies. Inhibitors of mutant *IDH1* and *IDH2* (~5% of MDS) have been approved in AML and are now being studied, both as single agents and in combination with HMA, in MDS. APR-246, which functions to restore wild-type p53 conformation and function, has shown robust activity in combination with AZA in *TP53*-mutated MDS, leading to breakthrough therapy designation by the FDA, with phase 3 study ongoing (NCT03745716). Immunotherapies have transformed the oncology landscape in recent years and are being explored in MDS. Initial studies have demonstrated activity with checkpoint inhibitors and anti-TIM-3 antibodies (MGG453) in combination with HMA. Magrolimab, a novel antibody targeting the anti-phagocytic macrophage immune checkpoint CD47, has shown RRs approaching 100% in combination with AZA in HR-MDS (NCT03248479).

▨ REFERENCES FOR SUPPLEMENTAL READING

1. Arber DA, Orazi A, Hasserjian R, et al. The 2016 revision to the World Health Organization classification of myeloid neoplasms and acute leukemia. *Blood*. 2016;127(20):2391–2405.
2. Bejar R, Stevenson K, Abdel-Wahab O, et al. Clinical effect of point mutations in myelodysplastic syndromes. *N Engl J Med*. 2011;364:2496–2506.
3. List A, Dewald G, Bennett J, et al. Myelodysplastic syndrome-003 study, lenalidomide in the myelodysplastic syndrome with chromosome 5q deletion. *N Engl J Med*. 2006;355(14):1456–1465.
4. Fenaux P, Mufti GJ, Hellstrom-Lindberg E, et al. Efficacy of azacitidine compared with that of conventional care regimens in the treatment of higher-risk myelodysplastic syndromes: a randomised, open-label, phase III study. *Lancet Oncol*. 2009;10(3):223–232.
5. Fenaux P, Platzbecker U, Mufti GJ, et al. Luspatercept in patients with lower-risk myelodysplastic syndromes. *N Engl J Med*. 2020; 382(2):140–151.

13 Aplastic Anemia

Jae Chung and Rami Komrokji

■ INTRODUCTION

Aplastic anemia (AA) is a specific cause of bone marrow failure characterized by pancytopenia and a markedly hypocellular bone marrow. It is a rare disorder, occurring at a rate of 2 to 4 individuals per 1 million people yearly (*Ann Intern Med.* 2002;136(7):534–546). Patients may present incidentally during routine laboratory evaluation or with symptoms related to the cytopenias. The most common presenting symptoms include fatigue, mucosal bleeding, heavy menstrual bleeding, or recurrent infections. Splenomegaly is absent, a useful feature that distinguishes AA from myelofibrosis. The most common proximate cause is injury to the pluripotent stem cell. Our refined understanding of underlying immune mechanisms helps explain why this disease responds to immunosuppressive therapy (IST). Improved understanding of molecular biology has led to new approaches in the treatment of refractory and relapsed cases.

■ PATHOGENESIS

Dividing AA into congenital and acquired cases is the first step in understanding the pathogenesis. Congenital causes include Fanconi anemia (FA), dyskeratosis congenita (DC), and Shwachman–Diamond syndrome, all of which are inherited disorders affecting important cellular functions, such as DNA repair, telomere preservation, and ribosome biogenesis. Commonly identified acquired causes include toxic chemical exposure, drug reactions, viral infections, and autoimmune disorders. More commonly, AA is idiopathic, and mounting evidence indicates that immune dysregulation is the underlying cause (*Blood.* 2012;119(9):2003–2043; *Blood.* 2012;120(8):1624–1632). For instance, one proposed mechanism involves regulatory T-cells. Decreased numbers of regulatory T-cells are seen in AA, diminishing the ability of the immune system to suppress effector T-cells. Interferon-gamma release from effector T-cells exerts an inhibitory effect on hematopoiesis through direct stem cell apoptosis. Additional work has demonstrated an association between *TERC* and *TERT* gene mutations with idiopathic and acquired cases of AA. These genes affect ribonucleic acid (RNA) subunits of telomerase and telomerase reverse transcriptase, respectively. They are commonly implicated in germline mutations in patients with DC. Haploinsufficiency may predispose individuals to the development

Table 13.1 Severity Criteria of AA

Nonsevere	Severe	Very Severe
<5% bone marrow cellularity	<25% bone marrow cellularity **OR** <50% *normal cellularity* with fewer than 30% of these cells being hematopoietic	Meets criteria for "severe" AA
Peripheral blood cytopenias not meeting criteria for "severe" or "very severe"	Two of the following three peripheral blood findings: 1. Neutrophils <500/mcL 2. Platelets <20,000/mcL 3. Reticulocytes <60,000/mcL	Neutrophils <200/mcL in the peripheral blood

AA, aplastic anemia.

of AA through impaired capacity to preserve telomere length (*Blood.* 2004;104(13):3936; *N Engl J Med.* 2005;352(14):1413).

■ DIAGNOSIS

An appropriate evaluation for AA should include a complete blood count (CBC), peripheral smear, vitamin B12/folate levels, human immunodeficiency virus (HIV)/hepatitis serologies, and a bone marrow aspiration/biopsy. The two most important findings from this evaluation include (a) pancytopenia and (b) a hypocellular bone marrow without infiltration or fibrosis (Table 13.1). Peripheral blood cytopenias must include at least two of the three following criteria: hemoglobin <10 g/dL, platelet count <50,000/mcL, or neutrophil count <1,500/mcL (*Br J Haematol.* 2007;136(4):549–564). Finally, patients with *TERC* and *TERT* mutations are at increased risk for liver cirrhosis and pulmonary fibrosis. Respiratory symptoms and abnormalities in liver testing should be immediately investigated.

■ KEY DIAGNOSTIC DILEMMA

The differential diagnosis of pancytopenia without splenomegaly is broad. The diagnostic approach includes a thorough history, including prior exposures, medications, and family history; physical exam assessing for the presence of organomegaly or congenital anomalies; CBC with peripheral smear; nutritional studies, flow cytometry, lactate dehydrogenase (LDH) and haptoglobin; and bone marrow aspirate and biopsy. Clinicians should consider myelodysplastic syndrome (MDS), T-large granular lymphocytic (LGL) leukemia, nutritional deficiency, and certain infections, such as HIV. Distinguishing

AA from MDS with hypoplastic features or paroxysmal nocturnal hemoglobinuria (PNH) is difficult and requires more comprehensive clinical and laboratory evaluation. In the setting of a hypoplastic marrow, dysplastic features in megakaryocytes are particularly useful clues to diagnosing MDS (see Chapter 9). In addition, certain cytogenetic findings are more consistent with MDS, such as del(7q), del(5q), del(13q), and del(11q), though cytogenetically abnormal clones can also be seen in AA (*Blood*. 2011;117(19):5019–5032). To diagnose PNH, one should use flow cytometry with the more sensitive FLAER antibody (fluorescently labeled aerolysin) for glycosylphosphatidylinisotol-linked (GPI-linked) proteins and GPI anchors (see Chapter 14).

PROGNOSIS

Unless treated, 70% of patients with severe or very severe disease will die within 1 year secondary to infections or hemorrhagic complications. The 5-year survival rate is 72% for patients under age 50 treated with ISTs. Prognosis worsens with age (57% 5-year survival for those ages 50–59 vs. 50% 5-year survival for those 60 and older) (*Ann Intern Med*. 1999;130(3):193–201). Patients with higher reticulocyte and lymphocyte counts had better response rates to treatment and had higher 5-year survival (*Br J Haematol*. 2009;144(2):206–216). In addition to the immediate morbidity and mortality associated with AA, about 15% of patients at 5 years will develop a related clonal disorder (i.e., PNH, MDS, or AML; *N Engl J Med*. 2015;373(1):35–47). This association is likely due to a high prevalence of clonal hematopoiesis in these patients. The most common karyotypic abnormalities that develop over time involve chromosomes 7 and 8. Isolated abnormalities in chromosome 7 or complex cytogenetic derangements are most frequently associated with leukemic transformation. Trisomy 8 predicts response to IST and is associated with improved survival compared to other chromosomal abnormalities (*Blood*. 2002;99(9):3129–3135). Interestingly, reduced telomere length has been associated with increased risk of relapse, clonal evolution, and inferior overall survival (*JAMA*. 2010;304(12):1358).

TREATMENT

The approach to treatment of AA depends on the severity of the disease. Patients with non-severe disease can be conservatively managed. Those with severe or very severe disease should receive definitive therapy in addition to supportive care, including leukocyte-reduced, irradiated transfusions, prophylactic antifungals, and antibiotics (*Bone Marrow Transplant*. 2013;48(2):168–173). Granulocyte-colony stimulating factor (G-CSF) and erythropoietin are not routinely used to treat cytopenias in patients with AA. Notably, unlike in other immune-mediated cytopenias, corticosteroids are ineffective.

FRONTLINE DEFINITIVE TREATMENT: TRANSPLANT CANDIDATES

- Allogeneic stem cell transplantation:
  - Increased overall long-term survival versus immunosuppression (*Haematologica*. 2007;92:11–18)
  - Recommended first line with a matched-sibling donor and younger than 40 years

FRONTLINE DEFINITIVE TREATMENT: NONTRANSPLANT CANDIDATES OR NO SIBLING DONOR

- High-dose, short-course IST (*Blood*. 2003;101(4):1236–1242; *N Engl J Med*. 2017;376(16):1540–1550):
  - Horse-derived anti-thymocyte globulin (ATG): 40 mg/kg daily on days 1 to 4:
    - ATG premedication: acetaminophen and diphenhydramine
  - Glucocorticoids: 1 mg/kg daily days 1 to 14 with a rapid taper until discontinuation on day 28
  - Cyclosporine: 10 to 12 mg/kg daily in two divided doses to start on day 1 and continued for 6 months (often initiated at time of discharge following completion of ATG)
  - Eltrombopag: 150 mg daily in individuals over 12 years of age of non-Asian ancestry to start on day 1 and continued for 6 months

RELAPSED/REFRACTORY DISEASE

- Allogeneic stem cell transplantation if a candidate
- Retreatment with IST if patient had previous response and potential use of rabbit ATG
- Eltrombopag: 50 mg daily to start and titrated up to maximum of 150 mg daily (using lowest effective dose)
- Alemtuzumab (*Blood*. 2012;119(2):345–354)
- Romiplostim (*Lancet Haematol*. 2019;6(11):e562)

Eltrombopag, a thrombopoietin mimetic, first demonstrated efficacy in the refractory setting in a 2014 prospective study. Forty percent of patients had responses, and counts remained durable after drug discontinuation (*N Eng J Med*. 2012;367(1):11–19). It was subsequently tested in combination with standard IST in previously untreated patients with severe AA and was associated with higher overall and complete response rates (*N Engl J Med*. 2017;376(16):1540–1550). Follow-up is limited, but rates of relapse and clonal evolution appear similar. While androgens have not been efficacious in severe AA, they are the standard of care for constitutional bone marrow failure syndromes. In a prospective trial, danazol, a synthetic androgen, induced hematologic responses and helped preserve telomere length in patients with telomere disease (*N Eng J Med*. 2016;374:1922–1931).

▓ POTENTIAL PRACTICE-CHANGING CLINICAL TRIALS

The SOAR trial (NCT02998645) is a phase II single-arm trial assessing the efficacy and safety of eltrombopag combined with cyclosporine as first-line treatment in patients with severe AA. Horse ATG was discontinued in most European, Asian, and South American countries, with only rabbit ATG (rATG) available. rATG has been shown to have inferior response rates and overall survival in prospective trials and may add little to first-line treatment, especially with the approval of eltrombopag. Another abstract presented at the American Society of Hematology 2019 annual meeting (*Blood* 2019;134(Suppl1):2503) retrospectively reviewed subcutaneous alemtuzumab in the first-line setting with calcineurin inhibitors in 80% of cases. Overall response rate in treatment-naïve patients younger than 60 years was 69% with no serious adverse events. This option may be a reasonable alternative for patients with limited access to horse ATG and more convenient, as patients would not longer require hospitalization.

▓ REFERENCES FOR SUPPLEMENTAL READING

1. Young NS. Acquired aplastic anemia. *Ann Intern Med*. 2002;136(7):534–546. PubMed PMID: 11926789.

2. Guinan EC. Diagnosis and management of aplastic anemia. *Hematology Am Soc Hematol Educ Program*. 2011; 2011:76–81. doi: 10.1182/asheducation-2011.1.76. PubMed PMID: 22160015.

3. Hochsmann B, Moicean A, Risitano A, et al. Supportive care in severe and very severe aplastic anemia. *Bone Marrow Transplant*. 2013; 48(2):168–173. doi: 10.1038/bmt.2012.220. PubMed PMID: 23208312.

4. Frickhofen N, Kaltwasser JP, Schrezenmeier H, et al. Treatment of aplastic anemia with antilymphocyte globulin and methylprednisolone with or without cyclosporine. The German Aplastic Anemia Study Group. *N Engl J Med*. 1991;324(19):1297–1304. doi: 10.1056/NEJM199105093241901. PubMed PMID: 2017225.

5. Frickhofen N, Heimpel H, Kaltwasser JP, et al. Antithymocyte globulin with or without cyclosporin A: 11-year follow-up of a randomized trial comparing treatments of aplastic anemia. *Blood*. 2003;101(4):1236–1242. doi: 10.1182/blood-2002-04-1134. PubMed PMID: 12393680.

14 Paroxysmal Nocturnal Hemoglobinuria

Hilda Ding

▨ INTRODUCTION

Paroxysmal nocturnal hemoglobinuria (PNH) is a rare acquired clonal hematopoietic stem cell disease. It is the result of the acquisition of the *PIG-A* (Xp22.1) mutation in multipotent hematopoietic stem cells. The reported incidence from limited studies of PNH is about 0.5 to 1.5 per million in the general population. The median age of diagnosis is in the thirties. While primarily a disease of adulthood, it can also occur in children and adolescents. The classic features of PNH include complement-mediated hemolytic anemia, bone marrow failure, thrombosis, and subsequent organ damage. Because this is a complement-mediated process, it is a Coombs-negative hemolytic anemia. Thrombosis in PNH often involves unusual sites (e.g., cerebral vein thrombosis, hepatic vein thrombosis, subdermal vein thrombosis). Therefore, for patients who present with thrombosis of an unusual site in the setting of cytopenias, PNH should be high on the differential diagnoses. Debilitating smooth muscle dystonia secondary to depletion of nitric oxide from plasma-free hemoglobin also commonly occurs in PNH. This condition results in abdominal pain, dysphagia, erectile dysfunction, and severe fatigue. Other symptoms include hemoglobinuria, renal dysfunction, and pulmonary hypertension. Clinical presentation can be variable, and disease course may change over time; therefore, treatment is often targeted at the individual patient's specific presentation. Given that this is a clonal disorder, there is a risk for clonal evolution to myelodysplastic syndrome (MDS) and malignant transformation to acute myeloid leukemia in PNH patients. Aplastic anemia can coexist with PNH as well. The only curative treatment for PNH is allogeneic hematopoietic stem cell transplantation, while complement inhibition is used for symptomatic management.

▨ PATHOGENESIS

The acquisition of the *PIG-A* mutation in hematopoietic stem cells drives the pathogenesis of PNH, with resultant proliferation and differentiation of these aberrant stem cells. The product of the *PIG-A* gene is an enzyme responsible in the first stage of glycosylphosphatidylinositol-anchored (GPI-anchored) protein synthesis. Deficient or mutant *PIG-A* hematopoietic stem cells lack glycosylphosphatidylinositol-anchored proteins (GPI-AP) on red blood cells and white blood cells. This condition subsequently leads to uncontrolled complement activity from complete or partial loss of complement-regulating surface proteins (i.e., decay-accelerating factor [DAF]/CD55 and membrane inhibitor of reactive lysis [MIRL]/CD59). CD55 inhibits C3 convertases, and CD59 inhibits the formation of the membrane attack complex (MAC). As a result, such unregulated complement activity on the red blood cells leads to severe intravascular and extravascular hemolytic anemia. As hemolysis ensues, the number of free hemoglobin and erythrocyte micro-particles released into the plasma increase. This situation culminates in the increase of reactive oxygen species, endothelial dysfunction, and monocyte activation as well as depletion of nitric oxide. The depletion of nitric oxide often leads to smooth muscle dystonia, which can cause significant disability and affect quality of life.

Thrombocytopenia may be present due to hypocellular bone marrow or coexisting aplastic anemia. Endothelial dysfunction, fibrinolytic defects, platelet activation, and inflammation from complement activation are thought to drive thrombosis in PNH.

▦ DIAGNOSIS

Initial laboratory evaluation includes complete blood count (CBC) with differential, reticulocyte count, peripheral blood smear review, total and direct bilirubin, lactate dehydrogenase (LDH), haptoglobin, direct antiglobulin test (DAT), and urine for hemoglobin or hemosiderin. Diagnostic workup should also include flow cytometry evaluation of GPI-AP, which is highly sensitive and specific for PNH. Fluorescein-labeled proaerolysin variant (FLAER) is the flow cytometric assay of choice in the confirmation of the diagnosis of PNH, because this assay uses reagents with specific binding to GPI and GPI-AP (Figure 14.1). Bone marrow aspirate and biopsy are recommended for all patients who have cytopenias of unknown etiology to determine their bone marrow cellularity and rule out other bone marrow failure syndromes, such as aplastic anemia, MDS, leukemia, or primary myelofibrosis (PMF). Studies report that up to 70% of patients with aplastic anemia exhibit PNH clones.[2] Additionally, some patients with MDS and aplastic anemia have small PNH clones. Flow cytometry must be done on at least two cell lineages with two independent reagents to ensure accurate diagnosis.

▦ KEY DIAGNOSTIC DILEMMA

The International Clinical Cytometry Society (ICCS) has published guidelines for the diagnosis and monitoring of PNH. The assessment of GPI-AP has high specificity and sensitivity for PNH. CD59 is the most common protein assessed, because it is universally expressed on all hematopoietic cells. CD55 is another commonly evaluated protein. Rare congenital deficiencies of CD55 and CD59 can yield false-positive results if only one monoclonal antibody is used in flow cytometric diagnostic evaluation. Therefore, at least two monoclonal

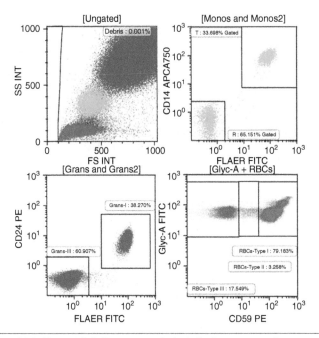

Figure 14.1 Characteristic flow cytometric analysis of a representative PNH patient. The flow cytometry study illustrates a significant loss of CD14/FLAER (monocytes, right upper panel) and CD24/FLAER (granulocytes, left lower panel) as well as a loss of CD59 expression on red blood cells.

Note: Type I: normal RBCs; type II: partial loss of CD59; type III: almost complete loss of CD59 on RBC membranes.

antibodies directed against two different GPI-AP on hematopoietic cells of at least two different lineages should be used during the diagnostic workup for patients with PNH. FLAER has become the standard flow cytometric assay in the diagnosis of PNH, as FLAER binds directly to GPI-AP, leading to more accurate results.

Please also refer to a typical immunophenotype of PNH for more extensive analysis.

The International PNH Interest Group (I-PIG) classifies PNH into three categories:

1. **Classic PNH:** Intravascular hemolysis with no other bone marrow failure abnormality

2. **PNH in the context of another bone marrow failure syndrome:** Intravascular hemolysis with another bone marrow failure abnormality (i.e., aplastic anemia, MDS, or PMF)

3. **Subclinical PNH:** No evidence of intravascular hemolysis with a small GPI-anchored clone (<10% GPI-AP–deficient granulocytes)

PROGNOSIS

PNH is a chronic illness with significant morbidity that negatively affects patients' quality of life due to clinical symptoms stemming from cytopenias, thrombosis, resultant organ damage, severe fatigue, and smooth muscle dystonia. The disease course can be variable, ranging from indolent to acutely life threatening. A multicenter study with long term follow-up of these patients has shown survival estimated at 65% at 10 years and 48% at 15 years from initial diagnosis; with the cumulative incidence at 8 years for pancytopenia, thrombosis, and evolution to MDS is 15%, 28%, and 5%, respectively (*Lancet*. 1996;348:573–577). Factors that confer worse prognosis include thrombosis, development of pancytopenia, thrombocytopenia at diagnosis, evolution to MDS or leukemia, and disease onset greater than 55 years of age. Thrombosis remains the major cause of death in PNH patients, but renal failure and clonal evolution also contribute significantly to morbidity and mortality.

TREATMENT

The decision to treat should be based on symptomatic disease. Asymptomatic patients can be observed. When patients become symptomatic, therapy should be targeted at the underlying bone marrow failure disorder and not the asymptomatic clone. Eculizumab, a humanized monoclonal antibody, has been shown to decrease hemolysis and risk of thrombosis in these patients via terminal complement C5 inhibition. It was Food and Drug Administration–approved (FDA-approved) in 2007 as an agent to treat PNH (*N Engl J Med*. 2006;355:1233–1243). The standard schedule is 600 mg intravenously weekly for the first 4 weeks, 900 mg intravenously the following week, and 900 mg intravenously every 2 weeks thereafter. Eculizumab has been shown to reduce transfusion requirements and hemolysis and to improve symptoms associated with anemia. However, some patients continue to experience breakthrough hemolysis on approved regimens. Until recently, this agent was the only FDA-approved option.

Ravulizumab, a long-acting C5 inhibitor approved in 2018, is now used for these patients. It has approximately four times the mean half-life of eculizumab (*Blood*. 2019;133(6):530–539). As a result, it is dosed based on weight and given over 8-week intervals, 2 weeks after the initial loading dose. In phase III clinical trials, ravulizumab led to fewer patients experiencing breakthrough hemolysis, and it was non-inferior to eculizumab. For patients with breakthrough hemolysis transitioning to ravulizumab, the ravulizumab loading dose should be administered 2 weeks after the most recent eculizumab.

Given that thrombosis is the leading cause of death in patients with PNH, initiating treatment with complement inhibition should be strongly considered in otherwise asymptomatic PNH patients who develop thrombosis. Anticoagulation should also be started immediately in these patients. Thrombolysis should be considered in certain circumstances, especially for patients with life- or limb-threatening thrombosis and/or in the setting of an extensive thrombus. Otherwise, careful consideration should be undertaken for patients with PNH. Limited studies exist to guide prophylactic anticoagulation, as it also carries significant risks of bleeding, given that some patients are also profoundly thrombocytopenic. Though partially effective in preventing thrombosis in some PNH patients, it is not known whether prophylactic anticoagulation should be implemented in all patients. Limited data exist to guide whether patients with history of thrombosis can discontinue anticoagulation once therapy with complement inhibitor has started.

Allogeneic hematopoietic stem cell transplantation remains the only curative option for PNH. It should be considered for patients who have clonal evolution to MDS, leukemia, or coexisting aplastic anemia.

■ POTENTIAL PRACTICE-CHANGING CLINICAL TRIALS

The PNH Registry continues to actively recruit patients to investigate clinical outcomes and progression for this rare disorder (NCT01374360). There are also several agents currently under investigation for PNH that may improve outcome and decrease treatment burden. Crovalimab is a SMART (Sequential Monoclonal Antibody Recycling Technology) antibody that inhibits complement C5 and is administered subcutaneously every 4 weeks to target such diseases as PNH where C5 regulation is crucial. In an ongoing phase I/II clinical trial, it has a non-inferior safety profile and has demonstrated complement pathway inhibition in patients with PNH who are naïve to C5 inhibition and in pretreated patients (NCT03157635). APL-2, a compstatin derivative inhibitor, is currently in a multicenter randomized phase III trial for patients with PNH as compared to eculizumab (NCT03500549). APL-2 is given subcutaneously and acts as a C3 inhibitor, thereby blocking the cleavage of C3 into C3a and C3b via C3 convertase. This in turn suppresses inflammation mediated by complement activation. For patients with suboptimal response to C5 inhibition, danicopan, a small molecule oral factor D inhibitor, has demonstrated improvement in transfusion dependence and decreased hemolysis via C3 convertase inhibition in a recent study (*Blood.* 2019;134(Suppl1):3514). It was granted breakthrough therapy designation by the FDA in 2019, with an ongoing phase II trial to evaluate its long-term safety and efficacy (NCT03181633).

■ REFERENCES FOR SUPPLEMENTAL READING

1. Borowitz MJ, Craig FE, Digiuseppe JA, et al. Guidelines for the diagnosis and monitoring of paroxysmal nocturnal hemoglobinuria and related disorders by flow cytometry. *Cytometry B Clin Cytom.* 2010;78B:211–230.

2. Brodsky R. How I treat paroxysmal nocturnal hemoglobinuria. *Blood.* 2009;113:6522–6527.

3. Brodsky R, Peffault de Latour R, Rottinghaus ST, et al. Characterization of breakthrough hemolysis events observed in the phase 3 randomized studies of ravulizumab versus eculizumab in adults with paroxysmal nocturnal hemoglobinuria. *Haematologica*. 2020 [Epub ahead of print]. doi: 10.3324/haematol.2019.236877

4. Hill A, Kelly RJ, Hillmen P. Thrombosis in paroxysmal nocturnal hemoglobinuria. *Blood*. 2013;121:4985–4996.

5. Lee JW, Kulasekararaj AG. Ravulizumab for treatment of paroxysmal nocturnal hemoglobinuria. *Expert OpinBiolTher*. 2020;20(3):227–237.

15 Myelodysplastic/ Myeloproliferative Overlap Syndromes

Virginia O. Volpe, Jennifer Eatrides, and

Eric Padron

▓ INTRODUCTION

Myelodysplastic/myeloproliferative overlap syndromes (MDS/MPN) are clonal disorders with coexisting dysplastic and proliferative features that do not meet the criteria for MDS or MPN individually. MDS/MPN subtypes are differentiated by their predominant myeloid subset in the peripheral blood and include the following disorders: (a) chronic myelomonocytic leukemia (CMML), (b) juvenile myelomonocytic leukemia (JMML), (c) atypical chronic myeloid leukemia (aCML), (d) MDS/MPN unclassifiable, and (e) MDS/MPN with ring sideroblasts and thrombocytosis (MDS/MPN-RS-T) (Table 15.1). Although the pathogenesis of these syndromes is unclear, in-depth molecular characterization of these diseases (i.e., next-generation sequencing [NGS]) has begun to shed light on the underlying molecular pathogenesis responsible for the apparent paradoxical clinical phenotype. As our understanding of CMML has most significantly advanced in recent years, it is discussed in detail in its respective section (see Chapter 16).

▓ DIAGNOSIS

DIAGNOSIS OF MDS/MPN REQUIRES EXCLUSION OF THE FOLLOWING:

1. Acute myeloid leukemia (AML): bone marrow (BM) blasts <20%
2. Chronic myelogenous leukemia (CML): lack of *BCR-ABL* rearrangement
3. Myeloid/lymphoid neoplasm with eosinophilia (MLN-Eo): lack of *PDGFR/FGFR* fusion
4. Reactive processes: clinical history and lack of clonality

▓ JUVENILE MYELOMONCYTIC LEUKEMIA (JMML)

CLINICAL PRESENTATION

JMML is a rare pediatric myeloid malignancy that predominantly affects children older than 3 years and accounts for 2% to 3% of childhood hematologic malignancies. Similar to CMML, JMML is characterized by a peripheral expansion of monocytes, with a required threshold

Table 15.1 2008 WHO Diagnostic Criteria for MDS/MPN Overlap Syndromes

Disease	Blood Findings	BM Findings	Common Molecular Mutations
CMML-0	• >1 ×10⁹/L monocytes • <2% blasts • ≥10% monocytes	Dysplasia ≥ 1 cell line + < 5% blasts	TET2, SRSF2, ASXL1, RUNNX1, NRAS, CBL
CMML-1	• >1 ×10⁹/L monocytes • <2% to 4% blasts • ≥10% monocytes	Dysplasia ≥ 1 cell line + <5% to 9% blasts	TET2, SRSF2, ASXL1, RUNNX1, NRAS, CBL
CMML-2	• >1 ×10⁹/L monocytes • <5% to 19% blasts or Auer rods • ≥10% monocytes	Dysplasia ≥ 1 cell line + <10% to 19% blasts	TET2, SRSF2, ASXL1, RUNNX1, NRAS, CBL
aCML	• WBC > 13 ×10⁹/L • Neutrophil precursors • ≥10% but <20% blasts • Dysgranulopoiesis	Hypercellular + <20% blasts	SETBP1, ETNK1
JMML	• >1 ×10⁹/L monocytes • <20% blasts • ≥10% monocytes • ↑ HbF	• >1 ×10⁹/L monocytes • <20% blasts • Ph– • GM-CSF hypersensitive	PTPN11, NF1, N/KRAS, CBL, SETBP1, JAK3
MDS/ MPN-U	• Dysplasia + myeloproliferative features • No prior MDS or MPN	Dysplasia + myeloproliferative features	TET2, NRAS, RUNX1, CBL, SETBP1, ASXL1
MDS/ MPN-RS-T	• Dysplasia + myeloproliferative features • Platelets ≥ 450× 10⁹/L • RS ≥15%	Dysplasia + myeloproliferative features	SF3B1, JAK2, MPL, CALR

aCML, atypical chronic myeloid leukemia; CMML, chronic myelomonocytic leukemia; GM-CSF, granulocyte macrophage colony stimulating factor; HbF, hemoglobin F; JMML, jueveline myelomonocytic leukemia; MDS/MPN-RS-T, myelodysplastic syndrome/myeloproliferative neoplasm ringed sideroblast and thrombocytosis; MDS/MPN-U, myelodysplastic syndrome/myeloproliferative neoplasm unspecified; RS, ringed sideroblasts; WBC, white blood count.

Source: Adapted from National Comprehensive Cancer Network. *Myelodysplastic Syndromes*. https://www.nccn.org/professionals/physician_gls/

of more than 1×10^9/L peripheral monocytes constituting greater than 10% of the differential. Patients typically present with symptoms associated with monocytic/granulocytic infiltration of various organs (i.e., splenomegaly, hepatomegaly, gastrointestinal tract), failure to thrive, cytopenias (anemia and thrombocytopenia), and leukocytosis (although white blood cells [WBC] rarely exceed 100×10^9/L). Markedly elevated levels of fetal hemoglobin can be seen in patients with normal karyotypes. Molecular mapping has identified an association of JMML with several congenital syndromes resulting from mutations in the RAS/MAPK pathways, including neurofibromatosis-1 (mutations in *NF1*) and Noonan syndrome (50% have mutations in *PTPN11*).

TREATMENT

Allogeneic hematopoietic stem cell transplantation (HSCT) is a potentially curative treatment and the treatment of choice in most patients with JMML (*PTPN-11, K-RAS, NF1,* and some *NRAS* mutation carriers), with an overall survival (OS) of 64% at 5 years. In those who require HSCT, if not treated, median survival is 10 to 14 months. A watchful waiting strategy is often used for patients with *CBL* mutations and some *NRAS* mutations (mutations associated with a self-limited phenotype of JMML). Bridging with hypomethylating agents (HMA) may be indicated and has shown to decrease the risk of complications prior to transplant.

▨ ATYPICAL CHRONIC MYELOID LEUKEMIA

CLINICAL PRESENTATION

aCML is characterized by a hypercellular BM with granulocyte dysplasia and peripheral leukocytosis ≥13 × 10^9/L with increased and dysplastic neutrophils. Patients typically present with anemia and thrombocytopenia, neutrophilic leukocytosis with profound dysplasia, and splenomegaly. Molecular and cytogenetics may be heterogeneous, with aneuploidy karyotypes, epigenetic and growth factor signaling mutations, and *BCR-ABL* always negative.

PROGNOSIS

aCML typically has an aggressive disease course and poor OS (12–22 months), with transformation to AML in about 40% of patients 18 months from diagnosis. Features contributing to shorter survival include age >65, female gender, leukocytosis >50 × 10^9/L, and peripheral blood myeloid precursors. Although they show no specific genetic abnormalities, about 24% of patients have a *SETBP1* mutation, which is typically associated with higher WBC count and worse OS.

TREATMENT

There is no standard treatment for aCML, but allogeneic HSCT can result in long-term remission. With the increased use of molecular testing, targetable mutations may be discovered and novel therapies used. JAK inhibitors (e.g., ruxolitinib) and Src TKI inhibitors (e.g., dasatinib) may have roles in patients with *CSF3R* mutations based on activation of these pathways via proximal or truncating mutations, respectively. Additionally, in RAS-activating mutations, trametinib may be considered. In patients who are not candidates for transplant or without targetable mutations, chemotherapeutics (e.g., pegylated interferon alpha and HMA) and cytoreductive agents, such as hydroxyurea, can improve blood counts but have not been shown to be disease modifying.

■ MDS/MPN-UNCLASSIFIED

CLINICAL PRESENTATION

This subtype is the most heterogeneous of the MDS/MPN syndromes and encompasses patients with mixed proliferative and dysplastic features who do not clearly fit into the other MDS/MPN subtypes. The 2016 World Health Organization (WHO) criteria require features of one MDS category as well as prominent myeloproliferative features without prior diagnosis of MDS or MPN. MDS/MPN-unclassified (MDS/MPN-U) may be difficult to distinguish from other Philadelphia chromosome negative myeloid neoplasms, because no specific karyotype or molecular findings can differentiate this entity. The diagnosis relies on expert morphologic examination in the context of the appropriate clinical and genetic background.

PROGNOSIS

The median OS has been reported at ranges from 11 to 47 months, depending on risk and treatment with HMA. Patients with increased platelet counts were found to have better outcomes. The following features have been found to correlate with inferior OS and AML-free survival: higher WBC count, higher peripheral and BM blast percentage, complex karyotype, and high LDH.

TREATMENT

Like other MDS/MPN syndromes, optimal treatment is with allogeneic HSCT. However, there is no current treatment consensus in patients who are ineligible for HSCT. HMA can improve symptoms, and in those with International Prognostic Scoring System (IPSS) high-risk disease, it may yield a modest increase in OS. Other treatment approaches may include interferon alpha and lenalidomide.

■ MDS/MPN-RS-T

CLINICAL PRESENTATION

MDS/MPN-RS-T is characterized with features with ring sideroblasts ≥15%, persistent thrombocytosis (≥450 × 10^9/L), anemia, normal blast count, and dyserythropoiesis in BM. Up to 60% of patients have the *SF3B1* mutation and frequently have a co-mutation with *JAK2V617F*.

BM may feature proliferation of large atypical megakaryocytes, which also appear similar to those seen in essential thrombocythemia (ET) and primary myelofibrosis. Similar to ET, MDS/MPN-RS-T can have vasomotor symptoms, thrombosis, and erythromelalgia.

PROGNOSIS
Unlike other cases of MDS/MPN-U, MDS/MPN-RS-T is an indolent disease with prognosis similar to low-risk MDS. Patients with *SF3B1* and/or *JAK2* mutations have improved OS compared to wild-type patients (6.9 versus 3.3 years).

TREATMENT
Recommended treatment for MDS/MPN-RS-T is similar to those with low-risk MDS, especially in the setting of ineffective erythropoiesis. In addition to HMA, erythopoiesus stimulating agents (ESA), and lenalidomide, luspatercept has recently been added to the arsenal of treatment options. Luspatercept is an activin receptor II ligand trap, leading to neutralization of the transforming growth factor betas (TGF beta) superfamily and ultimately inhibition of small mother against decapentaplegic homologue (SMAD) proteins to allow for effective erythropoiesis. This treatment has been approved for patients with MDS/MPN-RS-T in the setting of loss of response to ESA or patients predicted to not respond to ESA (i.e., erythropietin (EPO) level > 500 IU/L). Similar but less frequent than ET, patients with MDS/MPN-RS-T may be at risk for thrombosis. In those with low-risk disease (age <60 and no thrombotic events) and absence of extreme thrombocytosis, low-dose aspirin therapy may be appropriate to reduce the risk of arterial thrombosis.

▨ REFERENCES FOR SUPPLEMENTAL READING

1. Niemeyer CM. JMML genomics and decisions. *Hematol Am SocHematolEduc Program.* 2018;2018(1):307–312.

2. Schwartz LC, Mascarenhas J. Current and evolving understanding of atypical chronic myeloid leukemia. *Blood Rev.* 2019;33:74–81.

3. Smith BN, Savona M, Komrokji RS. Challenges in myelodysplastic/myeloproliferative neoplasms (MDS/MPN). *Clin Lymphoma Myeloma Leuk.* 2019;19(1):1–8.

4. Hendrix K, Alali N, Padron E, et al. Myelodysplastic/myeloproliferative neoplasms unclassified (MDS/MPN-U) overlap: can we alter the natural history? *Blood.* 2016;128(22):3125.

5. Patnaik MM, Tefferi A. Refractory anemia with ring sideroblasts (RARS) and RARS with thrombocytosis: 2019 update on diagnosis, risk-stratification, and management. *Am J Hematol.* 2019;94(4):475–488.

6. National Comprehensive Cancer Network. *Myelodysplastic Syndromes.* https://www.nccn.org/professionals/physician_gls/

16 Chronic Myelomonocytic Leukemia

Alexandra Gomez-Arteaga and Justin M. Watts

■ INTRODUCTION

Chronic myelomonocytic leukemia (CMML) is a clonal myeloid stem cell disorder with clinical, laboratory, and morphologic features that overlap those of myelodysplastic syndrome (MDS) and myeloproliferative neoplasms (MPN). CMML is a rare disease, and the incidence is estimated at 0.3 to 0.9 cases per 100,000 persons per year (*Blood.* 2008;112:45–52). The median age at diagnosis is in the seventh decade with a slight male preponderance. The classic features of CMML include a peripheral blood (PB) monocytosis with cytopenias (i.e., anemia ± thrombocytopenia) along with frequent hepatosplenomegaly and constitutional symptoms. The bone marrow (BM) is hypercellular, with myeloid predominance and dysplasia (specifically granulocytic dysplasia, which can be pronounced), ineffective hematopoiesis, and commonly increased blasts. The risk of transformation to acute myeloid leukemia (AML) is approximately 15% to 30%. Comprehensive molecular characterization has significantly advanced our understanding of this disease, which can aid in cases of diagnostic uncertainty as well as refine prognostication and ideally allow for the development of novel therapies. Until recently, treatment recommendations have been largely based on MDS literature, which often included few CMML patients (or excluded them completely, especially if proliferative). Also, these trials often did not include CMML-specific disease-response criteria. These factors have presented challenges in the development of CMML-specific disease-modifying therapies.

■ DIAGNOSIS

The 2016 revision of the World Health Organization (WHO) classification of myeloid neoplasms (*Blood.* 2016; http://dx.doi.org/10.1182/blood-2016-03-643544) include CMML in the MDS/MPN category along with atypical chronic myeloid leukemia (aCML), juvenile myelomonocytic leukemia (JMML), MDS/MPN neoplasm with ring sideroblasts and thrombocytosis (MDS/MPN-RS-T), and the MDS/MPN unclassifiable group (MDS-MPN-U; see Chapter 15).

WHO 2016 DIAGNOSTIC CRITERIA FOR CMML:

1. Persistent PB monocytosis $\geq 1 \times 10^3$/mcL (>3 months), with monocytes accounting for $\geq 10\%$ of the white blood cell (WBC) count

2. Not meeting WHO criteria for *BCR-ABL1*-positive CML, primary myelofibrosis, polycythemia vera, or essential thrombocythemia

3. No evidence of *PDGFRA*, *PDGFRB*, or *FGFR1* rearrangements or *PCM1-JAK2* fusion (should be specifically excluded in cases with eosinophilia)

4. Fewer than 20% blasts in the blood and BM

5. Dysplasia in one or more myeloid lineages:

   • Megakaryocytic dysplasia is seen in most cases.

   • If myelodysplasia is absent or minimal, the diagnosis of CMML may still be made if the other requirements are met **AND** an acquired clonal cytogenetic or molecular genetic abnormality is present in hemopoietic cells **OR** the monocytosis (as previously defined) has continued for at least 3 months **AND** all other causes of monocytosis have been excluded.

WHO recommends categorization into a "proliferative" variant (MPN-CMML), with WBC >13× 10^3/mcL, or "dysplastic" variant (MDS-CMML).

For prognostic purposes, CMML is also further subclassified according to blast percentage into:

1. **CMML-0**: <2% blasts in PB and fewer than 5% blasts in BM

2. **CMML-1**: 2% to 4% blasts in PB and/or 5% to 9% blasts in BM

3. **CMML-2**: 5% to 19% blasts in PB, 10% to 19% blasts in BM, and/or the presence of Auer rods irrespective of the blast count

Finally, secondary CMML is a described entity that constitutes <10% of new cases and is associated with a worse prognosis. It can include patients with treatment-related CMML (t-CMML), which occurs after chemotherapy or radiation exposure, or in patients with a preceding history of MDS, MPN, or another indolent myeloid or mast cell neoplasm (*Haematologica*. 2019; 104(10):1935–1949). Symptoms can be constitutional and/or relate to cytopenia and splenomegaly. CMML can present with leukemia cutis as an initial manifestation occurring before frank AML progression. Laboratory evaluation includes complete blood count (CBC) with differential, reticulocyte count, complete metabolic panel (CMP), uric acid, examination of the peripheral smear/BM aspiration and biopsy for morphologic assessment, cytogenetics by conventional karyotyping, MDS fluorescence in situ hybridization (FISH), flow cytometry, and molecular analysis by a next-generation sequencing (NGS) panel. Diagnostic workup should also include FISH for *BCR-ABL1* and *PDGFR* alpha and beta gene rearrangements. If patients are presenting with eosinophilia, the *ETV6(TEL)-PDGFRB* fusion oncogene [t(5;12)(q31–q32;p13)] should be excluded, as they are very sensitive to therapy with imatinib (although it can also occur in the absence of eosinophilia). MDS-related cytogenetic abnormalities are seen in approximately 30% of CMML patients, with common alterations including trisomy 8

(+8), −Y, abnormalities of chromosome 7 [monosomy 7 and del(7q)], trisomy 21 (+21), and complex karyotypes. When primary CMML cells were examined using whole-exome sequencing (WES), there was an average of 14±5 somatic mutations per patient (*Nat Commun.* 2016;7:10767). The most frequently mutated genes in CMML include those involved in epigenetic regulation (DNA methylation: ***TET2 ~60%***, *IDH1/2* ~5%; histone modification: ***ASXL1 ~40%***, *EZH2* ~5%), splicing machinery (***SRSF2~50%***, *SF3B1* ~10%, *U2AF1* ~10%), transcription factors (*RUNX1*~15%, *SETBP1*~15%), and signal transduction and cellular/receptor tyrosine kinase pathways (*RAS* ~30%, *CBL* ~15%, *JAK2* ~8%, *NPM1* ~3%, *FLT3* ~3%) (*Blood Cancer J.* 2016;6:e393; *J Clin Oncol.* 2013;31:2428–2436; *Blood.* 2016;127:2391–2405; *Nat Commun.* 2016;7:10767; *HemaSphere.* 2(6):e150). A comprehensive myeloid molecular panel is recommended for evaluating potential targetable mutations and to assess for mutations required for risk assessment (*ASXL1, NRAS, RUNX1,* and *SETBP1*) (see Prognosis).

▓ KEY DIAGNOSTIC DILEMMA

A key challenge in the diagnosis of CMML is to determine whether the PB monocytosis is reactive or clonal. Reactive monocytosis is commonly seen in a variety of viral infections, chronic infections, and inflammatory conditions. Clues in the history suggestive of infection and the timing of the laboratory findings as well as the absence of immature myeloid cells on the blood smear (myelocytes, promyelocytes, promonocytes, and blasts) can be useful in ruling out an infectious etiology. Clonal monocytosis is often persistent and can be associated with a variety of myeloid stem cell disorders, making pathologic evaluation a key step in diagnosis. More than 90% of patients will have at least one genetic mutation, so molecular analysis and cytogenetics are critical to diagnosing CMML. PB flow cytometry is essential in the routine workup of suspected CMML patients, not only to confirm the blast count but also to identify the presence of a distinct monocyte population. The fraction of "classical monocytes" expressing CD14(+)/CD16(−) are increased in patients with CMML, and a 94% cutoff has been reported to be both sensitive and specific in differentiating CMML from reactive monocytosis and other hematologic malignancies that express different monocyte phenotypes ("intermediate" CD14(+)/CD16(+) and "nonclassical" CD14(low)/CD16(+)) (*Blood.* 2015;125:3618–3626).

▓ PROGNOSIS

Recently, there has been significant advances in novel models to develop a CMML-specific risk stratification incorporating molecular genetics. The Groupe Francais des Myelodysplasies (GFM) (*JClin Oncol.* 2013;31(19):2428–2436) and the Mayo Molecular Model (MMM) (*Leukemia.* 2014;28:2206–2212) were the first to incorporate *ASXL1* mutations (only nonsense and frameshift mutations) into risk-classification models (Table 16.1). More recently, the new CMML-specific prognostic scoring system (CPSS) that incorporates molecular genetic data (CPSS-Mol) (Table 16.2) integrated clinical, cytogenetic, and somatic mutations (*RUNX1*, *NRAS*, *SETBP1*, and *ASXL1*), with clearly defined risk groups for overall survival (OS) and leukemic transformation (*Blood*. 2016;128(10):1408–1417).

◼ TREATMENT

Given the lack of specific disease-modifying agents for CMML and, until recently, no standardization of outcome evaluation, addressing both the MDS and MPN components of the disease has been challenging. Allogeneic hematopoietic stem cell transplantation (HSCT) continues to be the only curative option for eligible, fit patients. Unfortunately, it is only available for a small subset of patients. The biggest challenge remains the development of novel agents for CMML. The new international consortium proposal of a uniform response criteria for MDS/MPN has allowed standardized reporting in recent clinical trials and will foster reliable comparisons of the impact of new therapies (*Blood*. 2015;125:1857–1865). Hydroxyurea (HU) and other cytoreductive agents can be used successfully to control MPN-like features. Epigenetic modifiers, such as hypomethylating agents (HMA), have been used for MDS-like diseases (or more proliferative diseases) and offer some chance of remission, but it is often short-lived. In the only randomized controlled trial to date for CMML, HU was superior to etoposide (median OS 20 months vs. 9 months; $P =$ .02; *Blood*. 1996;88:2480–2487). HMA is an FDA-approved therapy for CMML. In two of the largest phase II trials of decitabine, the overall response rate (ORR) was 38% to 48%, the complete response (CR) rate was 10% to 17%, and the median OS was 17 to 19 months (*Blood*. 2011;118(14):3824–3831; *Leukemia*. 2018;32(2):413–418). In two of the largest phase II trials examining azacitidine, the CR rate was 13% to 17%, and the median OS was 12 to 29 months (*Leuk Res*. 2013;37(6):609–613; *Leuk Res*. 2014;38(4):475–483). Although they have not been compared head-to-head, these agents are essentially equivalent and have response rates similar to MDS. However, neither has been shown to significantly decrease the mutational allele burden (even in responding patients) or the risk of progression to AML (*Nat Commun*. 2016;7:10767). Combination therapy with azacitidine plus lenalidomide or vorinostat was evaluated in a randomized phase II study, with similar ORR to monotherapy (*JCO*. 2017;35(24):2745–2753). Other supporting agents include erythropoiesis-stimulating agents (ESA) that have shown an overall erythroid response rate of 64%, median duration of response of 8 months, and red blood cell transfusion independence in 31% of patients (*Eur J Haematol*. 2015;12679). The evidence supporting the use of HSCT in CMML is mainly from registry data. Analysis of the Center for International Blood and Marrow Transplant Research (CIBMTR) registry stratifying outcomes by CPSS risk group showed a

Table 16.1 GFM and MMM Prognostic Systems

GFM					MMM		
Risk Factors	Points	Risk Group Based on Risk Factors	Median OS (mo)	Risk Factors (1 point each)	Risk Group Based on Risk Factors	Median OS (mo)
ASXL1 mutations, excluding missense	2	Low = 0 to 4	Not reached	ASXL1 mutations, excluding missense	Low = 0	97
Age >65 years	2	Intermediate = 5 to 7	38.5	Absolute monocyte count >10 k/mcL	Intermediate-1 = 1	59
WBC count >15 k/mcL	3	High ≥ 8	14.4	Hemoglobin <10 g/dL	Intermediate-2 = 2	31
Hemoglobin <10 g/dL in female or 11g/dL in male	2			Platelets <100 k/mcL	High ≥3	16
Platelets <100 k/mcL	2			Circulating immature myeloid cells		

GFM, Groupe Francais des Myelodysplasies; MMM, Mayo Molecular Model; OS, overall survival; WBC, white blood cell.

Table 16.2 CMML CPSS-Mol: Two-Step Model

1. Define the genetic risk group.
2. Calculate the CPSS-Mol risk score.

A. Genetic risk group

Genetic Risk Variables		Points	Genetic Risk Group
CPSS Cytogenetic Risk Group*			Low = 0
	Low	0	
	Intermediate	1	
	High	2	
Mutated *ASXL1*		1	Intermediate-1 = 1
Mutated *NRAS*		1	Intermediate-2 = 2
Mutated *RUNX1*		2	High = ≥3
Mutated *SETBP1*		1	

*Cytogenetic Risk Group:
Low: Normal karyotype or isolated loss of Y chromosome
High: Trisomy 8, chromosome 7 abnormalities, or complex karyotype
Intermediate: All other abnormalities

B. CPSS-Mol Model

Risk Factors	Points	CPSS-Mol Risk Group	OS (mo)	48-mo Cumulative Incidence of AML Evolution
Genetic risk group		Low = 0	Not reached	0%
Low	0			
Intermediate-1	1			
Intermediate-2	2			
High	3			
BM blasts ≥5%	1	Intermediate-1: 1	64	9%
WBC >13 k/mcL	1	Intermediate-2: 2 to 3	37	16%
RBC transfusion dependency	1	High ≥4	18	51%

5-year disease-free survival (DFS) after HSCT of 26% in low/intermediate-1 versus 14% in intermediate-2/high-risk. The OS was 44% versus 18%, respectively (*Biol Blood Marrow Transplant.* 2017;23(5):767–775). Data from the European Bone Marrow Transplantation (EBMT) Society showed a 4-year DFS and OS after HSCT of 27% and 33%, respectively (*Eur J Haematol.* 2015;13576).

FRONTLINE TREATMENT

A. Lower-risk CMML:

1. Asymptomatic:
   - Patients with low blast count may be observed.
2. Symptomatic:
   - MPN-like: Clinical trials or HU
   - MDS like: Clinical trials, ESAs, or HMAs

B. Higher-risk CMML:

1. Available donor and acceptable HSCT comorbidity index:
   - Plan for Allogeneic HSCT.
   - Prior cytoreductive therapy should be considered for patients with high-disease burden.
2. No donor or high comorbidity index:
   - Consider clinical trials, HU, ESAs, HMAs, and supportive care.

*Modified from the Mayo Clinic risk-adapted algorithm (*Mayo Clin Proc.* 2016;91(2):259–272) and the EHA/ELN recommendations (*HemaSphere.*2(6):e150).

RELAPSE/REFRACTORY PATIENTS

There are limited options for these patients other than clinical trial and HSCT.

▓ POTENTIAL PRACTICE-CHANGING CLINICAL TRIALS

A phase 1 study of ruxolitinib (NCT01776723) showed promising preliminary activity, with a total response rate of 35% when combining International Working Group (IWG) response criteria and spleen response. Ten out of eleven patients who reported disease-related symptoms had clinically meaningful or complete resolution (*Clin Cancer Res.* 2016;22(15):3746–3754). A phase II study of ruxolitinib (NCT03722407) is ongoing. There is an ongoing randomized phase III trial of decitabine ± HU versus HU alone (NCT02214407) that will help determine whether HMA therapy should also be the standard of care in patients with proliferative CMML (in addition to MDS-type). Other targeted agents are being tested either alone or in combination with HMA for various stages of the disease. These include venetoclax (NCT04160052), anti-GM-CSF monoclonal antibody therapy (NCT02546284), farnesyltransferase inhibitor (NCT02807272), *SL-401* (NCT02268253), *FLT3/KIT/CSF1R* inhibitor (NCT03922100), and the neddylation inhibitor pevonedistat (NCT03268954).

▓ REFERENCES FOR SUPPLEMENTAL READING

1. Patnaik MM, Tefferi A. Chronic myelomonocytic leukemia: 2020 update on diagnosis, risk stratification and management. *Am J Hematol.* 2020;95(1):97–115. PubMed PMID: 31736132.

2. Itzykson R, Fenaux P, Bowen D, et al. Diagnosis and treatment of chronic myelomonocytic leukemias in adults: recommendations from the European Hematology Association and the European Leukemianet. *HemaSphere*. 2018;2(6):e150. PubMed PMID: 31723789.

3. Valent P, Orazi A, Savona M, et al. Proposed diagnostic criteria for classical chronic myelomonocytic leukemia (CMML), CMML variants and pre-CMML conditions. *Haematologica*. 2019;104(10):1935–1949. PubMed PMID: 31048353.

4. Merlevede J, Droin N, QinT, et al. Mutation allele burden remains unchanged in chronic myelomonocytic leukaemia responding to hypomethylating agents. *Nat Commun*. 2016;7:10767. PubMed PMID: 26908133.

5. Elena C, Gallì A, Such E, et al. (2016). Integrating clinical features and genetic lesions in the risk assessment of patients with chronic myelomonocytic leukemia. *Blood*. 128(10):1408–1417. PubMed PMID: 27385790.

17 Acute Myeloid Leukemia

David M. Swoboda and Kendra Sweet

▓ INTRODUCTION

Acute myeloid leukemia (AML) is a heterogeneous disorder of hematopoietic progenitor cells, which is characterized by an increase in the number of immature myeloid cells in the bone marrow (BM). It is the most common type of acute leukemia in adults, and the median age at diagnosis is 68. According to the Surveillance, Epidemiology, and End Results (SEER) data, the number of new AML cases has been rising at a rate of 2.0% per year since 2010.[4] Clinical features vary widely among individuals but are primarily due to the cytopenias resulting from disrupted hematopoiesis. Recently, our increased understanding of somatic mutations in AML has allowed us to not only better define prognosis but also discover novel agents able to target these mutations (ivosidenib for *IDH1*, enasidenib for *IDH2*, and midostaurin and gilteritinib for *FLT3*). Additionally, approval of novel therapies targeting *BCL2* (venetoclax), *CD33* (gemtuzumab), and the hedgehog pathway (glasdegib) as well as new formulations of chemotherapeutic agents (CPX-351) has vastly changed the landscape of AML.

▓ DIAGNOSIS

The initial workup for AML involves careful examination of the peripheral smear to look for circulating leukemic blasts. A BM aspiration and biopsy are needed to confirm the diagnosis and collect important prognostic information. Flow cytometry on the BM is an important aspect of the diagnostic workup; however, the immunophenotype varies among the different subtypes of AML. AML blasts most commonly express *CD13*, *CD33*, *CD34*, *CD117*, and *HLA-DR*. According to the World Health Organization (WHO), a diagnosis of AML requires at least 20% myeloblasts in the BM or peripheral blood or the presence of AML-defining cytogenetic abnormalities, such as t(15;17), t(8;21), t(16;16), or inv(16).[1] Fluorescence in situ hybridization (FISH) and cytogenetic and comprehensive molecular analyses (i.e., *FLT-3 ITD* and next-generation sequencing panels [~40–100 genes]) should be obtained on the BM for accurate risk stratification, prognostication, and treatment selection.

Table 17.1 Cytogenetic and Molecular Prognostic Factors in Acute Myeloid Leukemia

Risk Category	Cytogenetics	Molecular Abnormalities
Favorable risk	inv(16) or t(16;16)	Mutated *NPM1* without *FLT3*-ITD or with *FLT3*-ITD^{low*}
	t(8;21)	Biallelic mutated *CEBPA*
Intermediate risk	t(9;11); normal cytogenetics	Mutated *NPM1* with *FLT3*-ITD^{high*}
	Cytogenetic abnormalities not classified as favorable or adverse	Wild-type *NPM1* without *FLT3*-ITD or with *FLT3*-ITD^{low*} (without adverse-risk genetic lesions)
Adverse risk	Complex cytogenetics	Wild-type *NPM1* with *FLT3*-ITD^{high*}
	(≥3 clonal abnormalities)	Mutated *RUNX1*
	Monosomal karyotypes (−5, 5q−, −7, 7q−, −17, 17p−)	Mutated *ASXL1*
	11q23, inv(3), or t(3:3)	Mutated
	t(6;9) and t(9;22)	*TP53*

*FLT3-ITD^{high} is based on allelic ratio ≥0.5, whereas FLT3-ITD^{low} signifies allelic ratio <0.5.

■ PROGNOSIS

Risk stratification at diagnosis is required for prognostic purposes, and it may also guide treatment decisions (Table 17.1).[3] Prognosis in AML is extremely variable, depending on the biological features of the disease as well as patient-specific factors, including age ≥60, performance status, and coexisting medical conditions. Disease-specific factors include (a) white blood cell (WBC) count at time of diagnosis, (b) history of an antecedent hematologic disorder (i.e., MDS), (c) cytogenetics, (d) molecular aberrations, and (e) therapy-related disease from prior chemotherapy or radiation therapy (see Chapter 18).

■ TREATMENT

Treatment for AML has changed dramatically since 2017, such that standard 7 + 3 induction is no longer given to all patients newly diagnosed with AML. The initial treatment decision is now individualized and dictated by the patient's age, baseline functional status, and cytogenetic/molecular risk stratification. Critically, definitive treatment selection should be delayed in most cases until the above workup has been completed. Patients appropriate for induction chemotherapy generally receive cytarabine + anthracycline–based combinations. A

Table 17.2 Response Criteria in Acute Myeloid Leukemia

Response	Definition
CR without minimal residual disease (CR$_{MRD-}$)	CR with negativity for a genetic marker by real-time quantitative PCR or CR with negativity by multiparametric flow cytometry
CR	BM blasts <5%
	No evidence of extramedullary disease or Auer rods
	ANC ≥1.0 × 10⁹/L
	Platelet count ≥100 × 10⁹/L
CR with incomplete hematology recovery (CRi)	Meets criteria for CR except for neutropenia (ANC <1.0 × 10⁹/L) or thrombocytopenia (<100 × 10⁹/L)
MLFS	Meet criteria for CR except no hematologic recovery required
Partial remission	Decrease of BM blast percentage by 50%
	BM blast percentage of 5% to 25%
	Hematologic criteria of CR

ANC, absolute neutrophil count; BM, bone marrow; CR, complete response; MLFS, morphologic leukemia free state; PCR, polymerase chain reaction

baseline echocardiogram should be obtained in patients receiving anthracycline-based regimens. Patients ineligible for induction chemotherapy generally receive hypomethylating (HMA) or low-dose cytarabine (LDAC)–based combinations (ex-United States [ex-US] only), most frequently with venetoclax if they are able to tolerate it. The goal of therapy is to restore normal hematopoiesis (Table 17.2). A more detailed discussion regarding treatment regimens is included below.

▓ TREATMENT IN PATIENTS ELIGIBLE FOR INDUCTION CHEMOTHERAPY

- Induction chemotherapy options:
  - (7 + 3): cytarabine 100 to 200 mg/m² continuous intravenous infusion (CIVI) × 7 days + anthracycline [daunorubicin (60–90 mg/m²) or idarubicin (12 mg/m²)] × 3 days:
    - If *FLT3* ITD or TKD is mutated, add midostaurin 50 mg twice daily on days 8 to 21.
    - If CD33 positive and exhibits favorable risk cytogenetics, add gemtuzumab ozogamicin (GO) 3 mg/m² on day 1 or days 1, 4, and 7. Consider GO in CD33-positive intermediate-risk cytogenetic patients.
    - Liposomal cytarabine and daunorubicin (Vyxeos): daunorubicin 44 mg/m² on days 1, 3, 5 (secondary or therapy-related AML); see Chapter 18.

- Perform BM biopsy at nadir (day 14 or 21) to confirm hypoplastic marrow.
- Assess response to therapy with BM biopsy at the time of count recovery (~4–6 weeks/induction).
- If patient obtains remission, then consolidation chemotherapy is given based on initial risk status.
  - Favorable risk: Consolidation with high-dose cytarabine (HiDAC) 3 g/m^2 × 3 to 4 cycles followed by observation
  - Intermediate risk: Consolidation with intermediate or HiDAC and an allogeneic stem cell transplant if a suitable donor is available
  - Adverse risk: Consolidation followed by allogeneic stem cell transplant or alternative donor transplant.

TREATMENT IN PATIENTS INELIGIBLE FOR INDUCTION CHEMOTHERAPY

- Patients ineligible for induction chemotherapy, ECOG (>2), significant comorbidities, complex karyotype/*TP53* mutant, should receive HMA-based combinations if they are able to tolerate them.
  - Azacitidine 75 mg/m^2 on days 1 to 7 or Decitabine 20 mg/m^2 on days 1 to 5 in combination with venetoclax 400 mg daily (dose escalation needed in cycle 1) is the preferred option for most patients.[2]
- Additionally, lower intensity options included LDAC ± venetoclax or glasdegib, ivosidenib monotherapy (*IDH1* mutant), or HMA monotherapy.
- Allogeneic stem cell transplant should be considered in those patients who are thought to be candidates with intermediate- or high-risk disease when a suitable donor is available.

RELAPSED/REFRACTORY DISEASE

- Treatment options include salvage chemotherapy, targeted agents in patients with *FLT3* or *IDH1/2* mutations, HMA agents (monotherapy and combinations), LDAC combinations, or clinical trials (Table 17.3). Selection depends on the patient's age, performance status, and disease-specific features.
- No salvage chemotherapy regimen has been proven to be superior; thus, therapy should be tailored to each individual patient.

POTENTIAL PRACTICE-CHANGING CLINICAL TRIALS

Currently, many trials are underway in AML, but only a few of the most promising trials are highlighted here. With improvement in next-generation sequencing, many of the ongoing and future trials focus on targeting specific genetic changes in AML. Additionally,

Table 17.3 Summary of Salvage Acute Myeloid Leukemia Treatment Regimens

Indication	Regimens
Relapsed/refractory	1. Clinical trial
	2. CLAG (cladribine, cytarabine, G-CSF ± mitoxantrone), HiDAC ± anthracycline, FLAG-IDA (fludarabine, cytarabine, G-CSF ± idarubicin), or MEC (mitoxantrone, etoposide, cytarabine)
	3. Targeted therapy: Gilteritinib (*FLT3* mutant), Ivosidenib (*IDH1* mutant), Enasidenib (*IDH2* mutant)
	4. HMA or LDAC ± Venetoclax

G-CSF, granulocyte colony stimulating factor; HiDAC, high-dose cytarabine; HMA, hypomethylating agent; LDAC, low-dose cytarabine

novel formulations of HMA and immune-based therapies appear promising. Given the success of *IDH* inhibitors as monotherapy in relapsed/refractory AML, recent efforts have been made to test these in the front-line setting in combination with azacitidine (AZA). In ongoing phase Ib and phase II trials, the overall response rate (ORR) was 78% and 68%, with CR rates of 61% and 50% in ivosidenib + AZA and enasidenib + AZA, respectively (NCT02677922 and NCT02677922). Additionally, *TP53*-mutant patients are a very high-risk cohort with dismal outcomes and responses to induction chemotherapy. APR-246 is a molecule that restores wild-type function in mutant *TP53*. In the phase Ib/II trial of APR-246 + AZA in *TP53*-mutant MDS and oligoblastic AML, ORR was 87%, with CR rate of 53% (NCT03745716). Next, magrolimab is an antibody targeting *CD47*, a macrophage immune checkpoint and "don't eat me" signal on cancers. In the phase Ib trial of magrolimab, 88% of *TP53*-mutant patients, 5 AML and 2 MDS, achieved an objective response with 5/6 CR or CRi in the AML cohort (NCT03248479). These data have led to continued rapid advancement for both drugs. Finally, CC-486, also known as oral azacitidine, has recently been studied in the phase III QUAZAR AML-001 maintenance trial. Recent results presented in patients who had achieved CR after intensive chemotherapy but were not eligible for transplant showed median overall survival was 24.7 versus 14.8 months ($p < 0.001$) in patients who received CC-486 versus placebo.[5] The results of this trial are practice changing and will likely lead to an FDA approval for this indication.

▧ REFERENCES FOR SUPPLEMENTAL READING

1. Arber DA, Orazi A, Hasserjian R, et al. The 2016 revision to the World Health Organization classification of myeloid neoplasms and acute leukemia. *Blood*. 2016;127(20):2391–2405.

2. DiNardo CD, Pratz K, Pullarkat V, et al. Venetoclax combined with decitabine or azacitidine in treatment-naive, elderly patients with acute myeloid leukemia. *Blood*. 2019;133(1):7–17.

3. Döhner H, Estey E, Grimwade D, et al. Diagnosis and management of AML in adults: 2017 ELN recommendations from an international expert panel. *Blood*. 2017;129(4):424–447.

4. Surveillance, Epidemiology, and End Results (SEER) Program (www.seer.cancer.gov). *SEER*Stat Database: Populations - Total U.S.* (1969–2017), National Cancer Institute, DCCPS, Surveillance Research Program, released December 2018.

5. Wei AH, Döhner H, Pocock C, et al. The QUAZAR AML-001 maintenance trial: results of a phase III international, randomized, double-blind, placebo-controlled study of CC-486 (oral formulation of azacitidine) in patients with acute myeloid leukemia (AML) in first remission. *Blood*. 2019; 134(Suppl2):LBA-3–LBA-3.

18   Secondary AML and AML-MRC

Seongseok Yun, David A. Sallman,
and Jeffrey E. Lancet

▤ INTRODUCTION

Secondary acute myeloid leukemia (s-AML) is defined as acute myeloid leukemia (AML) in patients with prior exposure to environmental carcinogens, chemotherapy or radiation, or AML evolving from other myeloid stem cell disorders (e.g., myelodysplastic syndrome [MDS], myeloproliferative neoplasm [MPN], or mixed MDS/MPN). Accordingly, the 2016 World Health Organization (WHO) classification system categorized s-AML into AML with myelodysplasia-related changes (AML-MRC) and therapy-related myeloid neoplasms (t-MN) that include therapy-related AML (t-AML). s-AML accounts for 10% to 20% of total AML, and it is most commonly seen in elderly patients with previous chemotherapy. Although allogeneic stem cell transplant (SCT) is the only potentially curative treatment, many patients with s-AML are not eligible for aggressive treatment due to comorbidities, disease biology, advanced age, and/or lack of human leukocyte antigen–compatible (HLA-compatible) stem cell donors. Thus, new therapeutic approaches are needed for this distinct clinicopathologic entity.

▤ DIAGNOSIS

2016 WHO CLASSIFICATION T-AML AND AML-MRC

The diagnosis of t-AML or AML-MRC is made when patients with previous exposure to cytotoxic agents, radiation, or preceding MDS harbor morphologic and cytogenetic changes (Table 18.1) in the peripheral blood and bone marrow (BM) that are consistent with AML, including peripheral cytopenias and blasts ≥20%, and typically with associated multilineage dysplasia (defined as at least 50% dysplastic cells in 2 or more cell lines). Of note, multilineage dysplasia alone does not justify AML-MRC in AML cases with *NPM1* or *CEBPA* biallelic mutation.

▤ PATHOGENESIS

Previous studies showed that 8% to 12% of cancer patients developed t-AML within 20 years after treatment and that t-AML accounted for 10% to 20% of all AML cases. Although initial hypotheses were that chemotherapy directly induced mutations, recent data support that these clones can be present at very low levels and that therapy likely leads to their propagation over time. The risk of t-AML is high in patients treated

Table 18.1 Cytogenetic Abnormalities Sufficient to Diagnose AML-MRC	
Complex Karyotype	**3 or More Abnormalities**
Unbalanced abnormalities	−7/del(7q)
	del(5q)/t(5q)
	i(17q)/t(17p)
	−13/del(13q)
	del(11q)
	del(12p)/t(12p)
	idic(X)(q13)
Balanced abnormalities	t(11;16)(q23.3;p13.3)
	t(3;21)(q26.2;q22.1)
	t(1;3)(p36.3;q21.2)
	t(2;11)(p21;q23.3)
	t(5;12)(q32;p13.2)
	t(5;7)(q32;q11.2)
	t(5;17)(q32;p13.2)
	t(5;10)(q32;q21.2)
	t(3;5)(q25.3;q35.1)

AML-MRC, acute myeloid leukemia with myelodysplasia-related changes.

with higher dose chemotherapy and combinations of chemotherapy and radiation. The most common cytotoxic agents associated with t-AML are alkylating agents, such as cyclophosphamide and melphalan (Table 18.2). t-AML associated with alkylating agents or radiation therapy is often preceded by MDS, typically has a latency period of 5 to 10 years, and frequently is associated with unbalanced loss of chromosome 5 or 7. Other agents, including topoisomerase II inhibitors, antimetabolites, and mitotic inhibitors, are also known to be associated with high risk of developing t-AML (Table 18.2), and t-AML that arises after exposure to topoisomerase II inhibitors has a latency period of 1 to 5 years and is associated with 11q23 (*MLL*) or 21q22 (*RUNX1*) gene rearrangement. AML-MRC often has MDS-related cytogenetic abnormalities (Table 18.1). Also, several genes, including 40S ribosomal protein 14 (*RPS14*), enhancer of zeste homolog 2 (*EZH2*), catenin cadherin-associated protein α1 (*CTNNA1*), and adenomatosis polyposis coli (*APC*), have previously been shown to be involved in AML-MRC pathogenesis.

■ RISK STRATIFICATION

Previous studies showed relatively lower complete remission (CR) rates with induction chemotherapy in s-AML patients compared to de novo AML. Also, the median survival was shown to be lower than in

Table 18.2 Cytotoxic Agents Associated With t-AML

Category	Agents
Alkylating agents	Cyclophosphamide, cisplatin, carboplatin, dacarbazine, procarbazine, melphalan, mitomycin, chlorambucil, busulphan, thioTEPA, lomustine, bendamustine, carmustine
Topoisomerase II inhibitors	Doxorubicin, epirubicin, daunorubicin, mitoxantrone, etoposide, amsacrine, actinomycin
Cell cycle arresting agents	Vincristine, vinblastine, vinorelbine, paclitaxel, docetaxel, colchicines, discodermolide, fludarabine, thiopurines, 6-mercaptopurine
Ionizing radiation	Radiation therapy
Other	L-Asparaginase, hydroxyurea, benzene

t-AML, therapy-related acute myeloid leukemia.

patients with de novo AML, mainly due to poor performance status, older age, comorbidities, previous therapy, and a higher association with unfavorable cytogenetic abnormalities. Similar to de novo AML, karyotype remains an independent prognostic parameter in t-AML. Favorable cytogenetics include t(8;21), inv(16), and t(15;17), whereas del(5q), del(7q), t(6;9), monosomy 5 or 7, trisomy 8 or 13, 12p and 17p abnormalities, or complex karyotypes are known as unfavorable cytogenetics (Table 18.3).

▒ PROGNOSIS

Survival outcomes of t-AML patients with favorable karyotype are still lower than in those with de novo AML with favorable karyotype, suggesting that t-AML itself is an independent unfavorable prognostic factor. Additionally, prior chemotherapeutic agents seem to affect the prognosis of t-AML. Alkylating agent-related t-AML has a longer interval from chemotherapy to the development of t-AML as well as chromosome 5 or 7 abnormalities and complex karyotypes, which overall have a poor response to treatment. In topoisomerase II inhibitor-related t-AML, overt AML without preceding MDS is more common, and the interval to develop AML is typically shorter than with alkylating agent-related t-AML. Response to initial therapy is often better. Finally, AML-MRC is associated with worse prognoses than is de novo AML. The discovery of somatic mutations in both AML and MDS has helped further characterize the behavior and prognosis of these diseases, with important implications in s-AML. While the frequently observed mutations in MDS, including *IDH1*, *IDH2*, *ASXL1*, *DNMT3A*, *TP53*, *FLT3*, *RUNX1*, *SRSF2*, and *SF3B1*, were shown to

Table 18.3 Risk Stratification by Karyotype

Risk Group	Chromosomal Abnormalities
Favorable	t(8;21), inv(16), t(15;17)
Intermediate	Normal karyotype, t(9;11), other chromosomal abnormalities that do not belong to favorable or unfavorable group
Unfavorable	del(5q), del(7q), t(6;9), 3q21q26, 11q23, 12p, 17p abnormalities, monosomies 5 or 7, trisomies 8 or 13, complex karyotypes

del, deletion; inv, inversion; t, translocation.

be associated with poor prognoses, the prognostic impact of these mutations in AML-MRC needs further investigation. Recent data indicate that the presence of mutations in *SRSF2*, *SF3B1*, *U2AF1*, *ZRSR2*, *ASXL1*, *EZH2*, *BCOR*, or *STAG2* is highly specific for the diagnosis of s-AML. These mutations, when present in clinically defined de novo AML, confer a significantly inferior prognosis, similar to that of s-AML. These findings suggest that s-AML may be more accurately defined on a molecular basis than on a clinical one.

■ TREATMENT

Before treating patients with s-AML, multiple factors, including age, performance status, comorbidities, cytogenetic profile, and genetic mutations, should be considered to determine optimal treatment. A widely accepted standard of care for patients with s-AML does not exist.

PATIENTS ELIGIBLE FOR INTENSIVE CHEMOTHERAPY

- CPX-351, a liposomal formulation of fixed 5:1 molar ratio of cytarabine and daunorubicin, was recently approved by the FDA as the first-line standard therapy based on a phase 3 randomized trial that showed significantly improved overall survival (HR=0.69, $P = $ .003) in newly diagnosed t-AML and AML-MRC patients. Post-hoc analysis following allogeneic hematopoietic stem cell transplant (HSCT) showed improved overall survival (OS) in the CPX-351–treated cohort (OS not reached versus 10.3 months).
- Induction chemotherapy (7 + 3) followed by high-dose cytarabine (HiDAC) consolidation may be appropriate to treat s-AML in younger patients with good performance status.
- Younger and healthier patients with s-AML should be considered for allogeneic SCT during remission to allow for possible cure or extended survival, which may be achieved via a graft-versus-leukemia effect.

PATIENTS INELIGIBLE FOR INTENSIVE CHEMOTHERAPY

- Low-intensity chemotherapy, clinical trials, or supportive care is often used for elderly patients with comorbidities and poor performance status (due to a relatively high treatment-related mortality rate in this group) or for patients with an unfavorable karyotype.

- Previous phase 3 randomized trials that included patients with t-AML and AML-MRC have generally demonstrated a modest survival benefit of hypomethylating agents compared to low-dose cytarabine, intensive chemotherapy, or best supportive care (2-year OS 50% versus 16%, $P = .001$).

- Hypomethylating agents azacitidine and decitabine are commonly used for MDS and AML patients with reasonable outcomes, including some patients with complete response and durable survival.

- Venetoclax is a BCL-2 inhibitor, and recent phase 1 to 3 trials showed promising outcomes in combination with hypomethylating agents in newly diagnosed AML patients who are ages 75 years or older or not eligible for intensive induction chemotherapy. The s-AML subgroup in a recent large phase 1/2 clinical trial experienced a CR/complete response with incomplete count recovery (CRi) rate of 67%, with median OS not reached.

▧ POTENTIAL PRACTICE-CHANGING CLINICAL TRIALS

APR-246 is a novel molecule that selectively induces apoptosis in cancer cells harboring *TP53* mutations. A recent phase 1/2 trial showed 87% overall response rate and 53% CR rate in MDS and AML-MRC patients who were treated with APR-246 in combination with hypomethylating agents. Novel molecules attacking *FLT-3*, *IDH1/2*, or other targets may be viable options in the future. Immunotherapies targeting CD33, CD45, and CD123 are showing early signs of efficacy in relapsed or refractory AML patients. Further investigation of these agents may also be promising. The question of optimal first-line therapy for fit patients over the age of 60 is controversial, given good outcomes both with liposomal daunorubicin:cytarabine as well as venetoclax in combination with hypomethylating agents.

▧ REFERENCES FOR SUPPLEMENTAL READING

1. Kayser S, Döhner K, Krauter J, et al. The impact of therapy-related acute myeloid leukemia on outcome in 2853 adult patients with newly diagnosed AML. *Blood.* 2011;117:2137–2145.

2. Lindsley RC, Mar BG, Mazzola E, et al. Acute myeloid leukemia ontogeny is defined by distinct somatic mutations. *Blood.* 2015;125:1367–1376.

3. Rowe JM. Therapy of secondary leukemia. *Leukemia.* 2002;16:748–750.

4. Fenaux P, Mufti GJ, Hellström-Lindberg E, et al. Azacitidine prolongs overall survival compared with conventional care regimens in elderly patients

with low bone marrow blast count acute myeloid leukemia. *J Clin Oncol.* 2010;28:562–569.

5. Lancet JE, Uy GL, Cortes JE, et al. CPX-351 (cytarabine and daunorubicin) liposome for injection versus conventional cytarabine plus daunorubicin in older patients with newly diagnosed secondary acute myeloid leukemia. *J Clin Oncol.* 2018;36:2684–2692.

6. DiNardo CD, Pratz K, Pullarkat V, et al. Venetoclax combined with decitabine or azacitidine in treatment-naïve, elderly patients with acute myeloid leukemia. *Blood.* 2019;133(1):7–17.

19 Acute Promyelocytic Leukemia

Virginia O. Volpe and Jeffrey E. Lancet

▓ INTRODUCTION

Acute promyelocytic leukemia (APL) is a subtype of acute myelogenous leukemia (AML), comprising 4% to 15% of all AML cases and accounting for 600 to 800 new cases a year. There is a higher incidence among Hispanics, at 25% to 38% of new cases. The classic features of APL include promyelocytic marrow infiltrate, coagulopathy, and balanced translocations between chromosomes 15 and 17, t(15;17)(q22;q21), which result in a fusion of promyelocytic leukemia (PML) and retinoic acid receptor genes (*RARα*). This fusion protein PML-*RARα* blocks myeloid differentiation at the promyelocyte stage. Variant forms of APL are noted to have translocation t(11;17) or t(5;17). The implementation of targeted therapies, such as arsenic trioxide (ATO) and all-trans retinoic acid (ATRA), which promotes terminal differentiation of leukemic cells, has transformed APL from a highly fatal disease with long-term survival of <50% to one with a >95% cure rate. However, APL patients with high-risk disease still have a relapse rate of approximately 30%.

▓ DIAGNOSIS

The diagnosis of APL is made by the morphological appearance of the leukemic cells, but most importantly by cytogenetic and fluorescence in situ hybridization (FISH) analysis. APL patients normally present with fatigue, fever, and bruising secondary to cytopenias. Patients present with either leukopenia or leukocytosis and can frequently have mild bleeding from their abnormal coagulopathy to full-blown disseminated intravascular coagulopathy (DIC), resulting in spontaneous life-threatening bleeds, such as intracranial hemorrhage. This bleeding diathesis can also occur without abnormal coagulation parameters.

The most common morphological appearance of promyelocytes in APL is the hypergranular form, encompassing 75% to 80% of all APL cases (Figure 19.1). These cells are characterized by strong myeloperoxidase positivity. The cytoplasm has intense azurophilic granules and bundles of large Auer rods dispersed throughout the cytoplasm. The nuclei are bilobed or kidney shaped. The microgranular or hypogranular variant (10%–25% of APL) is characterized by a decrease in the quantity and microscopic size of azurophilic granules (Figure 19.1). The nuclei tend to be bilobed. Auer rods are also identified in these

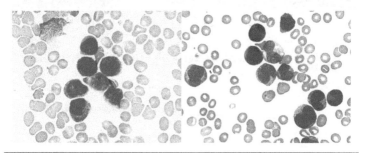

Figure 19.1 Comparison of hypergranular (left panel) and hypogranular promyelocytes (right panel).

cells. Patient with hypogranular APL tend to present with higher white blood cell (WBC) counts and rapid doubling times.

The immunophenotype of typical APL with t(15;17)(q22;q21) has a low or absence of expression of HLA-DR, CD34, CD11a, CD11b, and CD18. There is homogeneous expression of CD33 and heterogeneous expression of CD13. CD64 expression is also seen. Different from the typical APL, microgranular variant APL often coexpresses CD34 and CD2. Laboratory evaluation includes complete blood count (CBC) with differential, complete metabolic panel (CMP), lactate dehydrogenase (LDH), prothrombin time (PT), partial thromboplastin time (PTT), international normalized ratio (INR), fibrinogen and D-dimer levels, evaluation of peripheral smear, and evaluation of bone marrow (BM) aspirate and biopsy. Diagnostic workup includes cytogenetic analysis with reverse transcriptase polymerase chain reaction (PCR) for the PML-RARα fusion gene and FISH with probes for PML and RARα or an anti-PML antibody.

■ VARIANT FORMS

Rare variant forms of APL include t(11;17)(q23;21), resulting in PLZF-RARα; t(11;17)(q13;q21), creating a fusion of NuMA-RARα; t(5;17)(q35;q21), leading to a NPM1-RARα fusion protein; and t(17;17)(q11;q21), resulting in STAT5b-RARα. Variant forms such as these occur in <1% of APL cases, and responsiveness to therapy is based on small numbers of case reports only. NuMA-RARα and NPM1-RARα may be ATRA sensitive and could be managed with ATRA combined with anthracycline-based chemotherapy. The PLZF-RARα is typically resistant to ATRA and chemotherapy. STAT5b-RARα is exceedingly rare. The sensitivity of any of these variants to ATO is unclear.

■ PROGNOSIS

Patients were initially risk stratified into three groups: low, intermediate, and high. Stratified complete response (CR) rates ranged from 80% to 90%, dependent on the initial risk stratification. However, patients classified as low and intermediate were grouped together and treated as standard risk.

1. High risk: WBC >10,000/mcL
2. Intermediate risk: WBC ≤10,000/mcL and platelet count >40,000/mcL
3. Low risk: WBC ≤10,000/mcL and platelet count ≤40,000/mcL

▓ TREATMENT

Due to underlying coagulopathy and high risk of bleeding complications, it is imperative that treatment be initiated immediately. If there is any suspicion of APL from coagulation studies and morphological review of the leukemia cells, ATRA should be initiated prior to confirmatory diagnostic testing. Treatment for APL is divided into standard-versus high-risk disease. Course of treatment includes induction and consolidation therapy. It is important to note that with patients who are elderly or frail, anthracycline use should be avoided. If leukoreduction is necessary in this population, hydroxyurea or gemtuzumab ozogamicin should also be used.

INDUCTION THERAPY

- **Standard-risk APL:** Historically, APL was treated with ATRA plus anthracycline, which has been shown to induce high remission rates. A landmark phase 3 multicenter trial evaluated ATRA + ATO versus ATRA + chemotherapy in standard-risk patients. It found that ATRA + ATO was at least not inferior and may be superior, with lower risk of hematologic toxicity. Similar results were also found in the UK AML17 study, resulting in the development of ATRA + ATO as standard for standard-risk patients with APL.
- **High-risk APL:** More recently, studies have looked at an ATRA + ATO backbone in patients with high-risk disease. In the AML17 trial, ATRA+ ATO versus ATRA + anthracycline were studied in all risk groups. In high-risk patients, a dose of Gemtuzumab (6 mg/m^2) was given within the first 4 days of the first course. Among high-risk patients, ATRA + ATO + GO resulted in excellent and similar overall survival in comparison to ATRA + chemotherapy, with fewer serious adverse events. Other trials have shown similar results, suggesting ATRA + ATO (plus Gemtuzumab) as an acceptable frontline therapy in high-risk APL patients.

Duration of therapy is given every day until clinical remission. Tables 19.1 and 19.2 detail treatment further per risk stratification.

INTRATHECAL PROPHYLAXIS

Per the National Comprehensive Cancer Network (NCCN) guidelines, prophylaxis is recommended in patients with high-risk disease. Intrathecal (IT) chemotherapy may be given once peripheral blasts have cleared and upon count recovery.

Table 19.1 Standard Risk Treatment

Standard Risk Treatment			
			Contraindication to ATO
Induction therapy options	ATRA 45 mg/m² daily + ATO 0.15 mg/kg IV daily	ATRA 45 mg/m² daily + ATO 0.3 mg/kg IV on days 1 to 5 of week one and 0.25 mg/kg twice weekly in weeks 2 to 8	ATRA 45 mg/m² daily + idarubicin 12 mg/m² on days 2, 4, 6, 8
			Contraindication to ATO
Consolidation therapy options	ATO 0.15 mg/kg/d IV 5 d/wk for 4 weeks every 8 weeks for a total of 4 cycles; ATRA 45 mg/m²/d for 2 weeks every 4 weeks for a total of 7 cycles	ATRA 45 mg/m² for 2 weeks every 4 weeks cycles 1 to 4 + ATO 0.3 mg/kg IV on days 1 to 5 of week one in cycles 1 to 4 and 0.25 mg/kg twice weekly in weeks 2 to 4 in cycles 1 to 4	ATRA 45 mg/m² × 15 days + idarubicin 5 mg/m² × 4 days × 1 cycles, then ATRA × 15 days + mitoxantrone 10 mg/m²/d × 3 days × 1 cycle, then ATRA × 15 days + idarubicin 12 mg/m² × 1 cycle

ATRA, all-trans retinoic acid; ATO, arsenic trioxide.

CONSOLIDATION THERAPY

Although it is a highly curable disease, APL creates a significant risk of relapse without consolidation therapy. Therefore, multiple consolidation therapy strategies have been proposed and are dependent on the initial induction therapy choice based on the patient's characteristics. ATRA is used in all post-remission consolidation therapies, with the majority of patients receiving ATRA + ATO.

MAINTENANCE THERAPY

Maintenance therapy remains controversial in patients with APL. While some early trials have demonstrated event-free survival benefits, especially in high-risk patients, overall survival benefits are lacking. At present, maintenance therapy in standard-risk patients is not recommended, and its role in high-risk patients has not been determined, although single-agent ATRA as maintenance for patients who have received ATRA + ATO–based induction is often used. There have yet to be dedicated randomized trials with ATRA and ATO as maintenance.

Table 19.2 High-Risk Treatment

	High-Risk Treatment		
			Contraindication to ATO
Induction therapy options	ATRA 45 mg/m²/d + ATO 0.15 mg/kg/d + single dose gemtuzumab ozogamicin 6 to 9 mg/m²	ATRA 45 mg/m² days 1 to 36, idarubicin 6 to 12 mg/m² days 2, 4, 6, 8 + ATO 0.15 mg/kg days 9 to 36	ATRA 45 mg/m² daily + daunorubicin 60 mg/m² × 3 days + cytarabine 200 mg/m² × 7 days
			Contraindication to ATO
Consolidation therapy options	ATO 0.15 mg/kg 5 d/wk for 4 weeks every 8 weeks total of 4 cycles + ATRA 45 mg/m² for 2 weeks every 4 weeks for a total of 7 cycles. Consider maintenance ATRA 45 mg/m² daily for 2 weeks every 12 weeks for 2 years.	ATO 0.15 mg/kg 5 d/wk for 4 weeks every 8 weeks total of 4 cycles + ATRA 45 mg/m² for 2 weeks every 4 weeks for a total of 7 cycles. Consider maintenance ATRA 45 mg/m² daily for 2 weeks every 12 weeks for 2 years.	Daunorubicin 60 mg/m² × 3 days + cytarabine 200 mg/m² × 7 days × 1 cycle then cytarabine 2 g/m² every 12 hours × 5 days + daunorubicin 45 mg/m² × 3 days × 1 cycle

ATRA, all-trans retinoic acid; ATO, arsenic trioxide.

ASSESSMENT OF RESPONSE TO THERAPY

Unlike with other forms of AML, a day-14 BM biopsy in APL is not routine. After induction, a BM biopsy is obtained with count recovery to assess morphological recovery, which is usually seen between days 28 and 35. In addition to count recovery (ANC ≥1,000/mcL and platelets >100 k/mcL) to evaluate for CR, BM must show adequate cellularity, normal maturation of cell lines, and <5% blasts. Assessing for molecular response with FISH/RT-PCR may show persistence of APL/RARα; however, this is does not carry a prognostic role, as the clones, although detectable, may still be on a decline. BM biopsy and aspirate for RT-PCR of PML-*RAR*α should be performed at the completion of consolidation.

Once in remission, subsequent testing for PCR PML-*RAR*α can be performed on peripheral blood every 3 months for 2 years. For patients with high-risk APL, who are more than 60 years of age, or who have received an incomplete course(s) of treatment, periodic BM sampling for PML-RARα transcript (PCR) is recommended, typically every 3 months for 2 years following the completion of consolidation. If PCR is positive, an additional BM biopsy within 2 weeks is required to confirm a positive result. If repeat testing is negative, frequent monitoring every 3 months via BM sample is indicated to ensure the patient remains negative. If repeat testing is positive, the patient should be treated for relapsed APL.

MANAGEMENT OF RELAPSED APL

The rate of relapsed APL has been significantly reduced, between 10% and 30% with the treatment of ATRA + ATO–based regimens. As seen in Figure 19.2, patients are typically stratified by early or late relapse (<6 months or >6 months). In early relapse after ATRA + ATO without the use of prior anthracycline or gemtuzumab, typical regimens will add these medications to a ATRA + ATO reinduction or participation in clinical trial. Another consideration is single-agent Gemtuzumab. For relapse >6 months, reinduction with either ATO alone (if ATO-naïve) or combined with ATRA until count recovery with BM confirmation of remission should be considered. Autologous stem cell transplant (SCT) is suggested at the time of second molecular remission. Patients who relapse after autologous SCT or who fail to achieve molecular remission can be evaluated for allogeneic SCT.

MONITORING AND MANAGEMENT OF COAGULOPATHY

The majority of cases of fatal hemorrhage occur within the first month of therapy and are the primary cause of early mortality in APL. DIC panels should be monitored closely in each patient. Supportive guidelines

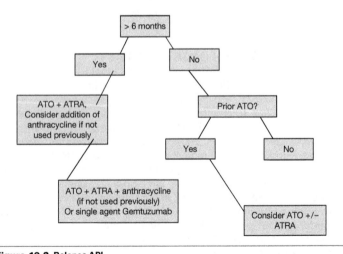

Figure 19.2 Relapse APL.

ATRA, all-trans retinoic acid; ATO, arsenic trioxide.

for APL patients include administration of fresh-frozen plasma (FFP) with PT or PTT elevation. Guidelines also indicate the need to administer platelets to maintain a platelet count ≥50,000/mcL and FFP or cryoprecipitate to maintain fibrinogen of >100 to 150 mg/dL until signs of coagulopathy have resolved.

MONITORING AND MANAGEMENT OF DIFFERENTIATION SYNDROME

Twenty-five to thirty percent of patients treated with ATRA will develop ATRA differentiation syndrome (DS), irrespective of risk category. Symptoms can present as dyspnea, weight gain, peripheral edema, congestive heart failure, and acute renal failure. Vigilant monitoring of APL patients treated with ATRA or ATO for these signs is imperative. DS is a potentially fatal complication of therapy and needs to be treated aggressively. At the first signs of symptoms, dexamethasone 10 mg IV twice a day should be started immediately and last at least 3 days until symptom resolution. There is no strong evidence to support prophylactic use of dexamethasone in the prevention of DS. Ideally, ATRA or ATO should be continued while the patient is undergoing management of DS. Temporary discontinuation of ATRA or ATO should take place if the patient is critically ill, such as requiring intensive care, intubation, or dialysis.

POTENTIAL PRACTICE-CHANGING CLINICAL TRIALS

Treatment strategies for high-risk patients remain challenging, as the trials comparing standard treatment options have not shown one to be superior. A current phase 3 clinical trial randomizes high-risk APL patients to standard chemotherapy with ATRA + IDA versus ATRA/ATO + low-dose idarubicin during induction (NCT02688140). In addition to this trial, another is randomizing high-risk APL with ATRA + ATO with or without gemtuzumab ozogamicin to evaluate for improved CR without increasing toxicities (NCT01409161).

REFERENCES FOR SUPPLEMENTAL READING

1. Wintrobe's Clinical Hematology. *Chapter 79: Acute Promyelocytic Leukemia* (14th ed.). Philadelphia: Wolters Kluwer; 2019: 1679–1697.

2. Burnett AK, Russell NH, Hills RK, et al. Arsenic trioxide and all-trans retinoic acid treatment for acute promyelocytic leukaemia in all risk groups (AML17): results of a randomised, controlled, phase 3 trial. *Lancet Oncol.* 2015;16(13):1295–1305.

3. Iland HJ, Collins M, Bradstock K, et al. Use of arsenic trioxide in remission induction and consolidation therapy for acute promyelocytic leukaemia in the Australasian Leukaemia and Lymphoma Group (ALLG) APML4 study: a non-randomised phase 2 trial. *Lancet Haematol.* 2015;2(9):e357–e366.

4. National Comprehensive Cancer Network. *Acute myeloid leukemia.* Updated 2020. https://www.nccn.org/professionals/physician_gls/

5. Lo-Coco F, Avvisati G, Vignetti M, et al. Retinoic acid and arsenic trioxide for acute promyelocytic leukemia. *N Engl J Med.* 2013;369(2):111–121.

20 Blastic Plasmacytoid Dendritic Cell Neoplasm

Justin Taylor and Andrew A. Lane

▦ INTRODUCTION

Blastic plasmacytoid dendritic cell neoplasm (BPDCN) is a rare, aggressive hematologic malignancy derived from plasmacytoid dendritic cells (pDCs) and classified as a unique hematologic malignancy in the 2016 update of the World Health Organization (WHO) Classification of Tumors.[1] The disease was previously called blastic NK-cell lymphoma or CD4+/CD56+ hematodermic neoplasm until the cell of origin was discovered. Now, unique pathologic markers, some derived from normal pDCs, are used to differentiate these tumors from other hematologic malignancies. The disease occurs at a median age of 65 years with a strong male predominance (>3:1 M:F), although it can occur at any age, including childhood. Clinically, BPDCN presents as skin lesions, usually with leukemic dissemination to the bone marrow (BM), lymph nodes, and spleen. Some cases are detected with only cutaneous involvement, but they invariably progress to systemic disease. A minority present with only features of acute leukemia (i.e., without skin or nodal involvement). Recently, investigation into the genetic mechanisms of leukemogenesis in BPDCN has revealed mutations commonly found in other hematologic malignancies, with particular similarity to myeloid diseases.[2,3]

▦ DIAGNOSIS

2016 WHO CLASSIFICATION OF TUMORS OF HEMATOPOIETIC AND LYMPHOID TISSUE

- Diagnosis is suspected in patients with violaceous plaques or tumors in the skin or with acute leukemia of ambiguous lineage.
- Skin biopsy shows infiltrating monomorphic medium-sized blasts. Immunohistochemical (IHC) staining is positive for CD4, CD56, CD123, BDCA-2/CD303, and TCL-1 and is typically negative for other myeloid markers, such as MPO and lysozyme.
- Rare cases of only leukemic presentation will have the same morphologic appearance and immunophenotype in the BM (Figure 20.1).

A BM evaluation is recommended for all patients with cutaneous disease. A contrast-enhanced computed tomography (CT) or positron emission tomography/computed tomography (PET/CT) scan of the chest, abdomen, and pelvis should be considered due to the frequent

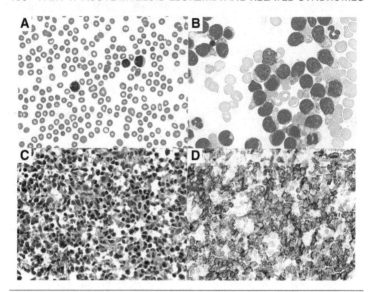

Figure 20.1 The peripheral blood film shows circulating blastic plasmacytoid dendritic cells with irregular nuclei and immature chromatin (A, Wright, ×600). The bone marrow aspirate demonstrates sheets of immature precursors with plasma-cytoid appearance, including round to oval or elongated nuclei, delicate chromatin, and abundant eccentrically located cytoplasm (B, Wright-Giemsa, ×1,000). The bone marrow core biopsy is interstitially infiltrated by the neoplasm and focally forms aggregates (C, Hematoxylin and Eosin [H&E], ×600), which stain positive for CD123 (D, Immunoperoxidase, ×600).

occurrence of splenic and lymph node infiltration. Cerebrospinal fluid (CSF) analysis is usually reserved for those with neurologic signs or symptoms at initial diagnosis, but CSF positivity is more frequent in relapse.

▨ KEY DIAGNOSTIC DILEMMA

BPDCN should be distinguished from other diseases with cutaneous involvement. Acute myeloid leukemia (AML) with CD56 positivity by IHC can present in the skin (myeloid sarcoma) and be mistaken for BPDCN. However, most cases also demonstrate positivity for myeloperoxidase (MPO) and other myeloid antigens, such as CD117. Conversely, those markers are absent in BPDCN, which instead has the pDC-associated antigen (for example, BDCA-2, CD123, and/or TCL-1). BPDCN is associated with the positive coexpression of CD56, TdT, or TCL-1 or negative staining for lysozyme, which myeloid sarcoma can also exhibit. Extranodal NK/T-cell lymphoma also frequently has skin manifestations with expression of the CD56+ immunophenotype, but BPDCN lacks Epstein–Barr virus positivity via in situ hybridization studies and shows CD123 positivity. Chronic myelomonocytic leukemia (CMML) can be associated with pDC proliferation but is instead mature morphologically and CD56 negative, thus differentiating it from BPDCN.

■ PROGNOSIS

Due to the aggressive clinical course, median survival of BPDCN is approximately 12 to 14 months, although aggressive treatments may be related with improved outcomes in a more modern cohort.[4] Most patients initially respond to chemotherapy, but relapse with resistant/refractory disease is common. Hematopoietic stem cell transplant as consolidation has been associated with improved outcomes.

■ TREATMENT

BPDCN is a rare disease; most treatment reports are small and retrospective. Patients have responded to AML, acute lymphocytic leukemia (ALL) (Hyper-CVAD), or lymphoma-like (cyclophosphamide, doxorubicin, vincristine, and prednisone [CHOP]) regimens. Allogeneic stem cell transplantation is the preferred consolidation therapy, although some long-term remissions have also been observed after autologous transplant (Figure 20.2).

The only prospective data are from a phase 1/2 trial of interleukin-3 (IL-3) conjugated to diphtheria toxin (tagraxofusp).[5] BPDCN expresses high levels of CD123, the IL-3 receptor, and SL-401, therefore delivering diphtheria toxin to the malignant cells. The researchers reported a clinical complete response rate of 72% in 29 previously untreated patients with BPDCN. Thirteen out of the 29 patients (45%) were bridged to hematopoietic stem cell transplant. The survival of the 29 previously untreated patients receiving tagraxofusp was 52% at 24 months, with a median follow-up of 25 months.

Relapsed/refractory BPDCN is less responsive to treatment. In the tagraxofusp trial, 15 previously treated patients achieved a complete response rate of only 33% and median survival of 8.5 months. Nonetheless, the Food and Drug Administration's (FDA's) approval of tagraxofusp, the first drug approved for use in BPDCN, is a major step forward for treatment of this previously neglected disease.

■ POTENTIAL PRACTICE-CHANGING CLINICAL TRIALS

An observation that BPDCN blasts express high levels of BCL2 led to an ongoing phase 1 dose-escalation trial of the BCL2 antagonist venetoclax in relapsed/refractory BPDCN (NCT03485547). Treatment-naïve patients will be included in the expansion portion of this study. Other trials are investigating venetoclax in combination with other therapies, such as hypomethylating agents, based on the successful use of the combination in AML. Lastly, trials of other CD123-targeted therapies, such as antibody-drug conjugates, chimeric antigen receptor (CAR) T-cells, and bi-specific antibodies, are being designed. It

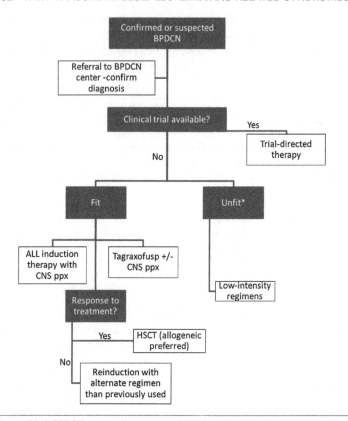

Figure 20.2 BPDCN proposed treatment algorithm.

*Patients on the tagraxofusp trial all had 0 to 1 Eastern Cooperative Oncology Group (ECOG) performance status and normal cardiac function.

BPDCN, blastic plasmacytoid dendritic cell neoplasm; CNS, central nervous system; HSCT, hematopoietic stem cell transplant.

is hoped that the future will hold a host of therapeutic options for patients with BPDCN and that combinations of these therapies can be studied with the goal of eradicating the disease.

■ REFERENCES FOR SUPPLEMENTAL READING

1. Arber DA, Orazi A, Hasserjian R, et al. The 2016 revision to the World Health Organization classification of myeloid neoplasms and acute leukemia. *Blood*. 2016;127(20):2391–2405.

2. Jardin F, Ruminy P, Parmentier F, et al. TET2 and TP53 mutations are frequently observed in blastic plasmacytoid dendritic cell neoplasm. *Br J Haematol*. 2011;153(3):413–416.

3. Menezes J, Acquadro F, Wiseman M, et al. Exome sequencing reveals novel and recurrent mutations with clinical impact in blastic plasmacytoid dendritic cell neoplasm. *Leukemia*. 2014;28(4):823–829.

4. Taylor J, Haddadin M, Upadhyay VA, et al. Multicenter analysis of outcomes in blastic plasmacytoid dendritic cell neoplasm offers a pretargeted therapy benchmark. *Blood*. 2019;134(8):678–687.

5. Pemmaraju N, Lane AA, Sweet KL, et al. Tagraxofusp in blastic plasmacytoid dendritic-cell neoplasm. *N Engl J Med*. 2019;380(17):1628–1637.

21 B-Lymphoblastic Leukemia/Lymphoma

Fernando Vargas and Bijal Shah

▨ INTRODUCTION

B-acute lymphoblastic leukemia/lymphoma (B-ALL) is a lymphoid neoplasm characterized by the proliferation and accumulation of immature B-cell precursors. B-ALL can present as B-cell lymphoblastic lymphoma (B-LBL) characterized by the presence of extramedullary disease with fewer than 25% marrow lymphoblasts. Alternatively, if >25% lymphoblasts are observed in the marrow, the disease is referred to as B-ALL, regardless of extramedullary manifestations. In contrast to T-ALL/T-LBL, B-ALL occurs more frequently than B-LBL, which constitutes approximately 10% of cases. B-ALL accounts for 85% and 75% of pediatric and adult ALL cases, respectively, while the remaining cases are those of the T-cell lineage (see Chapter 23). It also occurs more frequently in males than females, and there is an increased racial predisposition for Whites and Hispanics. ALL is considered a rare malignancy, with a total of 6,150 new cases and 1,520 deaths estimated for 2020; these numbers represent approximately 0.3% of all new cancer cases and 0.2% of all cancer-related deaths (American Cancer Society. *Cancer Facts & Figures 2020*). Although B-ALL accounts for only 10% to 15% of adult leukemia, it is the most common of childhood malignancy. ALL has a bimodal age distribution, with approximately 55% of cases occurring in those younger than 20 years old and then increasing again in those older than 45 years. According to the most recent Surveillance, Epidemiology, and End Results (SEER) data, the median age at diagnosis is 16 years. Although it is a disease predominantly seen in younger people, it is important to note that approximately 86% of ALL-related deaths occur in patients older than 20 years of age.

▨ DIAGNOSIS

Most patients present with evidence of bone marrow (BM) failure, including anemia, thrombocytopenia, and neutropenia. Given these abnormalities, patients present with anemia-related symptoms, bleeding, or infectious complications. Leukocytosis is not necessarily present, and symptoms of leukostasis are rare in patients with ALL. On the other hand, constitutional symptoms, such as fever, night sweats, and weight loss, are frequently present, and patients can also complain of significant bone pain and arthralgias. Hepatosplenomegaly and/or lymphadenopathy can be seen in about half of the cases. Clinicians must be vigilant for neurological deficits, as these may be related to central nervous system (CNS) involvement, which is not uncommon. A thorough history, physical exam, complete blood count (CBC) with differential, complete metabolic panel, uric acid, lactate dehydrogenase, peripheral smear, and BM biopsy should be performed promptly. In case of delay in obtaining a BM biopsy, a peripheral blood flow cytometry can establish the diagnosis. BM aspirate samples should be sent for cytogenetic analysis, fluorescence in situ hybridization (FISH), and next-generation sequencing (NGS), as it may be useful to identify specific mutations in cases of B-ALL. Additionally, FISH or ribonucleic acid (RNA) sequencing to identify *BCR-ABL1*–like B-ALL should be performed. Given its tendency for extramedullary involvement, particularly the CNS, a lumbar puncture (for delivering intrathecal chemotherapy and assessing involvement) should be performed. If extramedullary involvement is suspected, then imaging either by positron emission tomography/computed tomography (PET/CT) scan or contrast-enhanced CT scan should be performed. An echocardiogram or multigated acquisition (MUGA) scan to evaluate cardiac function should be performed in anticipation of anthracycline-based chemotherapy.

▓ KEY DIAGNOSTIC DILEMMA

Differentiating lymphoblasts from their morphologic mimic, normal B-cell precursors known as hematogones, can be challenging, especially in cases of minimal residual disease (MRD). Hematogone hyperplasia may be seen in settings, including post-BM transplantation or chemotherapy, viral infections, autoimmune diseases, or malignancies. Lymphoblasts may have a spectrum of morphologies ranging from small blasts with minimal amounts of cytoplasm, condensed chromatin, and nonvisible nucleoli to larger blasts with variable amounts of cytoplasm, fine chromatin, and prominent nucleoli. Atypical azurophilic granules may be observed in a small subset of cases. Hematogones, on the other hand, have a higher nuclear:cytoplasmic ratio, nonvisible nucleoli, and a uniform chromatin pattern. Hematogones have a spectrum of flow cytometric marker expression that reflects the progressive maturation of these precursors (Table 21.1), which may aid in distinguishing them from neoplastic lymphoblasts of B-ALL. B-ALL typically express the B-cell markers CD19, cytoplasmic CD79a (cyCD79a), cytoplasmic CD22 (cyCD22), CD10, surface CD22 (sCD22), PAX-5, CD24, and TdT. CD45, CD34, and CD20 are variable in expression, while CD13 and CD33 (myeloid markers) may be aberrantly expressed. B-ALL is further subdivided based on the level of differentiation of the B-lymphoblasts— namely, the early precursor B-ALL or pro-B-ALL, intermediate stage (or "common B-ALL"), and pre-B-ALL (most mature). Normal mature B-cell cells lack CD34 and TdT expression. Of note, a careful review of clinical history is necessary to help exclude the blast phase (lymphoid) of chronic myelogenous leukemia.

Table 21.1 Comparison of Flow Cytometric Marker Expression of B-ALL Lymphoblasts Versus Hematogones

Flow Cytometry Marker	B-ALL	Hematogones
CD45	±	Dim to moderate +
CD34	Variable +	Heterogeneous: + (most immature stage) to – (more mature stages)*
CD20	Variable +	Heterogeneous: – (most immature stage) to dim + (more mature stages) with characteristic "smearing" pattern*
CD19	+	+
CD10	Variable, but typically very bright +	Heterogeneous: Bright + (most immature stage) to moderate + (down-regulated in more mature stages)
TdT	+	Heterogeneous + (most immature stage) to – (more mature stages)
cyCD22	+	+
sCD22	Homogeneous +	Heterogeneous +
CD13/CD33	May be expressed in a subset of cases	–
CD38	±	Bright +

B-ALL, B-acute lymphoblastic leukemia; cy, cytoplasmic; s, surface; TdT, terminal deoxynucleotidyl transferase.

*The levels of expression of CD34 and CD20 are almost always mutually exclusive in normal hematogones. *Blood*. 2001;98(8):2498–2507.

▓ PROGNOSIS

In recent years, there has been a significant improvement in the outcome of pediatric patients with B-ALL, with cure rates exceeding 80% to 85%. On the other hand, adults have not enjoyed the same success, in part due to patient-related factors, and also because of a different disease biology. For example, adverse risk factors, such as the presence of *BCR-ABL1* or Ph-like genetic signature, are more prevalent in adults, while favorable markers such as hyperdiploidy and *ETV6-RUNX1* are more prevalent in children (Table 21.2). Appropriate risk stratification is critically important in developing an initial treatment plan and to guide the application of allogeneic stem cell transplantation in first complete remission (CR1).

A large retrospective study evaluating the outcome of 6,238 children with ALL defined four different risk groups; low, standard, high and very high. This was based on age, white blood cell (WBC) count, sex, extramedullary disease, cytogenetics, and rate of response to therapy. This study is the basis of risk-adapted therapy, which is currently standard practice in children oncology group (COG) trials (*Blood*. 2007;109(3):926–935). In adults, clinical factors associated with worse prognosis are age >35 and WBC >30 × 10^9 for B-ALL or >100 × 10^9 for T-ALL. These were defined in the largest prospective trial of adult ALL patients done to date, the MRC UKALL XI/ECOG E2993 (Table 21.3).

More recently, measurable residual disease (MRD) has shown to be the most important prognostic marker of long-term disease control and survival. Specifically, MRD assessment (negative ≤0.01% blasts) has become standard practice, as it is the most powerful predictor of potential relapse (*J Natl Compr Canc Netw*. 2015;(10):1240–1279). The impact of MRD was also shown in an extensive meta-analysis where the 10-year EFS in pediatric patients with MRD (–) and MRD (+) was 77% and 32%, respectively. In adults, the 10-year EFS for patients with MRD (–) and MRD (+) was 64% and 21%, respectively (*JAMA Oncol*. 2017;3(7):e170580. doi: 10.1001/jamaoncol.2017.0580).

■ TREATMENT

Treatment for B-ALL typically consists of multi-agent chemotherapy with intensive CNS chemoprophylaxis, resulting in a roughly 90% chance of CR1. Treatment typically consists of five chemotherapy stages: induction, consolidation, interim maintenance, delayed intensification, and maintenance. When choosing a treatment regimen, it is important to define the patient group being treated; adolescents

Table 21.2 Key Difference in Cytogenetic/Molecular Abnormalities Between Pediatric and Adult Patients

Cytogenetics	Gene	Frequency in Children	Frequency in Adults
Hyperdiploidy	–	25%	7%
Hypodiploid	TP53*	0.5%–1%	3%–4%
t(12;21)(p13;q22)	ETV6-RUNX1 (TEL-AML1)	22%	2%
t(1;19)(q23;p13)	TCF3-PBX1 (E2A-PBX1)	6%	3%
t(9;22)(q34;q11): Philadelphia Chromosome	BCR-ABL1	2%–4%	25%
BCR-ABL1–like/ Ph-like	Various	15%	10%–30%
Ikaros	IKZF1	12%–17%	25%–35%
t(v;11q23), t(11;19)	KMT2A	8%	10%

Adapted from NCCN Guidelines Version 1.2020 Acute Lymphoblastic Leukemia.

*TP53 mutations present in approximately 90% of low-hypodiploid ALL patients (*Cold Spring Harb Perspect Med*. 2017;7(3):a026286).

Table 21.3 Prognostic Factors in Adult and Pediatric ALL

Category	Variable	Favorable Factors	Adverse Factors
Patient-related factors	Age	1–10 years	<1 year
			>10 years
			>35 years
	Race	Asian, White	Hispanic, Black
	Sex	Female	Male
Disease-related factors	WBC count	<50,000/mcL (peds)	>50,000/mcL (peds), >30,000/ mcL (adult B-cell), >100,000/mcL (adult T-cell)
	CNS involvement	No	Yes
Genomic/ biologic features	Cytogenetics/ genomic rearrangements	Hyperdiploidy (>50); Trisomy 4, 10, and 17 (with hyperdiploidy); t(12; 21)/*ETV6-RUNX1,*	Hypodiploidy (<44), t(9;22)/*B-CR-ABL1, MLL* rearrangement, t(8,14), t(1,19), Ph-like ALL, TP53 mutations, IKZF1 abnormalities
Response to treatment	Post 1 week steroid prophase (peds)	<1,000 blasts/ mm^2	>1,000 blasts/mm^2
	Marrow blasts post 8- and 15-day induction	<5% blasts	>5% blasts
	Post-induction or post-consolidation MRD*	<0.01% in PB	≥0.01% in PB

and young adults (AYAs), adults, or older adults. Given the improved outcomes seen in pediatric patients, there has been increased interest in incorporating pediatric regimens into AYAs. In comparison to adult regimens, pediatric regimens incorporate more intensive dosing of glucocorticoids, vincristine, asparaginase, and anti-metabolites. Recently, CALGB 10403 reported the outcomes of patients 17 to 39 years of age when treated with a pediatric regimen, reporting a 3-year EFS of 59% and 3-year overall survival (OS) of 73% (*Blood.* 2019;133(14):1548–1559). Although these results compare favorably to historical controls, it is important to note that the tolerance of such regimens is challenging for patients older than 40 to 50 years; in such patients, alternative regimens (i.e., Hyper-CVAD, GRAALL-2005) can be considered. The OS of older adults with ALL has historically been dismal, but most recently the incorporation of anti-CD19 and anti-CD22 agents to multi-agent chemotherapy (mini-hyper-CVD) has led to encouraging outcomes and should be considered for older patients with Philadelphia chromosome–negative B-ALL.

For patients with Philadelphia chromosome–positive B-ALL, a tyrosine kinase inhibitor should be incorporated into their treatment regimen, preferentially second- or third-generation inhibitors with recent data strongly supporting ponatinib in the frontline setting (*Blood*. 2019;134(Suppl1):283; and see Chapter 22). Blinatumomab (see below for details) was recently approved by the food and drug administration (FDA) to treat patients with evidence of residual MRD who had received at least 3 blocks of chemotherapy. In the BLAST study, 1 cycle of blinatumomab led to MRD-negative status in 78% of patients treated, which was associated with an improved survival in comparison to patients who had persistent MRD (*Blood*. 2018;131(14):1522–1531). For a list of the most commonly used chemotherapy regimens, refer to Table 21.4.

REFRACTORY OR RELAPSE DISEASE

Refractory or resistant disease refers to patients who fail to obtain a CR with induction therapy, while relapsed disease refers to the reappearance of leukemia cells in the BM, peripheral blood, or extramedullary site after achieving CR. These two groups comprise more than 50% of adult ALL patients. The treatment goal in these patients is to achieve remission, followed by allogenic hematopoietic stem cell transplantation if they are transplant naïve. The choice of salvage therapy has historically been based on the patient's previous chemotherapy regimen and durability of prior response. More recently, novel immunotherapies, including bi-specific antibodies, antibody-drug conjugates (ADCs), and chimeric antigen receptor T-cells (CAR T-cells), have significantly improved outcomes and have been approved by the FDA. Blinatumomab is a first-in-class bi-specific T-cell engager (BiTE®), targeting CD19, and CD3. The drug engages cytotoxic T-cells through the CD3 receptor and B-cells in various stages of maturation through the CD19 receptor, leading to polyclonal T-cell activation and apoptotic cell death of target cells (B-lymphocytes). In a phase 3 randomized study, Blinatumomab proved to be superior to salvage chemotherapy, with an improvement in OS of 7.7 versus 4.0 months (*N Engl J Med*. 2017;376:836–847). In addition, inotuzumab ozogamicin, an anti-CD22 ADC, has shown considerable activity in relapse/refractory patients, leading to a CR/CRi rate of 80.7% compared to 29.4% in patients treated with salvage chemotherapy. Furthermore, patients treated with inotuzumab also achieved a higher rate of MRD- negative CR (78.4% vs. 28.1%) (*N Engl J Med*. 2016;375:740–753).

Additionally, B-ALL became the first disease to have an FDA-approved cellular therapy option. Initial studies at the Children's Hospital of Philadelphia evaluating an anti-CD19 CAR T-cell revealed significant response in pediatric patients with heavily pre-treated relapsed

Table 21.4 Most Common Induction Regimens for Adult B-ALL

Regimen	Induction	Post-Remission Therapy	CNS Prophylaxis/ Maintenance
CALGB (Cancer and Leukemia Group B) 10403	DR, VC, P, PEG	Consolidation: CP, CY, 6-MP, VC, PEG, IT MTX	Maintenance: VC, Dex, 6-MP, IT MTX, PO MTX (continue for 3 years from initiation of interim maintenance in males and 2 years in females)
	Extended induction (if required): DR, VC, P, PEG-ASP	Interim maintenance: C-MTX, PEG, IT MTX	
		Delayed intensification: VC, Dex, 6-MP, IT MTX, PO MTX	
DFCI ALL	VC, P, Dox, HD-MTX, ASP, IT Cy/MTX/HC (for 4 weeks)	Intensification: VC, Dex, Dox, 6-MP, ASP, C-MTX, IT Cy/MTX/HC (every 3 weeks for 30 weeks)	CNS prophylaxis: VC, 6-MP, Dox, IT MTX, cranial radiotherapy (given for 3 weeks after induction therapy)
			Continuation (every 3 weeks for 74 weeks): Same as intensification but without ASP and dose reduced Dex
Hyper-CVAD	Patients receive 1 cycle of arm A and B	Continue therapy for a total of 3 more cycles of arm A and B (total of 8 blocks of therapy)	CNS prophylaxis: Cy and IT MTX with every cycle of therapy
	-Arm A: VC, mesna, CP, Dox, Dex - Arm B: Cy, MTX every 21 days (+ rituximab for >20% + CD20 blasts)		Maintenance POMP (begins after 8 cycles of dose-intensive therapy): 6-MP, MTX, VC, and P for 30 months
French GRALL 2005	Corticosteroids prephase: P and IT MTX (for 7 days)	9 blocks of 2 weeks each: Block 1, 4, 7: Cy, Dex, ASP. Block 2, 5, 8: VC, IV MTX, ASP, 6-MP. Block 3, 6, 9: IV MTX, CP, VP-16	CNS prophylaxis: IT MTX/Cy/HC during induction, consolidation, and late intensification; cranial irradiation in non-SCT patients

(*continued*)

Table 21.4 Most Common Induction Regimens for Adult B-ALL (continued)

Regimen	Induction	Post-Remission Therapy	CNS Prophylaxis/ Maintenance
	Induction: P, DR, VC, ASP, CP for 28 days	Late intensification (between 6 and 7): P, VC, DR, ASP, CP	Maintenance: P, VC, 6-MP, IV MTX (for 2 years post consolidation)
	*Rituximab added if CD20 (+)		

Abbreviations: 6-MP, 6-mercaptopurine; ASP, asparaginase; CP, cyclophosphamide; Cy, cytarabine; Dex, dexamethasone; Dox, doxorubicin; DR, daunorubicin; MTX, methotrexate; P, prednisone; PEG, pegylated asparaginase; Th, thioguanine; VC, vincristine.

B-ALL. In 2017, the FDA approved Tisagenlecleucel, an anti-CD19 CAR T-cell, for children and adults younger than 26 years of age in second relapse or later. This was based on the ELIANA trial, where the remission rate for patients who received the infusion was 81% with a 1 year OS of 76% (*N Engl J Med.* 2018;378(5):439–448).

Therapeutic advancements in B-ALL continue to evolve, and studies evaluating how to best combine novel therapies and how to incorporate them in the frontline setting are ongoing. Additionally, more novel CAR T-cell studies looking at ways of minimizing toxicities and improving efficacy are ongoing.

▓ POTENTIAL PRACTICE-CHANGING CLINICAL TRIALS

Novel targeted and cellular immunotherapies have been one of the most exciting scientific advances in recent years. The success of these therapies in the relapse setting for patients with B-ALL led to increased interest in evaluating their role in the frontline. The Alliance for Clinical Trials in Oncology is conducting a randomized phase 3 trial evaluating in a randomized fashion whether the addition of inotuzumab ozogamicin to the CALGB 10403 backbone improves outcomes (NCT03150693). Additionally, the combination of inotuzumab and blinatumomab is being evaluated as frontline therapy for patients unfit for intensive induction therapy (NCT03739814). This novel strategy is foregoing cytotoxic chemotherapy with the goal of decreasing toxicities without compromising efficacy in this vulnerable patient population. Another recent breakthrough in B-ALL therapeutics has been CAR T-cells. Given the unprecedented responses seen in pediatric patients with relapsed B-ALL, several groups are investigating the safety and efficacy of CAR T-cells in adult patients. The ZUMA-3, a phase 1/2 clinical trial (NCT02614066), is evaluating the safety and efficacy of KTE-X19, an anti-CD19 CAR T-cell, in adults with relapsed B-cell ALL. The dose-finding phase of the study has been completed, and the phase 2 portion of the study is ongoing. It is important to note that despite the high CR rates achieved with cellular therapies, CD19-negative relapses remain a challenging clinical situation. To tackle this issue, studies targeting other markers on leukemic cells , such as CD22, are ongoing. The group at the University of Pennsylvania is evaluating an anti-CD22 CAR T-cell alone or in combination with an anti-CD19 CART (NCT03620058).

▓ REFERENCES FOR SUPPLEMENTAL READING

1. Gu Z, Churchman M, Mullighan CG, et al. PAX5-driven subtypes of B-progenitor acute lymphoblastic leukemia. *Nat Genet.* 2019;51(2):296–307.

2. Berry D, Zhou S, Higley H, et al. Association of minimal residual disease with clinical outcome in pediatric and adult acute lymphoblastic leukemia: a meta-analysis. *JAMA Oncol.* 2017;3(7):e170580. doi: 10.1001/jamaoncol.2017.0580

3. Hunger SP, Mulligan CG. Acute lymphocytic leukemia in children. *N Engl J Med.* 2015;373:1541–1552.

4. Sermer D, Brentjens R. CAR T-cell therapy: Full speed ahead. *Hematol Oncol.* 2019;37(Suppl1):95–100. doi: 10.1002/hon.2591

5. Basan R, Bourquin JP, DeAngelo D, et al. New approaches to the management of adult acute lymphoblastic leukemia. *J Clin Oncol.* 2018;21:JCO2017773648. doi: 10.1200/JCO.2017.77.3648

22 *BCR-ABL1*+ B-Lymphoblastic Leukemia

Yehuda Deutsch and Bijal Shah

■ INTRODUCTION

Philadelphia chromosome–positive acute lymphoblastic leukemia (Ph+ ALL), a clinically and biologically distinct form of ALL with *BCR-ABL1*, t(9;22)(q34;q11.2), was the first genetic abnormality associated with cancer. It is the result of a balanced translocation of the *ABL1* gene (from chromosome 9) onto the *BCR* gene (on chromosome 22). Although the function of *BCR* is largely unknown, *ABL1* is a multifunctional tyrosine kinase with multiple roles , including cell division, growth, survival, cytoskeletal remodeling, motility, adhesion, autophagy, DNA damage response, and apoptosis. This protein in its normal structure and function is tightly regulated by its SRC homology three domain. However, this domain is not expressed in the *BCR-ABL* fusion oncoprotein and thus acts as a constitutively "on" tyrosine kinase. The Ph chromosome is regarded as the genetic hallmark of chronic myelogenous leukemia (CML). The incidence of Ph+ in B-lymphoblastic leukemia/lymphoma (B-ALL) varies significantly by age, representing the most common genetic rearrangement in adult B-ALL (20%–30% of cases), but only 2% to 4% in childhood B-ALL (*Blood.* 2010;115:206). Historically, Ph+ ALL has been associated with a poor prognosis regardless of age; however, in the era of tyrosine kinase inhibitors (TKIs), the outcomes are similar to Ph-negative B-ALL.

■ DIAGNOSIS

Similar to acute myeloid leukemia, B-ALL commonly presents with an elevation of immature white blood cells (WBCs) compounded by anemia and/or thrombocytopenia. Flow cytometry is routinely performed in this setting to broadly delineate myeloid from B-cell acute lymphoblastic leukemias. Bone marrow (BM) biopsy is recommended to gauge morphology and disease burden and to facilitate cytogenetic, fluorescence in situ hybridization (FISH), and molecular studies. Together these studies help define ALL subtypes, refine prognosis, and guide treatment decision making (for specific diagnostic workup, see Chapter 21). Adult patients who present with B-ALL and significant leukocytosis, particularly with an aberrant myeloid antigen expression of CD13 and/or CD33, should raise suspicion for *BCR-ABL*+ disease. In addition to cytogenetics and FISH studies, quantitative polymerase chain reaction (PCR) for both p210 (M-BCR) and p190 transcripts (m-BCR) of *BCR-ABL1* can also be utilized to

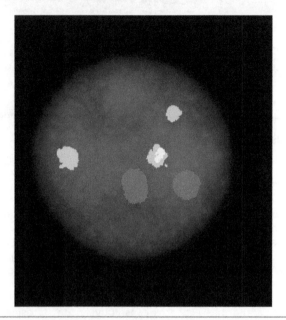

Figure 22.1 Representative positive FISH for *BCR-ABL1* gene rearrangement, t(9;22)(q34;q11.2). *BCR* (22q11.2) is shown in green, and *ABL1* (9q34) is shown in red. FISH shows two green signals and two red signals along with one fusion signal (yellow) that indicates the presence of *BCR-ABL* translocation.

confirm the diagnosis. These tests are also important for assessing the depth of remission on follow-up (see Key Diagnostic Dilemma; Figure 22.1).

▓ KEY DIAGNOSTIC DILEMMA

Making the distinction between *BCR-ABL1*+ B-ALL and CML in lymphoid blast crisis can prove challenging. Chemotherapy given together with TKI-based therapy, followed in turn by allogeneic hematopoietic stem cell transplant (allo-HSCT), has yielded significant and similar survival gains for both subtypes. To this end, the clinical relevance of this distinction may be more relevant in reconciling treatment-associated toxicities and monitoring post-remission. Some features that may warrant concern for CML in lymphoid blast crisis include:

- Age: *BCR-ABL*+ ALL more commonly presents in adults and appears to increase in incidence with each decade of life, where the frequency may be as high as 25% to 50%.
- Blood and BM at diagnosis: Those with CML in lymphoid blast crisis may present with basophilia, eosinophilia, preserved platelet counts, BM changes (myeloid bulge, dwarf megakaryocytes), and/or chromosomal complexity (e.g., trisomy 8 or 19; isochromosome 17).

- CBC data before diagnosis can suggest an antecedent CML, though such patients typically show a median time to transformation of only 25 months. CBC data following treatment may also prove helpful, as those with CML in lymphoid-blast phase tend to show more prolonged duration of neutropenia following high-dose chemotherapy and TKI-based treatment.

- Transcript size: The fusion of *BCR* and *ABL1* can culminate in three alternate transcripts: p190, p210, and p230—each labeled based on size in kD. The p190 transcript is more common to *BCR-ABL1*+ ALL, though it can also be rarely observed in CML (particularly in those prone to progress to blast phase). The p210 transcript is alternatively more common in CML and may accordingly suggest a higher likelihood of pre-existing CML when observed in B-lymphoblasts.

▓ PROGNOSIS

Historically, the presence of the Ph chromosome conferred a poor prognosis. Before the advent of TKI therapy, conventional chemotherapy trials reported no survivors at 5 years in adults with the rearrangement. Previous prospective studies have shown that with more dose-intensive regimens (without TKI), patients achieve similar Complete Remission (CR) rates as those with Ph-chromosome–negative B-ALL; nonetheless, they have on average shorter duration of remission, higher incidence of relapse, and shorter survival. However, with the use of TKIs, the prognosis is now similar to those with Ph-negative B-ALL. Higher-risk subtypes of Ph+ B-ALL include those with secondary mutations in the *ABL1* gene that affect TKI affinity as well as mutations or deletions involving chromosome 9p (*CDKN2A/B* and *PAX5*) and/or *IKZF1* on chromosome 7 (*N Engl J Med.* 2009;360(5):470–480).

▓ TREATMENT

The advent of TKIs to impair *BCR-ABL* signaling has changed the natural history of Ph+ ALL. The addition of Imatinib to the Ph+ arm of the UKALLXII/ECOG2993 study as well as other regimens, such as hyper-CVAD, has remarkably improved response and survival (*Blood.* 2014;123:843–850). Likewise, the benefit of second- and third-generation TKIs have been demonstrated. The choice of TKI remains controversial, as no randomized comparative trials exist to guide decision making. However, given the activity and potency of dasatinib (relative to imatinib) and central nervous system (CNS) penetrance, many favor its use (*Blood.* 2011;118:6521–6528). Ponatinib, a potent third-generation TKI with activity against the *T315I* mutation, is also favored (*Blood.* 2019;134(Suppl1):283). The role of chemotherapy intensity is similarly controversial (see Chapter 21). More recent clinical trials suggest that those unfit for high-dose therapy may still benefit from TKI given together with steroids with or without vincristine alone or with immunotherapy.

It is still standard practice to human leukocyte antigen (HLA) type the patient to begin the search for related and unrelated donors and proceed with Allo-HSCT for post-remission therapy, as many patients fail to achieve durable remission with TKI and chemotherapy alone. For those able to proceed to transplant, long-term remission and overall survival (OS) are approximately 60%. However, some patients, particularly those who achieve early molecular remission, may have long-term remission without undergoing allo-HSCT in first remission with ponatinib-based therapy (*Blood*. 2019;134(Suppl1):283). Emerging data suggest that there may be additional benefit for TKI maintenance following allogenic transplant, particularly for those with residual molecular disease before transplant.

Outcomes following relapse are poor and frequently occur on a background of secondary *BCR-ABL* mutations. In particular, the *T315I* mutation is commonly observed. Ponatinib is the only Food and Drug Administration–approved (FDA-approved) TKI that is functional in this context, although median remission durations with this agent are only around 6 months. Deep sequencing at diagnosis suggests that a clone of B-ALL with *T315I* may exist at diagnosis, expanding and culminating in relapse among those treated with alternative TKIs.

▨ POTENTIAL PRACTICE-CHANGING CLINICAL TRIALS

Studies combining second- or third-generation TKIs with intensive chemotherapy or immunotherapy are potentially practice changing. Hyper-cyclophosphamide, vincristine, adriamycin, and dexamethasone (Hyper-CVAD) and ponatinib demonstrated high response rates (CR 100%, CMR 84%) and impressive long-term survival (5-year OS 73%), even in patients who were not transplanted in first remission (*Blood*. 2019;134(Suppl1):283). Akin to conventional B-ALL, other combinations with novel therapies are being actively explored in this subgroup. Ponatinib is being studied in combination with low-intensity chemotherapy and Blinatumomab (NCT03147612) as well as chemotherapy-free regimens of TKI plus Blinatumomab (NCT04329325). In addition, chimeric antigen receptor (CAR) T-cell therapy is being evaluated in this patient population and holds significant promise.

BCR-ABL1–like disease has a very similar gene expression profile as *BCR-ABL1*+ disease (*N Engl J Med*. 2014;371(11):1005–1015). Of therapeutic importance, activating mutations in a limited number of pathways were found in 91% of patients, and in vitro data support targeted inhibition of these pathways. Specifically, gene fusions involved the *ABL1* pathway and rearrangements/mutations leading to *JAK/STAT* activation are the most common genetic events in this patient population and predict sensitivity to *ABL1* inhibitors (e.g., dasatinib) as well as *JAK* inhibitors (e.g., ruxolitinib), respectively. *ETV6–NTRK3* fusion is a rare event but predicts sensitivity to crizotinib. A phase 2 trial evaluating the combination of dasatinib or ruxolitinib with Hyper-CVAD in *BCR-ABL1*–like disease is ongoing (NCT02420717).

■ REFERENCES FOR SUPPLEMENTAL READING

1. Fielding AK, Rowe JM, Buck G, et al. UKALLXII/ECOG2993: addition of imatinib to a standard treatment regimen enhances long-term outcomes in Philadelphia positive acute lymphoblastic leukemia. *Blood.* 2014; 123(6):843–850.

2. Short NJ, Kantarjian HM, Ravandi F, et al. Long-term safety and efficacy of Hyper-CVAD plus ponatinib as frontline therapy for adults with Philadelphia chromosome-positive acute lymphoblastic leukemia. *Blood.* 2019;134(Suppl1):283.

3. Chalandon Y, Thomas X, Hayette S, et al. Randomized study of reduced-intensity chemotherapy combined with imatinib in adults with Ph-positive acute lymphoblastic leukemia. *Blood.* 2015;125:3711.

4. Fielding AK. Treatment of Philadelphia chromosome–positive acute lymphoblastic leukemia in adults: a broader range of options, improved outcomes, and more therapeutic dilemmas. *Am Soc Clin Oncol Educ Book.* 2015;35:e352–e359.

5. Strati P, Kantarjian H, Thomas D, et al. HCVAD plus imatinib or dasatinib in lymphoid blastic phase chronic myeloid leukemia. *Cancer.* 2014;120(3):373–380.

23 T-Cell Acute Lymphoblastic Leukemia/Lymphoma

Muhammad Sardar, Ravitharan Krishnadasan, and

Keri Maher

■ INTRODUCTION

T-cell acute lymphoblastic leukemia (T-ALL) is an aggressive malignancy responsible for 20% to 25% of adult ALL cases and is more common in males than females. With multiagent induction chemotherapy, more than 90% of patients achieve a complete remission, with a 50% 5-year overall survival (OS) rate. This is similar to, albeit perhaps better than, rates for B-ALL (see Chapter 21).[1] Importantly, T-ALL frequently has extramedullary involvement, including the central nervous system (CNS) and mediastinum, and often presents with marked leukocytosis (white blood cell [WBC] >100,000 cells/mcL).[2] The term "T-Cell lymphoblastic lymphoma" (T-LBL) is used when disease is limited to a extramedullary lesion with absent or minimal bone marrow (BM) or peripheral blood involvement. Conversely, the term "leukemia" refers to significant BM and/or peripheral blood involvement. However, these entities are pathophysiologically similar and, thus, share similar treatment paradigms, despite variation in clinical presentation. Even though no definitive blast percentage threshold exists for defining T-ALL, the terminology of T-ALL should not be used if blasts are <20%.

■ DIAGNOSIS

Diagnosis is typically achieved through a combination of clinical, radiologic findings, and tissue or BM biopsy with aspiration with appropriate ancillary studies (e.g., flow cytometry with adequate antibody marker panel, immunohistochemical studies). When possible, a next-generation sequencing panel covering prognostically significant genes should be performed. Thorough examination of disease phenotype through molecular and flow cytometric methods at diagnosis will aid in minimal residual disease detection throughout treatment course. Due to T-ALL's propensity to manifest in extramedullary locations, chest and brain imaging, testicular exam, and lumbar puncture should all be considered. Because T-ALL/T-LBL commonly involves the anterior mediastinum, other neoplasms that commonly involve this location should be excluded, such as thymoma, teratoma (or other germ-cell tumor), metastatic thyroid carcinoma, or nodular sclerosis classical Hodgkin lymphoma. Echocardiogram should be performed, as anthracyclines are used as part of therapy to ensure adequate cardiac reserve.

T-ALL is typically TdT, CD7, and cytoplasmic CD3 positive and can further be classified into pro-T, pre-T, cortical-T, and medullary-T leukemia/lymphoma. These subtypes are discernable by flow cytometry on the basis of different expression of other T-cell markers, including CD1a, CD34, CD4, and CD8.[2]

Early T-cell precursors (ETPs) were recognized as a new provisional entity in the 2016 update of the World Health Organization (WHO) classification. It has a distinct immunophenotypic and gene-signature profile, expressing CD7 and at least one myeloid or stem cell marker and the absence of CD1a or CD4/CD8. ETP is generally associated with a higher rate of induction failure and relapse compared to other T-ALL subtypes, although to date, there is no difference in upfront therapeutic regimen. Table 23.1 summarizes different categories of T-ALL based on immunophenotype.

▓ KEY DIAGNOSTIC DILEMMA

T-ALL must be differentiated from B-ALL and mixed-phenotype acute leukemia (MPAL), which can be achieved through flow cytometry and immunophenotyping using a panel of markers while excluding those of B and myeloid lineages that may lead to the diagnosis of MPAL (see Chapter 24). Of particular caution, ETP-ALL often co-expresses myeloid lineage markers and the stem cell marker CD34, which could lead to diagnostic ambiguitiy with MPAL (Table 23.1).

▓ PROGNOSIS

A number of clinical, cytogenetic, immunophenotypic, and molecular variables have been associated with prognosis; however, uncertainty remains about the prognostic role of many of the molecular markers (Table 23.2). *NOTCH* pathway mutations are present in approximately 60% of adult T-ALL patients (including mutations in *NOTCH1* and *FBXW7*) and are associated with improved OS.[3] *TP53*, *K-RAS*, and *PTEN* mutations are considered high risk. Although not statistically significant, a trend toward other poor prognostic features (higher WBC count, older age, CNS involvement) was seen more often in *NOTCH* wild-type cases.[3] The presence of minimal/measurable residual disease (MRD) after induction has a poor prognosis and is a strong indication to proceed with allogeneic hematopoietic stem cell transplant in eligible individuals. Likewise, relapsed T-ALL has a very poor prognosis, with a 5-year OS of 5%.[1] Assessment of MRD is of paramount importance, as it has significant impact on prognosis and will help guide the intensity of therapy (*Blood*. 2015;126(8):964–971; *Blood*. 2015;125(26):3996–4009).

▓ TREATMENT

FRONTLINE TREATMENT

Most of the available data to guide treatment combine B- and T-ALL; thus, the regimens are highly similar for these groups, especially in the frontline setting, with the exception of AALL0434, which was

Table 23.1 Immunophenotypic Differentiation of T-ALL Subtypes[2] and Their Respective Prognoses

	TdT	sCD3	cCD3	CD5	CD7	CD34	CD99	CD1a	CD4 or CD8	Prognostic Association
ETP-ALL*	+	–	+	Dim or –	+	±	±	–	Dual –	Adverse
Thymic (cortical T)	+	–	+	+	+	–	±	+	Dual +	Favorable
Mature (medullary T)	+	+	+	+	+	–	±	–	CD4+ or CD8+	Adverse

c, cytoplasmic; ETP, early T-cell precursor; s, surface; T-ALL, T-cell acute lymphoblastic leukemia.

*ETP-ALL must also express one or more myeloid or stem-cell markers (CD117, CD34, HLA-DR, CD13, CD33, CD11b, or CD65) (*Lancet Oncol.* 2009;10:147–156).

Table 23.2 Widely Accepted Prognostic Features in T-ALL and Their Associated OS

Prognostic Feature	Outcome	Effect on Survival
WBC >100 × 10⁹/L	Adverse	41% 5-year OS[1]
Age >35	Adverse	38% 5-year OS[1]
Complex karyotype (five or more abnormalities)	Adverse	10% 5-year OS[1]
CD1a + (cortical T immunophenotype)	Favorable	64% 5-year OS[1]
NOTCH1/FBXW7 mutations	Favorable	74% 3-year OS[3]

T-ALL, T-cell acute lymphoblastic leukemia; WBC, white blood cell.

designed for newly diagnosed T-ALL and T-LBL patients.[4] This regimen combines nelarabine into a multi-agent augmented-Berlin-Frankfurt-Munster (BFM) backbone and demonstrated an improvement in disease-free survival and OS, thus providing a new standard of care for this group. Pediatric and adolescent/young adult patients should receive a pediatric-inspired regimen. Common induction regimens in the fit adult population include the following (also see Chapter 21):

- CALGB 8811 (Larson regimen): *Blood.* 1995;85(8):2025–2037.
- Linker: *Blood.* 1991;78(11):2814–2822.
- Hyper-CVAD: *Cancer.* 2004;101(12):2788–2801.

As in B-ALL, prolonged treatment courses, including induction, consolidation, maintenance, and CNS prophylaxis/treatment, are necessary. Dosing and scheduling of chemotherapies for phases of chemotherapy and CNS prophylaxis vary by treatment protocol. All patients should receive CNS prophylaxis to minimize a high rate of CNS relapse. The role of allogeneic hematopoietic stem cell transplant (allo-HSCT) in first remission in T-ALL is currently being defined but can be considered for those with MRD and/or adverse genetics as well as for adults with T-ALL.[2] Allo-HSCT should be considered after relapse for those who attain a second complete remission (CR2).

RELAPSED/REFRACTORY PATIENTS

Relapsed T-ALL/LBL is associated with a poor prognosis. Clinical trials are encouraged when available. In addition to regimens using drugs similar to those listed earlier, single-agent chemotherapies have also been used. After salvage chemotherapy, clinical outcomes can be improved by alloHSCT in eligible patients:

- Clofarabine-based regimens—32% CR (combined B- and T-cell ALL data; *Am J Hematol.* 2012;87(6):631–634)
- Nelarabine—CR rate 31%, 1-year OS 28% (T-cell ALL only, relapsed/refractory setting after two lines of prior chemotherapy)[5]

- Liposomal Vincristine—20% CR (based on small phase 2 trial with 10 patients; currently Food and Drug Administration [FDA] approved for T-cell ALL in 2nd or greater relapse)

■ POTENTIAL PRACTICE-CHANGING CLINICAL TRIALS

Unfortunately, treatment of T-cell ALL/LBL has not experienced the same advancement as has B-ALL. Developing targeted and immune mediated therapy in T-cell ALL is difficult, as prolonged T-cell aplasia has an even greater risk of fatal opportunistic infection than does prolonged B-cell aplasia. Moreover, development of Chimeric-Antigen-Receptor T Cells (CAR-Ts), which have changed the landscape of B-ALL therapy, have been technically difficult due to CAR-T cell fratricide and disease contamination of therapeutic CAR-T manufacturing. Targeting of the *NOTCH* pathway, including gamma-secretase inhibition, has been studied, but there are currently no approved therapies in this domain. Table 23.3 summarizes key immune-based and targeted therapies currently being evaluated. Moreover, nelarabine is being incorporated into more up-front regimens as well (NCT00501826). There are also clinical trials incorporating bortezomib into BFM-type regimens (NCT02112916).

Table 23.3 Novel Therapeutic Options for T-ALL

IMMUNOTHERAPY		
CAR-T cells	There are two separate trials targeting:	
	• CD-7	NCT03690011
	• CD-5	NCT03081910
Monoclonal antibodies	Daratumumab (targeting CD-38) with chemotherapy	NCT03384654
Chemokine receptors	BL-8040 (short peptide antagonist of CXCR4) with nelarabine	NCT02763384
TARGETED AGENTS		
BCL2 inhibitor	Venetoclax in combination with:	
	• Navitoclax + chemotherapy	NCT03181126
	• Liposomal vincristine	NCT03504644
CDK inhibitors	Palbociclib in combination with sorafenib, decitabine, or dexamethasone	NCT03132454
JAK inhibitors	Ruxolitinib in combination with vincristine and prednisone	NCT03613428
MEK inhibitors	Selumetinib in combination with dexamethasone	NCT03705507

▥ REFERENCES FOR SUPPLEMENTAL READING

1. Marks D, Paietta E. T-cell acute lymphoblastic leukemia in adults: clinical features, immunophenotype, cytogenetics, and outcome from the large randomized prospective trial (UKALL XII/ECOG 2993). *Blood*. 2009;114(24):5136–5145.

2. LitzowM, Ferrando A. How I treat T cell acute lymphoblastic leukemia in adults. *Blood*. 2015;126(7):833–841.

3. Asnafi V, BuzynA, Le Noir S. NOTCH1/FBXW7 mutation identifies a large subgroup with favorable outcome in adult T-cell acute lymphoblastic leukemia (T-ALL): a group for research on adult acute lymphoblastic leukemia (GRALL) study. *Blood*. 2009;113(17):3918–3924.

4. Dunsmore K, Winter S, Devidas M. COG AALL0434: a randomized trial testing nelarabine in newly diagnosed T-cell malignancy. *JClin Oncol*. 2018;36(Suppl15):10500.

5. DeAngelo D. Nelarabine for the treatment of patients with relapsedor refractoryT-cell acute lymphoblastic leukemia of lymphoblastic lymphoma. *Hematol Oncol Clin North Am*. 2009;23:1121–1135.

24 Acute Leukemia of Ambiguous Lineage

Muhammad Sardar, Ravitharan Krishnadasan, and

Keri Maher

▓ INTRODUCTION

Acute leukemia of ambiguous lineage includes mixed-phenotype acute leukemia (MPAL) and acute undifferentiated leukemia (AUL). MPAL has markers from different linages—for example, both myeloid and lymphoid lineages (further described below)—whereas undifferentiated leukemia does not have lineage-defining markers.[1] Both of these entities are rare malignancies and together are estimated to comprise 3% to 5% of all acute leukemia cases in both pediatric and adult populations.[2,3] Because of their rarity, relatively little is known about these types of leukemia, including optimal treatment strategies.

▓ DIAGNOSIS

The World Health Organization (WHO) revised the diagnostic categorization of Acute Leukemias of Ambiguous Lineage in 2016 to include AUL and MPAL with t(9;22)(q34.1;q11.2); *BCR-ABL1 and* MPAL with t(v;11q23.2); KMT2A rearranged; MPAL B/Myeloid Not Otherwise Specified (NOS); and MPAL T/myeloid NOS (Arber et al., *Blood*, (2016) 127(20):2391–2405).

Important cell lineage–specific markers to aid in classification are as follows:

- Markers in MPAL (coexpression of markers from different lineages):
    - i. Myeloid lineage: Myeloperoxidase (MPO) + or monocytic differentiation (nonspecific esterase, CD11c, CD14, CD64, lysozyme)
    - ii. T lineage: Cytoplasmic CD3 (epsilon chain) or surface CD3
    - iii. B lineage: CD19 with CD79a, cytoplasmic CD22, CD10 (note: if CD19 is strongly expressed, only one other B-cell marker is needed; if CD19 is weakly expressed, two of the other B-cell markers are necessary)
- Markers in AUL:
    - i. No cell lineage–specific markers; often express CD34, HLA-DR, CD38, TdT

Similar to other acute leukemias, 20% or greater blasts in the bone marrow (BM) or peripheral blood are needed for diagnosis. Extensive immunophenotypic, cytogenetic, and molecular studies should be performed to exclude other types of leukemia.

▨ KEY DIAGNOSTIC DILEMMA

MPAL and AUL must be differentiated from acute myeloid leukemia (AML), B- or T-cell acute lymphoblastic leukemia (ALL), chronic myelogenous leukemia (CML) in blast phase, and rarer entities, such as blastic plasmacytoid dendritic cell neoplasms (see Chapters 17, 21, 23, 8, and 20). It is important to note that leukemia due to specific, recurrent genetic alterations aside from *BCR-ABL1* or *MLL* rearrangements are excluded from MPAL.[1] For example, acute leukemia with t(8;21), t(15;17), and inv(16) (p13.1;q22) is classified as AML, even if the immunophenotype is consistent with MPAL.[3] Similarly, therapy-related leukemia and CML in blast phase are excluded, even when an MPAL immunophenotype is present.[4]

▨ PROGNOSIS

Acute leukemia of ambiguous lineage is believed to have a worse prognosis than either AML or ALL, perhaps due to increased frequency of poor-prognostic cytogenetics and more frequent extramedullary presentations.[3] Prognosis varies based on age (children more than adults), therapy type (ALL-based regimens more than AML-based regimens), and genetics (e.g., *BCR-ABL1* positivity is a poor prognostic feature).[2,3] In a retrospective review of pediatric patients with MPAL, 5-year survival was estimated at 67%.[2] Patients with measurable residual disease (MRD) at >10^{-3} following induction had a marked reduction in their 5-year event-free survival (51% vs. 90%, p = .0002).[2] This is far superior to adult data, with 37% 5-year survival.[4] Prognostic studies of AUL patients are lacking, although a case series of AUL patients (n = 13) showed a 3-year survival rate of 44%.[5] Allogeneic hematopoietic stem cell transplant may improve prognosis over chemotherapy alone, but prospective data on patient selection are lacking.

▨ TREATMENT

Because of the rare nature of acute leukemia of ambiguous lineage, no prospective studies have been completed to guide therapy. Retrospective series have revealed that those treated with ALL regimens tend to have a higher complete remission (CR) and perhaps better overall survival (OS) than those treated with AML regimens.[2,3] This may even hold true for patients with more myeloid features (such as high MPO expression).

FRONTLINE TREATMENT: MPAL

Typically, patients are treated with ALL-based regimens according to their age and functional status (see Chapter 21). Pediatric-inspired regimens have proven to be feasible alternatives for adults with ALL up to the age of 40. These more intensive regimens are now being explored in MPAL as well. When there is hope that this intensification will yield improved outcomes. In those cases where *BCR-ABL1* translocation is present, a tyrosine kinase inhibitor (TKI), such as dasatinib, is a necessary part of therapy. Consolidative allogeneic stem cell transplant is considered for functionally fit patients. Elderly patients harboring the Ph chromosome or patients not able to undergo traditional chemotherapy may benefit from a TKI with steroids to improve disease control. Similar to ALL, MPAL can manifest in the central nervous system (CNS), and thus prophylaxis should be completed according to the ALL-based protocol chosen for the patient (Wolach et al., *Blood*, (2015) 125(15):244–2485).

FRONTLINE TREATMENT: AUL
There is currently no standard treatment regimen for those diagnosed with AUL. Small retrospective reviews suggest better outcomes with ALL-based regimens.[5] AUL lacks targetable mutations (in contrast to MPAL with *BCR-ABL1*, as discussed earlier).[5]

RELAPSED/REFRACTORY PATIENTS
Clinical trials should be considered in relapsed or refractory patients. For MPAL patients, there has been some suggestion that those treated with an ALL-based regimen upfront might be salvaged with an AML-based regimen, and vice versa. If remission is achieved, these patients should proceed to allogeneic stem cell transplant.

▨ POTENTIAL PRACTICE-CHANGING CLINICAL TRIALS
Few clinical trials specifically for acute leukemia of ambiguous lineage exist. Currently, a multi-agent regimen including clofarabine, cytarabine, vincristine, and dexamethasone is underway in the upfront or relapsed setting specifically for MPAL (NCT02135874). Other trials include the MPAL diagnosis in B-ALL trials and may include immunotherapy agents, such as inotuzumab ozogamicin (NCT03959085), blinatumomab (NCT02879695), and CAR-T therapy (NCT02529813) when the target is present. Other trials include the BCL-2 inhibitor venetoclax with combination chemotherapy in patients with AML or acute leukemia of ambiguous lineage (NCT03194932). There is an early-phase study of SNDX-5631, a small molecule inhibitor of the Menin-*MLL* binding interaction for acute leukemias, including MPAL patients harboring the *MLL/KMT2A* gene rearrangement (NCT04065399).

▨ REFERENCES FOR SUPPLEMENTAL READING

1. Vardiman J, Thiele J, Arber D, et al. The 2008 revision of the World Health Organization (WHO) classification of myeloid neoplasms and acute leukemia: rationale and important changes. *Blood*. 2009;114(5):937–951.

2. Hrusak O, Haas V, Luks A, et al. Acute leukemia of ambiguous lineage: a comprehensive survival analysis enables designing new treatment strategies. *Blood*. 2016;128(22):584.

3. Van den Anker W, Terwijn M, Westers T, et al. Acute leukemias of ambiguous lineage: diagnostic consequences of the WHO 2008 classification. *Leukemia*. 2010;24:1392–1396.

4. Matutes E, Pickl W, Veer M, et al. Mixed-phenotype acute leukemia: clinical and laboratory features and outcome in 100 patients defined according to the WHO 2008 classification. *Blood*. 2011;117(11):3163–3171.

5. Heesch S, Neumann M, Schwartz S, et al. Acute leukemias of ambiguous lineage in adults: molecular and clinical characterization. *Ann Hematol*. 2013;92(6):747–758.

25 T-Cell Prolymphocytic Leukemia

Pei Zhang and Abhijeet Kumar

▦ INTRODUCTION

T-cell prolymphocytic leukemia (T-PLL) is a rare, mature T-cell leukemia that accounts for approximately 2% of all T-cell leukemias. T-PLL mainly affects the elderly, with a mean age at presentation of 65 years. It is rarely diagnosed in those under the age of 30 years. Patients with ataxia telangiectasia have a greatly increased incidence of T-PLL, with a much earlier median age of presentation. Patients typically present with widely disseminated disease at diagnosis manifesting as significant leukocytosis, hepatosplenomegaly, lymphadenopathy, skin lesions, and serous effusions. Despite advances in therapeutic approaches, the response and prognosis of these patients remain poor, with a median survival of less than 1 year.

▦ DIAGNOSIS

Morphology and immunophenotyping are the primary means of diagnosing T-PLL:

- Peripheral blood smear (PBS): A PBS is a key test to diagnose T-PLL, which reveals a population of prolymphocytes (Figure 25.1). The typical cytology of prolymphocytes consists of medium-size cells with condensed nuclear chromatin, a single prominent nucleolus, and intensely basophilic nongranular cytoplasm with cytoplasmic protrusions or "blebs." The nuclei can be round to oval in 50% of cases. A "cerebriform" variant can be seen in about 5% of cases (Sézary cell–like).

- Bone marrow (BM): Infiltration of the marrow with prolymphocytes creates a mixed pattern (diffuse and interstitial). Reticulin fibrosis is almost always present.

- Other tissues: Spleen histology shows infiltration of the red pulp, with involvement of blood vessels, capsule, and white pulp. Infiltration of the lymph nodes is diffuse (predominantly para cortical). The skin involvement reveals dermal infiltration with prolymphocytes but lacks epidermotropism.

- Immunophenotype: T-PLL cells express CD2, CD3, CD7, and CD52. CD7 expression is strong in contrast to other mature T-cell neoplasms. CD52 expression is strong as well, which renders the disease susceptible to alemtuzumab (see the following). Terminal

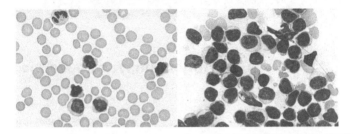

Figure 25.1 Atypical lymphocytosis in T-PLL. PBS shows atypical lymphoid cells that display condensed chromatin, prominent nucleoli, and a certain amount of amphophilic cytoplasm, compatible with prolymphocytes (left, ×1,000 total magnification). A touch imprint of bone marrow core biopsy reveals sheets of atypical lymphocytes with morphologic features similar to those in peripheral blood (right, ×1,000).

deoxynucleotidyl transferase (Tdt) is not expressed. CD3 may be expressed on the cell membrane at low or high levels. Expression of CD4 and CD8 is variable: 60% of cases are CD4+/CD8−, 25% of cases are CD4+/CD8+, and 15% of cases are CD4−/CD8+. T-PLL cells overexpress TCL1, as demonstrated by immunohistochemistry.

GENETICS

The most common characteristic chromosome abnormality is inversion of chromosome 14 (inv 14(q11;q32)) followed by t(14;14)(q11;q32) occurring in 80% and 10% of cases, respectively. Both rearrangements juxtapose the *TCL1* locus with oncogenes *TCL1A* and *TCL1B* at chromosome 14q32.1, resulting in activation and expression of the proto-oncogene *TCL1*. *TCL1* can also be detected by flow cytometry. Other genetic abnormalities include t(X;14)(q28;q11), trisomy 8/iso8q, 12p13, and 11q23, with the latter being the locus for the ataxia telangiectasia mutated gene. Abnormalities of chromosomes 6 and 17, including deletion of the *TP53* gene, have also been observed.

KEY DIFFERENTIAL DIAGNOSES

B-cell prolymphocytic leukemia (B-PLL) has a similar clinical presentation and cytologic appearance to T-PLL. However, skin infiltration and lymphadenopathy, which are unusual in B-PLL, are much more common in T-PLL. In addition, these two entities differ in their immunophenotype. Both T-PLL and mycosis fungoides (MF)/Sézary syndrome are T-cell neoplasms that can involve the blood and skin. The morphology of the cerebriform variant resembles the Sézary cells seen in MF (see Chapter 49). Leukemic manifestation of peripheral T-cell lymphoma and the CD4+ variant of large granular lymphocytic leukemia should also be included in the differential diagnosis.

▓ TREATMENT

A minority of patients (10%–15%) who present with stable or slowly progressive lymphocytosis without symptoms can be monitored closely without therapeutic interventions. It is generally prudent to follow these patients much more closely than patients with chronic lymphocytic leukemia. However, the majority of patients present with aggressive disease requiring treatment. Alemtuzumab, a humanized monoclonal IgG1 antibody, has significantly improved outcomes in T-PLL patients. Serious infusion reactions can occur and thus the initial dose is 3 mg followed by titration to the standard dose of 30 mg, three times weekly. Patients require *Pneumocystis jiroveci* and herpes virus prophylaxis along with weekly cytomegalovirus (CMV) monitoring. Referral for BM transplantation should be made up front for all patients who are candidates.

FRONTLINE TREATMENT

Alemtuzumab + consolidation with a hematopoietic stem cell transplant (*J Clin Oncol.* 1997;15(7):2667–2672):

- IV administration of alemtuzumab is preferable in T-PLL versus subcutaneous (SC) route. IV patients experience a 91% overall response rate (ORR) (29/32; 81% complete response [CR]) versus 33% (3/9) with SC route (*Blood.* 2011;118(22):5799–5802).
- Allogenic stem cell transplant offers a chance of cure and should be considered in the first remission whenever possible. Autologous stem cell transplant provides a longer duration of remission and lower toxicity profile but does not cure the disease (*Br J Haematol.* 2010;149(6):907–910).
- Allografted patients do still have a risk of relapse, and when relapsed, they have a very poor prognosis, with no established treatment available. However, tapering of immunosuppressive therapy or donor lymphocyte infusion after re-induction therapy can result in remission.

ALTERNATIVE FRONTLINE TREATMENTS

- Pentostatin (*J Clin Oncol.* 1994;12(12):2588–2593): Although there have been no head-to-head comparisons, pentostatin monotherapy appears to have a lower response rate than alemtuzumab monotherapy.
- Alemtuzumab + pentostatin (*J Clin Oncol.* 2009;27(32):5425–5430).
- Fludarabine, mitoxantrone, and cyclophosphamide (FMC) × four cycles, followed by consolidation with IV alemtuzumab 3×/week × 12 weeks in responding patients (*Cancer.* 2013;15;119(12):2258–2267).

  - FMC-A had an ORR of 92% (12 CR, 11 partial remission [PR]) with median progression-free survival (PFS) and OS of 17 and 12 months, respectively. Higher *TCL1* protein expression was associated with inferior PFS.

RELAPSED REFRACTORY T-PLL

- For those patients who received induction therapy with alemtuzumab, with response duration of at least 6 months, re-treatment can be successful in achieving a second remission.
- Nelarabine, with or without fludarabine (*J Clin Oncol.* 2008; 26(7):1098–1110).
- Bendamustine, ORR of 53% (*Br J Haematol.* 2015;168(6):916–919).
- Ibrutinib and venetoclax (*Blood.* 2019;134(Suppl1):3965): Two patients with relapsed/refractory T-PLL who failed at least two prior lines of therapy (including alemtuzumab) were treated with this combination and experienced significant improvement in their leukocytosis, lactate dehydrogenase (LDH), and clinical symptoms.

▧ POTENTIAL PRACTICE-CHANGING CLINICAL TRIALS

There is a paucity of randomized clinical trials in T-PLL due to the rarity of the disease. There are clinical trials looking at maintenance romidepsin, an histone deacetylase (HDAC) inhibitor, after stem cell transplant (NCT02512497). Trials are also looking at alemtuzumab in combination or in sequence with purine analogs, JAK inhibitors, and other agents. The use of chimeric antigen receptor NK cells targeting CD7 has also recently emerged as an area of exploration.

▧ REFERENCES FOR SUPPLEMENTAL READING

1. Damlaj M, Sulai NH, Oliveira JL, et al. Impact of alemtuzumab therapy and route of administration in T-prolymphocytic leukemia: A single-center experience. *Clin Lymphoma Myeloma Leuk.* 2015;15(11):699–704.

2. Dearden C. How I treat prolymphocytic leukemia. *Blood.* 2012;120(3):538–551.

3. Herbaux C, Genet P, Bouabdallah, K, et al. Bendamustine is effective in T-cell prolymphocytic leukaemia. *Br J Haematol.* 2015;168(6):916–919.

4. Hopfinger G, Busch R, Pflug N, et al. Sequential chemoimmunotherapy of fludarabine, mitoxantrone, and cyclophosphamide induction followed by alemtuzumab consolidation is effective in T-cell prolymphocytic leukemia. *Cancer.* 2013;119(12):2258–2267.

5. Kornauth C, Herbaux C, Boidol B, et al. Combination of venetoclax and ibrutinib increases bcl2-dependent apoptotic priming, reduces ITK-phosphorylation and is clinically promising in relapsed/refractory T-prolymphocytic leukemia. *Blood.* 2019;134(Suppl1):3965.

26 T-Cell Large Granular Lymphocytic Leukemia

Ning Dong, Magali Van den Bergh,
and Lubomir Sokol

▓ INTRODUCTION

T-cell large granular lymphocytic leukemia (T-LGLL) is a rare malignancy arising from aberrant proliferation of mature post-thymic large granular lymphocytes in the peripheral blood (PB), bone marrow (BM), and spleen. Its incidence is estimated at 0.2 cases per 1 million individuals per year in the United States and affects males and females equally. The median age of diagnosis is in the 60s, and 25% of patients present before age 50. Chronic antigenic stimulation with putative autoantigens or unknown viruses is hypothesized to contribute to its pathogenesis. A constitutive activation of signal transducer and activator of transcription (STAT) pathways plays a pivotal role in the pathobiology of LGLL. Somatic-activating mutation of *STAT3* was identified in 28% to 75% of patients, and *STAT5b* mutation was reported in about 2% of cases. Patients often present with lymphocytosis, neutropenia, anemia, or splenomegaly. LGLL is associated with autoimmune conditions, most notably rheumatoid arthritis (11%–32%), Sjögren syndrome, systemic lupus erythematosus, and others. Hematologic disorders, such as myelodysplastic syndrome, aplastic anemia, paroxysmal nocturnal hemoglobinuria, pure red cell aplasia (PRCA), and B-cell malignancies, have been reported in T-LGLL patients.

▓ DIAGNOSIS

Diagnosis of T-LGLL is made with findings of increased clonal T-lymphocytes in PB for more than 6 months. The presence of at least 2.0×10^9/L (normal <0.3 10^9/L) LGL cells is no longer required for diagnosis, and LGL $>0.4 \times 10^9$/L in blood with matching clinical features is consistent with diagnosis.

Workup starts with a complete blood count (CBC) with differential, complete metabolic panel (CMP), and review of PB smear. PB smear shows large lymphocytes with abundant cytoplasm containing azurophilic granules (Figure 26.1A). However, LGLL cells are undifferentiable from reactive LGL cells morphologically.

PB flow cytometry demonstrates a typical cytotoxic T-cell immunophenotype with co-expression of surface CD3, CD8, CD57, TIA1, granzyme B, granzyme M, and CD16. CD56 and CD28 antigens are usually absent. Characteristic for T-LGLL is dim or aberrant expression of

CD5 and/or CD7 (Figure 26.1). The majority of T-LGLL patients are CD8+ and alpha/beta TCR-positive. A small percentage of patients are CD4+ or gamma/delta TCR-positive.

PCR for TCRβ and/or TCRγ gene arrangement to confirm a clonal origin of malignant cells is an essential test for diagnosis.

BM biopsy is not mandatory for diagnosis of LGLL but can help confirm diagnosis in patients with low T-LGLL counts in PB (<0.5 × 10⁹/L) and in patients suspicious for concomitant BM failure syndromes. BM demonstrates an interstitial and intrasinusoidal T-LGLL

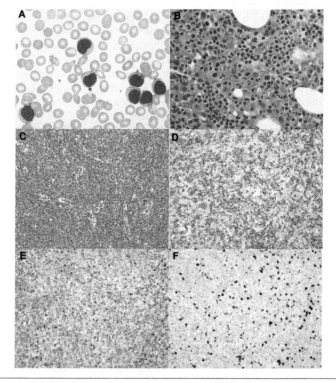

Figure 26.1 The peripheral blood smear shows increased circulating large granular lymphocytes with atypical morphology, including visible nucleoli and vaguely visible cytoplasmic cytotoxic granules (A, wright, ×1,000). The corresponding bone marrow core biopsy demonstrates interstitial and sinusoidal infiltrate by these neoplastic lymphoid cells, significantly increased in number (B, H&E, ×600). A section from splenectomy reveals a diffuse, atypical lymphoid infiltrate, resulting in expansion of splenic red pulps (C–E, ×200). The infiltrating cells are stained positive for CD3 (D, immunoperoxidase, ×200), dim CD5 and dim CD7 (not shown), and a cytotoxic marker perforin (E, immunoperoxidase, ×200) with a low proliferation index highlighted by Ki67, estimated at 5%–10% (F, immunoperoxidase, ×200), distinguishing it from aggressive hepatosplenic gamma/delta T-cell lymphoma.

infiltrates (Figure 26.1B). *STAT3* mutations, if present, support the diagnosis of T-LGLL.

Viral studies are typically performed to rule out reactive LGL lymphocytosis to viral infections, including HIV-1/2, human T-lymphotropic virus types 1/2 (HTLV-1/2), hepatitis B virus, hepatitis C virus, Epstein–Barr virus (EBV), and cytomegalovirus (CMV).

In selected cases, rheumatological workup, including rheumatoid factor, antinuclear antibody (ANA), and erythrocyte sedimentation rate (ESR), and ultrasound of spleen to evaluate splenomegaly can be considered. Differential diagnoses include reactive polyclonal, oligoclonal, or even small clonal LGL lymphocytosis secondary to a viral infection, autoimmune conditions, or aging. Reactive lymphocytosis in setting of viral infection is only transient in contrast to a persistent clonal LGL lymphocytosis that exceeds 6 months in patients with LGLL. Both hepatosplenic gamma delta T-cell lymphoma (HSTCL) and T-LGLL can express TCR gamma/delta, but they clinically behave very differently. While T-LGLL often has an indolent course with cytopenias in older individuals, HSTCL is very aggressive, with marked hepatosplenomegaly and B-symptoms in young males. An estimated proliferative index by Ki-67 immunohistochemistry will be highly elevated in HSTCL, in comparison to lower Ki-67 expression (typically <10%) in T-LGLL (Figure 26.1).

■ PROGNOSIS

LGLL takes an indolent course. A large registry study showed a 5-year overall survival (OS) of 89%. The median survival is 9 years according to a US registry study. Disease-related mortality is most commonly due to severe neutropenia with infection, which happens in ~10% of patients.

A prognostic scoring system for T-LGLL has been suggested that estimates the median OS based on the initial manifestation of 1, 2, or 3 cytopenias (anemia, severe neutropenia, or lymphopenia) at 105, 55, and 5 months, respectively (Table 26.1).

■ TREATMENT

Asymptomatic patients do not need treatment and can be closely observed. Approximately half of patients do not need treatment at first diagnosis. However, the majority of patients will need treatment at some point. Indications for treatment include absolute neutrophil count (ANC) <0.5 × 10^9/L, neutropenia with frequent infections, hemoglobin <10 g/dL or symptomatic anemia, platelets <50 × 10^9/L, associated autoimmune diseases requiring therapy, symptomatic splenomegaly, or severe B-symptoms.

FRONTLINE TREATMENT

The optimal frontline treatment for LGLL is unknown. Accepted first-line therapy includes a sequential use of low-dose methotrexate (MTX) ± corticosteroids, cyclophosphamide (Cy) ± corticosteroids, or cyclosporine

Table 26.1 Prognostic Scoring System for T-LGLL

Number of Cytopenias (Anemia, Severe Neutropenia, or Lymphopenia)	Median Overall Survival
1	105 months
2	55 months
3	5 months

T-LGLL, T-cell large granular lymphocytic leukemia.

Cytopenic parameters: hemoglobin <12 g/dl, severe neutropenia (absolute neutrophil count <0.1 × 10^9/L), and lymphopenia (absolute lymphocyte count <1 × 10^9/L).

A (CSA). Patients who achieve a partial response (PR) or complete response (CR) to MTX or CSA after 4 months of treatment should continue their treatment until progression of the disease (Table 26.2). Due to increased risk of secondary malignancies, the administration of Cy should be limited to fewer than 12 months. The addition of steroids during the first month of immunosuppressive therapy can aid in the resolution of constitutional symptoms and accelerate improvement of cytopenias or symptoms.

Bareau et al. reported on treatment response rates in 229 T-LGLL patients.[3] Specifically, the overall response rate (ORR) to MTX was 55%, with a CR rate of 21% and a mean response duration of 21 months. The ORR to Cy was 66%, with a CR rate of 47% and a mean response duration of 31 months. The ORR to CSA was 21%, with a CR rate of 4% and a mean response duration of 12 months. If a patient does not respond to a drug after 4 months, switching to a different one is reasonable. In a phase 2 trial conducted by the Eastern Cooperative Oncology Group (ECOG), patients treated with MTX as an initial therapy achieved ORR of 38%, and in those not responding to MTX, 64% responded to Cy.

Table 26.2 Response Criteria in T-LGLL

Response	Hemoglobin	Absolute Neutrophil Count	Platelets	Other
CR	>12 g/dL	>1.5 × 10^9/L	>150 × 10^9/L	Lymphocytes <4 × 10^9/L LGL <0.5 × 10^9/L
PR	>8 g/dL	>0.5 × 10^9/L	>50 × 10^9/L	Absence of transfusions

CR, complete response; T-LGLL, T-cell large granular lymphocytic leukemia; PR, partial response.[3]

Commonly used doses of drugs:

- MTX 10 mg/m^2 orally weekly × 4 months
- Cy 50 to 100 mg orally daily × 4 months
- CSA 3 to 5 mg/kg or 5 to 10 mg/kg orally daily or 100 to 150 mg orally daily × 4 months
- Prednisone 1 mg/kg orally daily × 1 month with tapering off by the end of the second month

RELAPSED/REFRACTORY PATIENTS

Treatment for progressive or refractory LGLL is challenging. Options include a clinical trial, alemtuzumab, purine analogs (pentostatin, cladribine, and fludarabine), or splenectomy. Among those, only alemtuzumab has been evaluated in a clinical trial. In a phase 2 single-arm trial using low-dose alemtuzumab in previously heavily treated LGLL patients, 14 of the 25 patients had a hematologic response at 3 months.

▓ POTENTIAL PRACTICE-CHANGING CLINICAL TRIALS

The optimal therapy for initial treatment of LGLL is unknown. A multi-center French randomized trial comparing methotrexate versus cyclophosphamide as initial therapy for LGLL has been completed, and final results are pending (NCT01976182). A multi-center, single-arm phase I/II study of BNZ-1, an injectable PEGylated peptide antagonist that binds to the common gamma chain (γc) signaling receptor for the cytokines interleukin (IL)-2, IL-9, and IL-15, completed accrual of 20 patients with LGLL (NCT03239392). Preliminary report revealed no dose-limiting toxicities and ORR of 20%. Given the presence of gain-of-function mutations in *STAT3* and *STAT5b* genes in LGLL patients, future clinical trials with JAK/STAT pathway inhibitors or STAT protein degraders could potentially be novel targeted therapeutic options for these patients.

▓ REFERENCES FOR SUPPLEMENTAL READING

1. Sokol L, Loughran TP. Large granular lymphocyte leukemia. *Oncologist*. 2006;11:263–273.
2. Lamy T, Moignet A, Loughran TP. LGL leukemia: from pathogenesis to treatment. *Blood*. 2017;129(9):1082–1094.
3. Bareau B, Rey J, Hamidou M, et al. Analysis of a French cohort of patients with large granular lymphocyte leukemia: a report on 229 cases. *Haematologica*. 2010;95(9):1534–1541.
4. Loughran TP Jr, Zickl L, Olson TL, et al. Immunosuppressive therapy of LGL leukemia: prospective multicenter phase II study by the Eastern Cooperative Oncology Group (E5998). *Leukemia*. 2015;29(4):886–894.
5. Munoz J, Dhillon N, Janku F, et al. STAT3 inhibitors: finding a home in lymphoma and leukemia. *Oncologist*. 2014;19(5):536–544.

27 Aggressive Natural Killer Cell Leukemia

Emilie Wang, Mintallah Haider,

and Lubomir Sokol

▮ INTRODUCTION

Lymphoproliferative disorders of natural killer (NK) cells comprise less than 5% of lymphoid neoplasms. There are three disease entities originating from NK cells, according to the 2008 World Health Organization (WHO) classification of hematologic neoplasms: chronic lymphoproliferative disorders of NK cells; extranodal NK/T-cell lymphoma, nasal type; and aggressive NK-cell leukemia (ANKCL), with the latter being most rare, at 0.1% of lymphoid neoplasms (see Chapter 48). ANKCL manifests as a fulminant systemic disease leading to multi-organ failure, with the involvement of peripheral blood, bone marrow (BM), spleen, liver, and lymph nodes. Central nervous system (CNS) involvement is also very common at presentation. The clinical presentation can include fever, jaundice, splenomegaly, hepatomegaly, lymphadenopathy, cytopenias, coagulopathy, and hemophagocytic lymphohistiocytosis (HLH) (see Chapter 52). HLH can be frequently found at diagnosis or during the course of the disease and is a result of uncontrolled monocyte/macrophage activation due to cytokine release by the NK cells. The incidence of ANKCL is highest in East Asia, followed by Central and South America, and it is very low in Europe and North America. There does not seem to be gender predominance, with both males and females being equally affected. The median age is between 30 and 40 years. There is a limited understanding of etiology, but the disease is almost always found in association with a clonal episomal Epstein–Barr virus (EBV), suggesting that this virus plays a pathogenic role in ANKCL. The rarity of the disease presents a diagnostic and therapeutic challenge for hematologists. ANKCL is often primary refractory to chemotherapy, and thus prognosis remains poor.

▮ DIAGNOSIS

The initial workup includes morphologic evaluation of the peripheral blood smear and flow cytometry, complete metabolic panel (CMP) with lactate dehydrogenase (LDH), coagulation studies, EBV DNA titer by polymerase chain reaction (PCR), imaging studies with contrast computed topography (CT) scan or positron emission tomography/computed tomography (PET/CT), and BM aspiration and biopsy.

Standard T-cell gene-rearrangement analysis often shows germline status, and thus other methods, such as cytogenetic evaluation, are needed. In addition, advanced molecular studies are being increasingly used in the evaluation of ANKCL. As discussed earlier, HLH is commonly associated with ANKCL and can be a part of the initial presentation (see Chapter 52).

CYTOMORPHOLOGY

Circulating leukemic cells can be morphologically heterogeneous, spanning from large granular lymphocytes to atypical larger cells with pale cytoplasm, irregular nuclear contours, and azurophilic granules. BM often reveal s the angiocentric and angiodestructive infiltration associated with frequent necrosis and apoptosis. Hemophagocytosis can also be observed.

IMMUNOPHENOTYPE

ANKCL cells are clusters of differentiation 2+ (CD2+), CD56+, CD16+, CD7+, and cytoplasmic CD3ε+ (although surface CD3 negative). They are also positive for the cytotoxic molecules TIA-1, granzyme B, and perforin. These cells may express CD11b, but CD57 is often negative (in contrast to T-large granular lymphocyte [LGL]). As mentioned previously, the T-cell receptor is in germline configuration. Ki-67 is frequently high. ANKCL cells are positive for CXCR1 and CCR5, the ligands of which are interleukins and chemokines. More than 90% of the cases will be positive for EBV (in situ hybridization tested on formalin-fixed paraffin-embedded tissue via EBV-encoded small RNAs [EBER] probe).

GENETICS

The most common recurrent chromosomal aberrancy is loss of chromosomes 6q (deletion 6q21q25 followed by deletions of 11q, 13q, and 17p). *PRDM1* and *FOXO3* are tumor-suppressor genes that map to 6q21 and play an important role in the pathogenesis of NK-cell malignancies, including ANKCL (*Blood*. 2011, 118(12):3195–3204). Recent study elucidating genetic landscape in 14 patients with ANKL using whole-exome sequencing (WES) identified mutations in genes for *STAT3* in 21%, *RAS-MAPK* pathway in 21%, *DDX3X* in 29%, and epigenetic modifiers in 50% of tested samples (*Nat Commun*. 2018;9:1567).

■ KEY DIAGNOSTIC DILEMMA

Extranodal NK/T-cell lymphoma, nasal type, can also present with peripheral blood involvement (see Chapter 48). Similarly, ANKCL, which primarily involves peripheral blood, BM, spleen, and liver, can sometimes present with lymphadenopathy. In these cases, among other clinical factors as aforementioned, CD16 status is important to distinguish between the two entities, as it is positive in 75% of ANKCL cases while negative in ENKTL.

▨ PROGNOSIS

A highly aggressive and fulminant clinical course results in a median survival of 2 months. Most patients die within 24 months regardless of treatment. Prognostic indices used in aggressive T-cell and NK-cell lymphomas, such as International Prognostic Index (IPI), Prognostic Index for T-Cell Lymphoma (PIT), or the Korean Index for NK/T-cell lymphoma, have not been validated in patients with ANKCL. In a small retrospective study, patients with EBV-negative ANKCL had significantly better prognoses compared to EBV-positive patients (*Acta Haematol.* 2008;120(4):199–206).

▨ TREATMENT

Due to the rarity of the disease, there is a paucity of controlled prospective clinical trials to guide treatment decisions. Chemotherapy is the mainstay of treatment, followed by consolidation therapy with allogenic hematopoietic stem cell transplantation (allo-HSCT) after complete response (CR) is achieved. Unfortunately, ANKL has poor CR rates (<20%). However, those who receive allo-HSCT after CR exhibited significantly superior survival rates compared to those who did not. Often at diagnosis, patients may not be treatment candidates due to multi-organ failure and poor performance status (PS), although intensive therapy represents the only treatment option for a durable response. The disappointing CR rates may also be explained by the fact that NK cells express a high concentration of P-glycoprotein due to overexpression of multidrug resistance-1 (MDR-1). The NK P-glycoprotein has a smaller molecular weight compared to the classic P-glycoprotein, which does not allow the transportation of anthracycline into cancer cells, making anthracycline-based regimens typically ineffective. Such agents as methotrexate and L-asparaginase, not affected by P-glycoprotein, have demonstrated efficacy, but administration of L-asparaginase may be difficult for patients with hepatic failure. Currently, the treatment recommendations are based on the patient's overall condition and may need modifications to address organ failure at presentation. Younger patients should be treated through coagulopathy and HLH. In patients with concomitant HLH, etoposide can be added to the induction regimen. Monitoring of the EBV DNA titer by PCR is also helpful in response assessment and can alert the clinician of progressive disease. CNS prophylaxis should be incorporated into the induction regimen due to a high risk of CNS involvement.

FRONTLINE TREATMENT

1. SMILE: dexamethasone, methotrexate, ifosfamide, L-asparaginase, and etoposide (*J Clin Oncol.* 2011;29:4410–4416)

2. AspaMetDex: L-asparaginase, methotrexate, and dexamethasone (*Blood.* 2011;117:1834–1839)

3. VIDL: etoposide, ifosfamide, dexamethasone, and L-asparaginase (*Hematol Oncol.* 2016;9:41)

RELAPSED/REFRACTORY PATIENTS

Patients resistant to multiple chemotherapies have limited therapeutic options and, as a result, short life expectancies. Most regimens used in the relapsed or refractory setting have been based on case reports or case series. In patients with relapsed or refractory disease, an L-asparaginase–containing regimen should be administered if not included in the initial therapy. If L-asparaginase has been used, such regimens as ifosfamide, carboplatin, etoposide (ICE); dexamethasone, cisplatin, cytarabine (DHAP); or etoposide, solumedrol, cytosine arabinoside, and cisplatin (ESHAP), as used in refractory lymphoma, could also be considered in the second-line setting. Immune checkpoint inhibitors have shown some efficacy in patients with NK/T-cell lymphoma. In a small case series, all seven patients with NK/T-cell lymphoma who failed a median of two regimens demonstrated responses based on clinical, radiologic, morphologic, and molecular (circulating EBV DNA) criteria after administration of pembrolizumab for a median of seven cycles. Five of these patients achieved CR (*Blood.* 2017;129(17):2437–2442). In a case series of three patients who failed an L-asparaginase–containing regimen, low-dose nivolumab demonstrated a response in relapsed/refractory disease after just one dose (*Ann Hematol.* 2018;97(1):193–196). In a patient with relapsed disseminated CD30+ NK/T-cell lymphoma after an L-asparaginase–based regimen, combination therapy with brentuximab vedotin and bendamustine resulted in CR (*Ann Hematol.* 2016;95(5):847–849).

HEMATOPOIETIC STEM CELL TRANSPLANTATION

Consolidation with allo-HSCT should be offered to every patient eligible for transplant who achieves CR or has only minimal residual disease (MRD). The data regarding transplantation in ANKCL are limited to fewer than two dozen patients. In the Center of International Blood and Marrow Transplant Research database study, 21 patients with ANKL who received allo-HSCT were included. At the time of transplant, 14 patients were in CR, and 5 had active disease. The 2-year progression-free survival (PFS) and overall survival (OS) rates were 20% and 24%, respectively, with a reported 2-year relapse/progression rate of 59%. Patients who achieved CR did better compared to those who had active disease at the time of transplant. The 2-year PFS and OS for those in CR were 30% and 38%, respectively, compared to 0% in both categories for those with active disease prior to allo-HSCT. This study highlights the important role of allo-HSCT in achieving a durable response in patients with ANKL prior to transplant (*Biol Blood Marrow Transplant.* 23(2017):853–856).

▒ POTENTIAL PRACTICE-CHANGING CLINICAL TRIALS

Currently, there are not any active clinical trials conducted specifically for ANKL, according to www.clinicaltrials.gov. However, there are numerous early clinical trials open for patients with other NK or T-cell neoplasms that allow enrollment of ANKL patients. Due to similarities in pathobiology between ANKL and the more common extranodal NK/T-cell lymphoma, nasal type, treatment approaches for ANKL are often derived from the latter.

There have been four clinical trials studying the safety and efficacy of sintilimab, a novel anti-PD1 antibody, in treating relapsed/refractory NK/T-cell lymphoma. Sintilimab has been combined with PEG-asparaginase (NCT04096690), decitabine (NCT04279379), lenalidomide (NCT04231370), and PEG-asparaginase plus a receptor tyrosine kinase inhibitor, anlotinib (NCT03936452). Several potentially breakthrough novel immunotherapeutic approaches, including anti-CD30 CAR T-cell (NCT04008394) and anti-CD7 universal CAR T-cell (NCT04008394), have been tested in clinical studies for patients with relapsed, refractory NK/T-cell lymphomas expressing CD30 and CD7 antigens, respectively. EBV-specific antigens expressed by malignant cells of NK/T-cell lymphomas have been therapeutically targeted in early clinical trials using EBViNT cell, an EBV latent membrane protein-2a [LMP2A] specific eutil autologous blood-derived T lymphocytes (NCT03789617) and EBV human cytotoxic T-cells, VT-EBV-N (EBV-CTL) (NCT03671850).

Several agents, such as decitabine (hypomethylating agent), ruxolitnib (JAK1/2 inhibitor), and navitoclax (BCL2 inhibitor), were found to have in vitro activity against ANKL cells. The efficacy against ANKL and safety of these agents must be proven in future studies before they can be incorporated into clinical practice. Additionally, the discovery and characterization of cancer driver genes and the identification of druggable targets in individual patients will most probably be necessary to improve outcomes of this aggressive disease.

▧ REFERENCES FOR SUPPLEMENTAL READING

1. Hamadani M, Kanate AS, DiGilio A, et al. Allogeneic hematopoietic cell transplantation for aggressive NK cell leukemia: a center for international blood and marrow transplant research analysis. *Biol Blood Marrow Transplant*. 2017;23(5):853–856.

2. Jung KS, Cho SH, Kim SJ, et al. L-asparaginase-based regimens followed by allogeneic hematopoietic stem cell transplantation improve outcomes in aggressive natural killer cell leukemia. *J Hematol Oncol*. 2016;9:41.

3. Yamaguchi M, Kwong YL, Kim WS, et al. Phase II study of SMILE chemotherapy for newly diagnosed stage IV, relapsed, or refractory extranodal natural killer (NK)/T-cell lymphoma, nasal type: the NK-cell tumor study group study. *J Clin Oncol*. 2011;29:4410–4416.

4. Gao LM, Zhao S, Liu WP, et al. Clinicopathologic characterization of aggressive natural killer cell leukemia involving different tissue sites. *Am J Surg Pathol*. 2016;40:836–846.

5. Ishida F. Aggressive NK-cell leukemia. *Front Pediatr*. 2018;6:292.

28 Monoclonal Gammopathy of Unknown Significance, Smoldering Myeloma, and Plasmacytomas

Hannah Asghari and Brandon Blue

▓ INTRODUCTION

Plasma cell (PC) dyscrasias are disorders characterized by clonal proliferation of PCs with or without elevated levels of monoclonal protein (M protein) and immunoglobulin fragments. It encompasses a number of disorders, including monoclonal gammopathy of unknown significance (MGUS), smoldering myeloma (SMM), solitary plasmacytoma (SP), multiple myeloma (MM), PC leukemia, Waldenström macroglobulinemia (WM), and amyloidosis (AL). In this chapter, we focus on MGUS, SMM, and plasmacytoma (see Chapters 28–31).

▓ MONOCLONAL GAMMOPATHY OF UNKNOWN SIGNIFICANCE

MGUS is an asymptomatic clonal PC disorder and a precursor for MM. The incidence and prevalence of MGUS increase with age, with a prevalence in the United States estimated to be slightly greater than 3% in individuals ages 50 years or older. In a population-based study from Olmstead County, Minnesota, the annual incidence of MGUS was noted to be 120 per 100,000 and 60 per 100,000 in men and women older than 50 years, respectively (*Mayo Clin Proc.* 2012;87(11):1071–1079). In men and women older than 90 years, the incidence of MGUS increased to 530 per 100,000 and 370 per 100,000, respectively. A large population-based study by the National Health and Nutritional Examination Survey noted significantly higher prevalence of MGUS in Black individuals compared to White individuals (*Leukemia.* 2014;28(7):1537–1542).

▓ DIAGNOSIS

The 2014 International Myeloma Working Group (IMWG) definition for MGUS is summarized in Table 28.1.[1] By definition, patients with MGUS are asymptomatic. Commonly, patients are diagnosed incidentally while being worked up for other disorders. Considering the lack of proven benefit, health care burden, and psychological implications, universal screening for MGUS is not advocated. The workup for MGUS needs to incorporate the tests to rule out more serious conditions, such as SMM or MM (Figure 28.1). The term "monoclonal gammopathy of clinical significance" (MGCS) has

Table 28.1 IMWG Definitions

MGUS (non-IgM)
- Serum non-IgM M protein <3 g/dL
- Clonal BM PCs <10%
- *Absence of end organ damage, such as CRAB features or AL, that can be attributed to a PC disorder

MGUS (IgM)
- Serum IgM M protein <3 g/dL
- BM lymphoplasmacytic infiltration <10%
- No evidence of anemia, constitutional symptoms, hyperviscosity, lymphadenopathy, hepatosplenomegaly, or other end organ damage that can be attributed to the underlying lymphoproliferative disorder

SM
- Serum M protein (IgG or IgA) ≥3 g/dL or urinary M protein ≥500 mg per 24 hr and/or clonal BM PCs 10%–60%
- *Absence of end organ damage (CRAB), myeloma-defining events** or AL

SP
- Biopsy-proven solitary lesion of bone or soft tissue with evidence of clonal PCs
- Clonal BM PCs <10%
- Normal skeletal survey and MRI (or CT scan) of spine and pelvis (except for the primary solitary lesion)
- *Absence of end-organ damage (CRAB) that can be attributed to a lymphoplasma cell proliferative disorder

AL, amyloidosis; BM, bone marrow; CRAB, hypercalcemia, renal insufficiency, anemia, and bone lesions; CT, computed tomography; IgA, immunoglobulin A; IgG, immunoglobulin G; IgM, immunoglobulin M; IMWG, International Myeloma Working Group; MGUS, monoclonal gammopathy of unknown significance; M protein, monoclonal protein; MRI, magnetic resonance imaging; PC, plasma cell; SM, smoldering myeloma; SP, solitary plasmacytoma.

*Evidence of end organ damage that can be attributed to the underlying PC proliferative disorder (hypercalcemia: serum calcium >1 mg/dL higher than the upper limit of normal or >11 mg/dL; renal insufficiency: creatinine clearance <40 mL/min or serum creatinine >2 mg/dL; anemia: hemoglobin value of >2 g/dL below the lower limit of normal or <10g/dL; one or more osteolytic lesions on skeletal radiography, CT scan, or positron emission tomography–computed tomography [PET-CT] scan).

**Myeloma-defining events: (a) clonal BM PC percentage ≥60%; (b) involved: uninvolved serum-free light chain ratio ≥100; (c) >1 focal lesion on MRI studies.

Source: Rajkumar SV, Dimopoulos MA, Palumbo A, et al. International Myeloma Working Group updated criteria for the diagnosis of multiple myeloma. *Lancet Oncol.* 2014;15(12):e538–e548.

been used to categorize several conditions classified by end-organ damage secondary to monoclonal immunoglobulin or other processes (*Blood.* 2018;132(14):1478–1485). Bone marrow (BM) biopsy can be considered for patients who are younger than 65 years and/ or have high-risk MGUS (Figure 28.1).

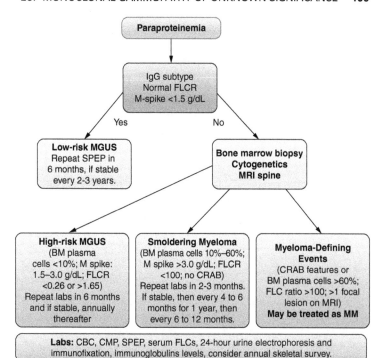

Figure 28.1 Diagnostic workup and surveillance for paraproteinemia.

BM, bone marrow; CBC, complete blood count; CMP, complete metabolic panel; FCLR, free light chain ratio; IgG, immunoglobulin G; M-spike, monoclonal spike; MGUS, monoclonal gammopathy of unknown significance; MM, multiple myeloma.

Based on the immunoglobulin heavy and light chains involved, MGUS can be subclassified into three different types:

1. **Non-IgM MGUS**—Immunoglobulin G (IgG), immunoglobulin A (IgA), or immunoglobulin D (IgD) are the immunoglobulins involved. IgG MGUS is the most common subtype. The rate of progression for this subtype is 1% per year and usually progresses to SMM, SP, MM, or AL.

2. **IgM MGUS**—About 15% of MGUS cases are of this subtype. Patients with IgM MGUS can progress (1%–5% per year) to smoldering or symptomatic WM, IgM MM, and AL.

3. **Light-chain MGUS**—This subtype is characterized by clonal proliferation of immunoglobulin light chains only and absence of heavy chains. Light-chain MGUS can progress to light-chain MM and AL (<1% per year).

*Basic workup includes serum protein electrophoresis (SPEP) with immunofixation (IFE), 24-hour urine for urine protein electrophoresis

Table 28.2 Risk Model for Progression of MGUS	
Risk Factors	• **Non-IgG MGUS** • **Serum M protein >1.5 g/dL** • **Abnormal serum-free light chain ratio (i.e., ratio of kappa to lambda free light chains <0.26 or >1.65)**
No Risk Factors	5% risk for progression in 20 years
1 of 3 Risk Factors	21% risk for progression in 20 years
2 of 3 Risk Factors	37% risk for progression in 20 years
All 3 Risk Factors	58% risk for progression in 20 years

IgG, immunoglobulin G; MGUS, monoclonal gammopathy of unknown significance; M protein, monoclonal protein.

Source: Kyle RA, Durie BG, Rajkumar SV, et al. Monoclonal gammopathy of undetermined significance (MGUS) and smoldering (asymptomatic) multiple myeloma: IMWG consensus perspectives risk factors for progression and guidelines for monitoring and management. *Leukemia.* 2010;24(6):1121–1127.

(UPEP) with IFE, serum light chains and free light chain ratio (FCLR), complete metabolic panel (CMP), complete blood count (CBC), immunoglobulin levels, and a skeletal survey (quantification of paraprotein and evaluation of hypercalcemia, renal insufficiency, anemia, and bone lesions [CRAB] criteria).

PROGNOSIS

Multiple studies have evaluated risk factors that can predict the progression of MGUS to MM. The risk prediction model (Mayo Clinic Model) from the 2010 IMWG consensus statement is summarized in Table 28.2.[2]

SURVEILLANCE

After initial diagnosis, a follow-up evaluation with SPEP in 6 months is recommended for patients at low risk of MGUS. If they are stable, subsequent testing and surveillance can be done every 2 to 3 years (Figure 28.1). For patients at high risk of MGUS, a follow-up evaluation with SPEP and CBC in 6 months are recommended. Subsequent testing can be done annually. A large retrospective population-based study noted that the highest rate of MGUS progression to a lymphoplasmacytic malignancy was during the first year of follow-up (*Haematologica.* 2018;103(3):e123–e125).

SMOLDERING MYELOMA

SMM is an asymptomatic monoclonal gammopathy, intermediate between MGUS and MM. SMM is estimated to represent approximately 8% to 20% of patients with MM.

DIAGNOSIS

The 2014 IMWG definition for SMM is summarized in Table 28.1. Like MGUS, SMM patients are asymptomatic. The basic diagnostic workup for SMM is similar to that of patients at high risk of MGUS (see earlier). In addition, all SMM patients should undergo BM biopsies to assess the level of marrow infiltration with abnormal PCs, cytogenetics, and fluorescence in situ hybridization (FISH) for high-risk genetic abnormalities and whole-body MRI or PET-CT scans to identify bone lesions (Figure 28.1).

PROGNOSIS AND RISK STRATIFICATION

Patients with SMM progress to MM or AL at a rate of 10% per year for the first 5 years, 3% per year for the next 5 years, and 1% per year for the next 10 years. However, SMM is heterogeneous, and certain risk factors predict a faster rate of progression. The Mayo Clinic criteria and the Programa para et Tratamiento de Hemopatias Malignas (PETHEMA) Spanish group criteria are two well-known models for prediction of SMM risk (*N Engl J Med.* 2007;356(25):2582–2590; *Blood.* 2007;110(7):2586–2592). The Mayo 2018 risk stratification model incorporates the revised 2014 IMWG diagnostic criteria for SMM. Risk factors for progression include BM PCs >20%, M protein ≥2 g/dL, or involved/uninvolved serum-free light chain (SFLC) ratio > 20. Low-risk patients (no risk factors present) had an estimated median time to progression (TTP) of 110 months, intermediate-risk (1 risk factor present) median TTP of 68 months, and high-risk (2–3 risk factors present) median TTP of 29 months.[3] Multiple other factors that predict higher risk for SMM progression have also been identified (Table 28.3).

TREATMENT

Lenalidomide-based therapy has been shown to have survival benefits in SMM patients (*N Engl J Med.* 2013;369(5):438–447). Follow-up analysis of a phase 3 open-label randomized trial of patients at high

---

Table 28.3 Risk Factors Associated With High Risk of SMM

- M protein >3 g/dL
- IgA subtype
- Involved to uninvolved FLCR >8 but <100
- Decreased levels of >1 uninvolved immunoglobulin
- BM PC >20%, >95% of PC in BM aberrant
- t(4;14), del(17p), add(1q)
- Gene expression profiling: 70 score ≥0.26, 4 score >9.28
- MRI showing diffuse BM abnormalities or > 1 focal lesion
- Increased circulating PCs

BM, bone marrow; FLCR, free light chain ratio; IgA, immunoglobulin A; M protein, monoclonal protein; MRI, magnetic resonance imaging; PC, plasma cell; SMM, smoldering myeloma.

Sources: *N Engl J Med.* 2007;356(25):2582–2590; *Blood.* 2007;110(7): 2586–2592; Blood. 2014;123(1):78–85.

risk of SMM evaluating lenalidomide/dexamethasone followed by lenalidomide monotherapy noted improved overall survival (OS; 3-year OS 94% vs. 80%; hazard ratio [HR], 0.43; 95% confidence interval [CI], 0.20 to 0.90; median OS not reached) and improved median progression-free survival (PFS; not reached vs. 23 months; HR, 0.24; 95% CI, 0.14 to 0.41; $p < .0001$) compared to observation.[4] An additional study evaluating single-agent lenalidomide in SMM patients at intermediate or high risk per Mayo Clinic 2018 criteria noted improved 2-year PFS, particularly those at high risk on subgroup analysis (*J Clin Oncol.* 2020;38(11): 1126–1137). Of note, there is currently a lack of long-term OS data for the use of lenalidomide in patients at high risk of SMM, and observation remains the standard of care for those at lower risk of SMM currently outside the context of a clinical trial. One such clinical trial, the ASCENT trial, will address whether adding carfilzomib, lenalidomide, daratumumab, and dexamethasone to treatments for patients at high risk of SMM will potentially cure them prior to their developing active myeloma disease.

■ SURVEILLANCE

After initial diagnosis, CBC, creatinine, calcium, SPEP, SFLC, and UPEP should be repeated in 2 to 3 months (Figure 28.1). If results are stable, then follow-up testing should be conducted every 4 to 6 months for 1 year, and then every 6 to 12 months.

■ PLASMACYTOMA

SP is a disorder characterized by the presence of a localized clonal PC mass without evidence of systemic disease. SP involving bone is called solitary bone plasmacytoma (SBP), and SP involving soft tissues is called extramedullary plasmacytoma (EMP). In a Surveillance, Epidemiology, and End Results (SEER) database review, the incidence rate of SP is about 0.34 per 100,000 person-years, and SP is estimated to represent 6% of all PC disorders. SBP is more common than EMP, and a vast majority of EMP involve the upper aerodigestive tract. Bone pains, pathological fracture, and symptoms of nerve compression are some of the common presenting symptoms from SBP. Based on the location of the EMP, a variety of presenting symptoms can occur, including nasal congestion, obstruction, cough, epistaxis, hemoptysis, and other gastrointestinal symptoms.

■ DIAGNOSIS

The 2014 IMWG definition for SP is summarized in Table 28.1. Preliminary workup for SP is similar to that for MGUS or SMM. CBC, calcium, creatinine, SPEP, UPEP, IFE, and FLCR should be obtained. Biopsy of the suspected lesions is critical in diagnosis. Furthermore, imaging with whole-body MRI or PET-CT scan is recommended.[5]

PROGNOSIS

The risk for progression of SP to MM is about 10% within 3 years. However, the rate of progression to MM is higher, and the survival rate is worse in patients with SBP compared to those with EMP. In general, patients with SP were noted to have median OS ranging from 86.4 months to 156 months in different studies. Patients who had clonal PCs in marrow less than 10% or persistent M spike more than 1 year after radiation therapy (RT) had a higher risk of progression to MM (*Cancer*. 2002; 94(5):1532–1537).

TREATMENT

Plasmacytomas are radiosensitive tumors, and RT is the treatment of choice for both SBP and EMP. A minimum cumulative radiation dose of 40 to 50 Gy (45 Gy for EMP) administered over 4 weeks is recommended. RT results in excellent local disease-control rates of 90% to 100% (*Int J Radiat Oncol Biol Phys*. 2006;64(4):1013–1017; *Radiother Oncol*. 1990;17(4):293–303). Primary surgical resection is not a recommended treatment modality. The role of further RT is unclear if a complete resection of the lesion is achieved during initial diagnostic workup. Adjuvant radiation is recommended for partially or incomplete resected lesions. The role of adjuvant chemotherapy/systemic therapy is not well established.

POTENTIAL PRACTICE-CHANGING CLINICAL TRIALS

A phase 2 study of patients at high risk of SMM and ages younger than 65 investigated carfilzomib, lenalidomide, dexamethasone induction (KRd) followed by high-dose melphalan with autologous stem cell transplant and subsequent consolidation KRd followed by maintenance Rd. This study noted that 64% of patients receiving KRd and transplant achieved complete response (56% minimal-residual disease undetectable), but larger studies with longer follow-up are indicated to evaluate the role of transplant in patients at high risk of SMM (*Blood*. 2019;134(Suppl1):781–781). A randomized phase 3 study (NCT02544308) is evaluating the role of lenalidomide and dexamethasone in patients at high risk of SBP compared with RT only. The emergence of monoclonal antibodies in the treatment of MM (see Chapter 29) has raised the possibility of using them as monotherapy or in combination for SMM, given their excellent side-effect profile. These clinical trials along with the aforementioned ASCENT trial for patients at high risk of SMM (NCT03289299) will likely change the practice landscape for years to come.

REFERENCES FOR SUPPLEMENTAL READING

1. Rajkumar SV, Dimopoulos MA, Palumbo A, et al. International Myeloma Working Group updated criteria for the diagnosis of multiple myeloma. *Lancet Oncol*. 2014;15(12):e538–e548.

2. Kyle RA, Durie BG, Rajkumar SV, et al. Monoclonal gammopathy of undetermined significance (MGUS) and smoldering (asymptomatic) multiple myeloma: IMWG consensus perspectives risk factors for progression and guidelines for monitoring and management. *Leukemia.* 2010;24(6):1121–1127.

3. Lakshman A, Rajkumar SV, Buadi FK, et al. Risk stratification of smoldering multiple myeloma incorporating revised IMWG diagnostic criteria. *Blood Can J.* 2018;8(6):59.

4. Mateos MV, Hernández MT, Giraldo P, et al. Lenalidomide plus dexamethasone versus observation in patients with high-risk smouldering multiple myeloma (QuiRedex): long-term follow-up of a randomised, controlled, phase 3 trial. *Lancet Oncol.* 2016;17(8):1127–1136.

5. Hillengass J, Usmani S, Rajkumar SV, et al. International myeloma working group consensus recommendations on imaging in monoclonal plasma cell disorders. *Lancet Oncol.* 2019;20(6):e302–e312.

29   Multiple Myeloma

Shonali Midha, Patrick Griffin, and Rachid Baz

▓ INTRODUCTION

Multiple myeloma (MM) is a neoplastic disorder of plasma cells. Patients often present with symptoms of end-organ dysfunction, including unexplained anemia, renal failure, hypercalcemia, and/or painful osteolytic bone lesions, although some patients are asymptomatic. MM accounts for about 1% to 2% of all malignancies and 17% of all hematologic malignancies, with a median age at diagnosis of 66 and decreasing incidence by decade (age <50 approximately 10% and age <40 approximately 3%). There is a higher incidence among men (1.4:1). African Americans have an incidence of 2 to 3 times that of Caucasians. Interestingly, there is also a small cluster of familial cases, with persons having a 3.7 times increased risk with a first-degree relative diagnosed with the disease.

▓ EVALUATION

1. History and physical exam.
2. Labs: Complete blood count (CBC), complete metabolic panel (CMP), lactate dehydrogenase (LDH), beta 2-microglobulin (B2M), serum protein electrophoresis (SPEP) with immunofixation (IFE), quantitative immunoglobulins, serum-free light chains (SFLC), 24-hour urine protein electrophoresis with IFE (Figure 29.1).
3. Imaging: Skeletal survey; consider magnetic resonance imaging (MRI) for unexplained pain; consider positron emission tomography–computed tomography (PET-CT) to rule-out occult bone lesions absent other evidence of end-organ dysfunction (Figure 29.2).
4. Bone marrow (BM) biopsy: Including immunohistochemistry (IHC), flow cytometry, cytogenetic analysis, and fluorescence in situ hybridization (FISH) for recurrent cytogenetic abnormalities (e.g., t(4;14), t(14;16), t(14;20), del(17p), hypodiploidy); consider gene-expression profiling and next-generation sequencing (NGS) identification of trackable clones, especially in young and fit patients.

▓ DIAGNOSIS

MORPHOLOGY

The peripheral blood can show rouleaux formation of red blood cells. In BM, ≥10% clonal plasma cells are present. In contrast to normal BM plasma cells, which are in perivascular regions, neoplastic plasma

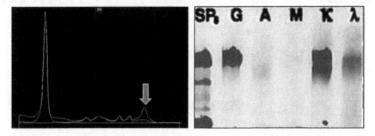

Figure 29.1 Serum protein electrophoresis (SPEP) with immunosubtraction shows a monoclonal spike (M-spike) in the gamma region measuring 0.6 g/dL (Left Panel). Immunofixation (IFE) demonstrates an IgG (kappa) monoclonal gammopathy (Right Panel).

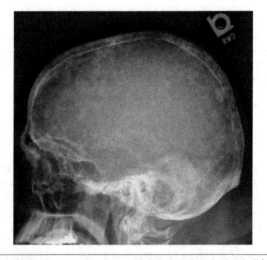

Figure 29.2 Skeletal survey showing multiple lytic lesions in the skull (arrows).

cells form clusters, large aggregates, or sheets. Neoplastic plasma cells have a spectrum of morphologies. They are typically oval with a round, eccentrically located nucleus; characteristic "clock-face" chromatin; and an abundant basophilic cytoplasm with a perinuclear "hof" (clearing zone containing the Golgi apparatus). Occasionally, plasma cells with cytoplasmic (Russell bodies) or nuclear (Dutcher bodies) inclusions are identified (representing excess production of immunoglobulin). Malignant plasma cells are typically CD138+, CD38+, CD79a+, or CD19−, with aberrant CD56+ in most cases.

INTERNATIONAL MYELOMA WORKING GROUP (IMWG) DIAGNOSTIC CRITERIA 2014[1]

Clonal BM plasma cells ≥10% or biopsy-proven bony or extramedullary plasmacytoma **AND** any one or more of the following myeloma defining events and CRAB features:

1. Evidence of end-organ damage that can be attributed to the underlying plasma-cell proliferative disorder:
   a. Anemia: Hemoglobin <10 g/dL, or >2 g/dL below baseline
   b. Renal insufficiency: Glomerular filtration rate (GFR) <40 mL/min or serum creatinine (Cr) >2.0 mg/dL
   c. Bone lesion: One or more osteolytic lesions on skeletal radiography, CT, or PET-CT scan
   d. Hypercalcemia: Serum-corrected calcium >11 mg/dL or >1 mg/dL higher than the upper limit of normal
1. **OR any one or more of the following biomarkers of malignancy (MDEs)** predicting a high rate of progression to symptomatic disease:
1. Clonal BM plasma cell percentage ≥ 60%
2. Serum-involved-to-uninvolved SFLC ratio ≥100 (involved free light chain level must be ≥ 100 mg/L)
3. >1 focal lesion on MRI (at least 5 mm in size)

Note that for patients with MDE as the sole indication of therapy, systemic therapy can be considered after a careful discussion with the patient regarding risks, as the benefits of early therapy have not been conclusively demonstrated.

▓ KEY DIAGNOSTIC DILEMMA

The differential diagnosis for a patient presenting with a newly identified monoclonal gammopathy includes monoclonal gammopathy of undetermined significance (MGUS), smoldering myeloma (SM), symptomatic MM, Waldenström macroglobulinemia (WM), and immunoglobulin light chain amyloidosis (AL). Lytic lesions should be biopsied to exclude metastatic carcinoma before a diagnosis of nonsecretory myeloma is made in patients with no M protein in the serum or urine.

▓ PROGNOSIS

The Revised International Staging System (R-ISS) incorporates the original ISS criteria (based on serum albumin and B2M), high-risk FISH abnormalities, and serum LDH (Table 29.1).[2] Specific cytogenetic features have been associated with effects on prognosis. One primary dichotomy that differentially affects outcomes is hyperdiploid and non-hyperdiploid subtypes; hyperdiploid MM, characterized by numerous chromosomal trisomies typically involving chromosomes 3, 5, 7, 9, 11,

Table 29.1 R-ISS Staging for MM

R-ISS Stage	Criteria	OS
I	ISS stage I and standard-risk FISH and normal LDH	Median NR, 5-year OS 82%
II	Not R-ISS stage I or III	Median 83 months, 5-year OS 62%
III	ISS stage III and either high-risk FISH or LDH > ULN	Median 43 months, 5-year OS 40%

FISH, fluorescence in situ hybridization; LDH, lactate dehydrogenase; MM, multiple myeloma; NR, not reached; OS, overall survival; R-ISS, revised international staging system; ULN, upper limit of normal.

Definitions: ISS stage I: B2M <3.5 mg/L and serum albumin ≥3.5 g/dL; ISS stage II not I or III; ISS stage III: B2M ≥5.5 mg/L; high-risk FISH: del(17p), t(4;14), or t(14;16).

Source: Palumbo A, Avet-Loiseau H, Oliva S, et al. Revised International Staging System for multiple myeloma: a report from International Myeloma Working Group. *J Clin Oncol.* 2015;33(26):2863–2869.

15, 19, and 21 and a low prevalence of IgH translocations, confers a favorable prognosis. However, hyperdiploidy with gain of 1q or loss of chromosome 13 has been associated with a poorer prognosis. Another important cytogenetic factor conferring poor prognosis is deletion 17p13, the locus of the p53 tumor-suppressor gene. Deletions of 17p13 are associated with shorter overall survival (OS) rates, more aggressive disease, higher prevalence of extramedullary disease (such as plasmacytomas), and hypercalcemia. It also predicts a short duration of response after transplant and involvement of the central nervous system. 12p deletion, which occurs in about 12% of patients, is associated with both a short event-free survival and short OS, likely related to the decreased expression of CD27. A number of other genetic abnormalities demonstrate conflicting data: Chromosome 13 monosomy or deletions were thought to be associated with a worse prognosis, similar to deletion 13 by metaphase analysis, but the poor prognosis is likely due to its close association with other high-risk genetic features. Similarly, some reports have shown chromosome 1 abnormalities, specifically 1q21+ and deletion of 1p, to be independent adverse prognostic factors (*Leukemia.* 2009;23(12):2210–2221). Other high-risk features include circulating plasma cells or high-risk gene-expression profiles (e.g., GEP70).[3]

▓ MONITORING

Response to therapy is assessed using the International Myeloma Working Group uniform response criteria (see Table 29.2 for response criteria). Recently, the assessment of minimal residual disease (MRD) has become crucial to assessing treatment effectiveness, as the depth of response is correlated to survival. MRD may be detected by Ig allele-specific oligonucleotide-based quantitative polymerase chain

Table 29.2 IMWG Response Criteria for MM

Response	Serum SPEP	Serum IFE	24-hr UPEP	Urine IFE	Involved and Uninvolved SFLC Difference*	BM Plasma cell Percentage	BM IHC and/or Flow Cytometry	Plasmacytoma
CR	(−)	(−)	(−)	(−)	Normal	≤5%	(+)	Disappearance
sCR	(−)	(−)	(−)	(−)	Normal	≤5% and not clonal	(−)	Disappearance
VGPR	(−) or ≥90% decrease	(+)	≤100 mg/24h	(+)	≥90% decrease	NA	(+)	NA
PR	≥50% decrease	(+)	≥90% decrease or ≤200 mg/24h	(+)	≥50% decrease	≥50% decrease	(+)	≥50% reduction
PD (at least one of the following)	≥25% increase and at least 0.5 g/dL increase	(+)	≥25% increase and ≥200 mg/24 h increase	(+)	≥25% increase and an absolute increase of 100 mg/L	≥25% increase	(+)	New or increase in size of existing plasmacytomas

BM, bone marrow; CR, complete response; IFE, immunofixation; IHC, immunohistochemistry; IMWG, International Myeloma Working Group; MM, multiple myeloma; PD; progressive disease; PR, partial response; sCR, stringent complete response; SFLC, serum-free light chains; SPEP, serum protein electrophoresis; VGPR, very good partial response; UPEP, urine protein electrophoresis.

*sFLC is used to monitor disease in patients who don't have a "measurable" M-spike in the serum (≥1 g/dL) and urine (≥200 mg/24 h), provided that the involved sFLC is ≥100 mg/L and the ratio is abnormal.

Source: Durie BG, Harousseau JL, Miguel JS, et al. International uniform response criteria for multiple myeloma. *Leukemia.* 2006;20(9):1467–1473.

reaction (ASO-PCR), multiparameter flow cytometry (MFC), or NGS. ASO-PCR utilizes the unique junctional sequences resulting from rearrangements of germ-line V, (D), and J gene segments in the Ig gene complexes (IGH, IGK, and IGL) to identify a detectable signature with which to establish MRD. While this approach is sensitive, with the ability to detect down to 1 in 10^5 to 10^6 malignant cells, it is time-consuming and not reliably reproducible due to somatic hypermutation of functional V(D)J exons. Highly sensitive MFC, utilizing the simultaneous assessment of ≥ 8 markers, allows for the characterization and identification of a high number of plasma cells based on both cell surface and intracellular antigens within a few hours, down to 1 in 10^5 malignant cells. This fast and cost-effective method takes advantage of the highly conserved plasma-cell maturation process to identify aberrant plasma-cell phenotypes without requiring patient-specific diagnostic phenotypic profiles; however, it may miss MM cancer stem cells with immature phenotypes. Next-generation flow (NGF) using an optimized 2-tube 8-color antibody panel for highly sensitive (close to 10^{-6}) MRD detection has been standardized by EuroFlow/International Myeloma Foundation (IMF). Similar to ASO-PCR, high-throughput screening (HTS) and NGS using multiplex primer sets to detect all potential rearrangements of antigen receptor genes has been applied to the detection of clonal Ig gene rearrangements to define MRD, with a sensitivity of 1 in 10^6 malignant cells. However, like PCR, NGS also requires a characteristic diagnostic sample, and detection may be hampered by somatic hypermutation. In addition, quantitation of MRD is highly variable, as the defined clonal rearrangements must be detected between polyclonal Ig rearrangements derived from the remaining normal B-cells of varying frequency. NGS has not yet been standardized and lacks regular quality-assurance monitoring. Persistence of MRD as measured by MFC or NGS has been identified as an adverse prognostic feature and validated as a surrogate for PFS or OS in clinical trials, although currently no specific changes in therapy are recommended based on MRD status (*Blood*. 2015 May 14;125(20):3059–3068).

■ TREATMENT

Outcomes for patients with MM have improved with the development of novel agents, including immunomodulatory drugs (IMiDs) and proteasome inhibitors and higher use of autologous hematopoietic stem cell transplantation (auto-HSCT) with median OS of >7 years for patients with standard-risk disease and median OS of approximately 3 years for those with high-risk disease.[4] Despite these gains, MM remains incurable; relapsed disease has been proposed to be mediated by clonal heterogeneity of MM with the emergence of subclonal populations undetectable at diagnosis that may be selected by treatment, differentially proliferative capacity, or BM niche microenvironment or induced by newly acquired mutations in myeloma drivers

(*Leukemia*. 2018;32(12):2636–2647). The presence of a second MGUS has also been described, occurring in up to 6% of people with plasma cell dyscrasias, or up to 24% to 29.8% of patients undergoing autologous stem cell transplant, that may confer a survival advantage, especially in post-transplant patients with prolonged latency periods (>10 months) (*Biol Blood Marrow Transplant*. 2014;20(3):319–325; *Bone Marrow Transplant*. 2012;47(9):1212–1216). Current treatment strategies have focused on driving down disease burden with multiagent regimens, while attempting to minimize toxicity. High-dose therapy (Melphalan 200 mg/m^2) and autologous stem cell transplant continues to play a crucial role, and evidence suggests that continuous and/or maintenance therapy may result in improved survival (*J Clin Oncol*. 2015;33(30):3459–3466).

NEWLY DIAGNOSED MULTIPLE MYELOMA (NDMM)

Three-drug induction regimens result in deep and prolonged responses when compared to those seen with two-drug regimens, as noted by significantly higher rates of CR and VGPR when comparing bortezomib-thalidomide-dexamethasone versus thalidomide-dexamethasone (74% vs. 58%, *p* = .02; *Blood*. 2011;118(22):5752–5758) and similarly noted improved responses in the SWOG S0777 trial, in which patients in the bortezomib-lenalidomide-dexamethasone group noted an overall response rate (partial response or better) of 81.5% vs. 17.5% in the lenalidomide-dexamethasone group (*p* = .02) (*Lancet*. 2017;389(10068):519–527). Several prospective randomized trials have shown that these improvements translate into an OS benefit (*Lancet*. 2017;389(10068):519–527). The introduction of daratumumab, an anti-CD38 monoclonal antibody, has been shown to improve depth of response and progression-free survival (PFS). However, patient comorbidities, tolerability, and prognosis must be considered when determining a treatment regimen. Common first-line induction regimens in the United States include the following:

YOUNG AND FIT PATIENTS

1. Lenalidomide-bortezomib-dexamethasone (VRd): Improved OS (75 months in the VRd group vs. 64 months in the Rd group, HR 0·709, 95% CI 0·524–0·959; two-sided *p* value .025) and PFS (43 months in the VRd group vs. 30 months in the Rd group; stratified hazard ratio [HR] 0·712, 96% Confidence Interval (CI) 0·56–0·906; one-sided *p* value .0018) was seen for VRd versus Rd in the SWOG S0777 trial (*Lancet*. 2017;389(10068):519–527). Additional support for IMID-based combinations comes from the IFM2013-14 study, which demonstrated superior responses for VTD as compared to VCD, with 66.3% of the patients in the VTD arm achieving at least a VGPR vs. 56.2% in the VCD arm (*p* = .05) prior to high-dose chemotherapy and auto-HSCT in NDMM (*Blood*. 2016;127(21):2569–2574). Lenalidomide requires dose adjustment for renal dysfunction.

2. Bortezomib-cyclophosphamide-dexamethasone (VCD-modified, a.k.a. CyBorD): (EVOLUTION trial; *Blood.* 2012 May 10;119(19):4375–4382). VCD-modified (with cyclophosphamide delivered on days 1, 8, and 15) led to an overall response rate (ORR) of 100%, with rates of VGPR or better observed in 53% of patients. This regimen shows that VCD has significant activity with high rates of deep responses comparable to VRD (although the study was not powered for direct comparison), does not require renal dosing, and may be easier to administer if a response is needed quickly (e.g., acute renal insufficiency). Subcutaneous and/or weekly dosing of bortezomib offers similar activity with less peripheral neuropathy.

3. Carfilzomib-lenalidomide-dexamethasone (KRD): The FORTE trial revealed greater depth of response to the second-generation proteasome inhibitor carfilzomib in KRD over carfilzomib-cyclophosphamide-dexamethasone (KCD), with higher rates of ≥VGPR of 88% with KRd and 74% with KCD (p = .002) (*Blood.* 2018;132(Suppl1):121), and significantly increased rates of MRD negativity after four cycles of KRd therapy (56% compared to four cycles of KCD of 30%). This is recommended in young patients with high-risk cytogenetics and especially patients with pre-existing neuropathy. The ENDURANCE trial comparing KRd to VRd initial therapy did not show superior PFS in newly diagnosed standard- or intermediate-risk MM (mPFS 34.6 mos for KRd vs 34.4 mos for RVd, with HR = KRd/VRd in a stratified analysis of 1.04 (95% CI = 0.83–1.31, P = .742), but it does not include high-risk patients. More severe cardiac, pulmonary and renal toxicities were observed with carfilzomib, while neuropathy was more common in those receiving bortezomib (*Lancet.* 2020 Oct;21(10):1317–1330).

4. Daratumumab: The addition of daratumumab to bortezomib-thalidomide-dexamethasone (VTD) (CASSIOPIEA; *Lancet.* 2019; 394(10192):29–38) and lenalidomide-bortezomib-dexamethasone (GRIFFIN; ASH. 2018 Nov 21. Abstract #151) compared to the respective three-drug regimens has shown improved depth of response, higher rates of MRD negativity and, in the case of the CASSIOPIEA trial, significantly improved PFS (median PFS rate at 18 months was 92.7% with daratumumab vs. 84.6% without [HR, 0.47; 95% CI, 0.33–0.67; p < .0001]). In the United States, however, the VTD backbone is not commonly used.

OLDER OR FRAIL PATIENTS

1. Lenalidomide-dexamethasone (RD): Continuous RD resulted in superior PFS and OS compared to melphalan-prednisone-thalidomide (MPT) among transplant-ineligible patients in the FIRST trial (*N Engl J Med.* 2014;371(10):906–917). Dose reduction may be required for elderly/frail patients.

2. Bortezomib-dexamethasone (VD): Neither bortezomib-melphalan-prednisone (VMP) nor bortezomib-thalidomide-dexamethasone

(VTD) was superior to VD alone in the UPFRONT trial of transplant-ineligible patients, with no significant difference in mPFS at median follow-up of 42.7 months (14.7, 15.4, and 17.3 months with VD, VTD, and VMP, respectively) or mOS (49.8, 51.5, and 53 months for VD, VTD, and VMP, respectively) (*J Clin Oncol.* 2015; 33(33):3921–3929).

3. Melphalan no longer appears necessary in the management of older patients: As stated earlier, trials have demonstrated that VD is equivalent to VMP, with no significant difference in mPFS (14, 16, and 16 months in the VP, VCP, and VMP group, respectively) or 1-year OS that was observed in 80%, 82%, and 80% of patients 75 or older in the VP, VCP, and VMP groups, respectively (*Blood.* 2013;122(21):539).

4. Daratumumab: Similar to use in transplant-eligible patients, the addition of daratumumab to bortezomib-melphalan-prednisone (VMP) in the ALCYONE trial (*N Engl J Med.* 2018;378:518–528) and RD in the MAIA trial (*N Engl J Med.* 2019;380:2104–2115) compared to respective comparator arms led to deeper responses, higher rates of MRD negativity, and significantly improved mPFS and mOS. In the ALCYONE trial, the mPFS was not reached (95% CI, could not be estimated) in the daratumumab group versus 18.1 months (95% CI, 16.5 to 19.9) in the control group ($p < 0.001$). Similarly, in the MAIA trial, mPFS was not reached in the daratumumab group and was 31.9 months (95% CI, 28.9 to not reached) in the control group. However, the VMP backbone is not commonly used. While the addition of daratumumab doesn't seem to add much to the toxicity profile of RD, it does add to the inconvenience, given the requirements for parenteral administration.

FRAILTY

Several tools are currently available to assess frailty, including that of the IMWG, which has been correlated with survival, treatment discontinuation, and non-hematologic toxicity. However, while several of these tools provide prognostic information, chronological age automatically increases frailty without taking biologic or functional age into account. Mian et al. have developed an updated index of frailty based on the accumulation of aging-associated deficits rather than on chronological age alone (*JCO Clin Cancer Inform.* 2018;2:CCI.18.00043). The deficit-accumulation frailty index (DAFI) includes 25 variables related to health, function, and activities of daily living; each incremental increase in the DAFI was found to correlate to an increased risk of death and serve as a better predictor of adverse outcomes. This tool allows clinicians to more safely assess and recommend appropriate treatment regimens.

SUPPORTIVE CARE

- Patients receiving IMiDs require appropriate risk assessment of venous thromboembolism and prophylaxis with aspirin if lower/ standard risk. Low molecular weight heparin (LMWH), warfarin with target International Normalized Ratio (INR) of 2 to 3, or a direct oral anticoagulant (DOAC), such as apixaban, should be considered for high-risk patients.[5]

- Patients receiving proteasome inhibitors or monoclonal antibodies require herpes zoster prophylaxis with acyclovir or equivalent for the duration of administration, although it may be discontinued 3 months following discontinuation of proteasome inhibitor.

- The TEAMM study recently showed prophylaxis with levofloxacin 500 mg orally once daily significantly reduced the risk of febrile episodes and death in patients receiving treatment for newly diagnosed MM (*Lancet Oncol.* 2019;20(12):1760–1772).

- All patients with adequate renal function should receive bisphosphonates (zoledronic acid preferred) based on improved OS seen in the MRC IX trial (*Lancet.* 2010;376(9757):1989). Patients with impaired renal function could receive denosumab (*Lancet Oncol.* 2018;19(3):370). The optimal frequency is yet to be defined, but every 3 months is recommended for patients without bone disease and those who have completed a few years of therapy, whereas monthly antiresorptive therapy is indicated for most patients. Patients in sustained complete response (CR) could potentially discontinue such therapy.

- Patients should be up to date on influenza, shingles, and pneumococcal vaccinations.

FRONTLINE CONSOLIDATION

High-dose therapy and autologous stem cell transplant continue to play roles in the treatment of MM (*N Engl J Med.* 2014;371(10):895). Per the IFM/DFCI 2009 DETERMINATION trial, transplant-eligible patients randomized to receive induction therapy with three cycles of RVD followed by high-dose melphalan and auto-HSCT versus 5 additional cycles of RVD experienced improved PFS and deeper responses; however, it did not lead to a significant difference in OS, although follow-up is limited. Transplant-eligible patients should have stem cells collected after 4–6 cycles of induction therapy. Patients may then proceed directly to high-dose therapy and autologous transplant. Moreau et al. have shown that myeloablative conditioning with melphalan 200 mg/m^2 confers a survival advantage, with a 45-month survival of 65.8%, as compared to nonmyeloablative conditioning with melphalan 140 mg/m^2 and 8 Gy TBI, with a 45-month survival of 45.5% (p = .05)(*Blood.* 2002;99(3):731–735). Given that newer regimens are providing deeper, more durable responses, one may defer transplant until first relapse, especially if the patient achieves an excellent response. The StaMINA trial was a phase 3 trial that revealed that tandem auto-HSCT or auto-HSCT followed by RVD consolidation did not provide a PFS or OS benefit compared to single auto-HSCT and lenalidomide maintenance (*J Clin Oncol.* 2019;37(7):589–597). The role of allogeneic transplant in high-risk and/or refractory patients is considered investigational, with no difference in PFS or OS compared to single or tandem auto-HSCT and increased rates of treatment-related mortality (TRM) and graft-versus-host disease (GVHD).

MAINTENANCE

Post-transplant maintenance therapy with lenalidomide improves PFS and improves OS, based on a meta-analysis (*N Engl J Med.* 2012;366:1770–1781). Bortezomib-based maintenance regimens have also been evaluated, with a suggestion of favorable PFS in high-risk patients (*J Clin Oncol.* 2012;30(24):2946). Ixazomib maintenance does improve PFS, but the magnitude of the benefit is limited (*N Engl J Med.* 2016;374(17):1621–1634).

RELAPSED REFRACTORY MULTIPLE MYELOMA (RRMM)

The selection of regimens must take into account the pattern of relapse: slow versus indolent, symptomatic versus biochemical, high risk versus standard risk, prior therapies, and patient preference. Despite the availability of many therapeutic options, clinical trials should be considered whenever possible. In the early relapsed setting, the following regimens have demonstrated superiority over lenalidomide and dexamethasone alone:

- Carfilzomib-lenalidomide-dexamethasone (ASPIRE, *N Engl J Med.* 2015;372(2):142).
- Elotuzumab-lenalidomide-dexamethasone (ELOQUENT-2, *N Engl J Med.* 2015;373(7):621).
- Ixazomib-lenalidomide-dexamethasone (TOURMALINE-MM1, *N Engl J Med.* 2016;374(17):1621–1634).
- Daratumumab-lenalidomide-dexamethasone (POLLUX, *N Engl J Med.* 2016;375(14):1319–1331).

For patients who have already progressed on >2 prior lines of therapy, pomalidomide-dexamethasone (PD) has become the standard backbone. Subsequent trials have shown the benefit of pomalidomide-containing triplet therapies, such as pomalidomide-cyclophosphamide-dexamethasone (PCD), with improved response rates and mPFS of 9.5 months with PCD compared to 4.4 months with PD ($p = .106$), although this was not statistically significant, as the study was powered to evaluate ORR (*Blood.* 2016;127(21):2561–2568). Other pomalidomide-containing triplets, such as daratumumab-pomalidomide-dexamethasone (DPD) and carfilzomib-pomalidomide-dexamethasone (KPD), have also shown benefits in phase I/II trials.

Carfilzomib demonstrated superior response and PFS to bortezomib in a prospective randomized trial of previously treated patients, with mPFS of 18.7 months in the carfilzomib group versus 9.7 in the bortezomib group ($p < .0001$) (ENDEAVOR, *Lancet Oncol.* 2016;17(1):27). Ixazomib offers the convenience of oral administration, but its activity has not been directly compared to that of bortezomib or carfilzomib.

Elotuzumab is a humanized monoclonal antibody targeted against signaling lymphocytic activation molecule F7 (SLAMF7), a glycoprotein expressed on myeloma and natural killer cells, that was evaluated in the ELOQUENT trials in combination with RD and PD and showed improved PFS compared to the respective doublet regimens, with mPFS of 19.4 months in the elotuzumab group versus 14.9 with lenalidomide-dexamethasone in ELOQUENT-2 (*N Engl J Med*. 2015;373:621–631) and mPFS of 10.3 months in the elotuzumab group versus 4.7 months with PD in ELOQUENT-3 (*N Engl J Med*. 2018;379:1811–1822).

Panobinostat is a pan-histone deacetylase (HDAC) inhibitor without significant single-agent activity. However, the PANORAMA1 trial revealed improved PFS with panobinostat-bortezomib-dexamethasone over bortezomib-dexamethasone alone (*Blood*. 2016;127(6):713–721). The triplet therapy was associated with increased rates of diarrhea and thrombocytopenia.

Selinexor, an oral selective inhibitor of the nuclear exporter protein Exportin 1 was evaluated in the STORM trial in combination with dexamethasone in patients with triple-class refractory disease (proteasome inhibitors, IMiDs, and an anti-CD38 monoclonal antibody) and found to have an overall response rate of 26%, with mPFS of 3.7 months and mOS of 8.6 months, in this single-arm study (*N Engl J Med*. 2019;381:727–738). This agent is associated with significant gastrointestinal GI toxicity (nausea, diarrhea), thrombocytopenia, fatigue, and hyponatremia.

▧ FUTURE THERAPIES

There are several promising emerging targeted therapies currently being evaluated in clinical trials.

Venetoclax is a potent, selective oral small molecule *BCL-2* inhibitor that was found to have a response rate of 40% in patients with t(11,14). A high response rate was noted in combination with bortezomib in unselected patients, which led to the BELLINI trial, a phase 3 trial of venetoclax-bortezomib-dexamethasone versus bortezomib-dexamethasone in RRMM, which demonstrated an improvement in PFS. This trial was suspended due to an increased number of deaths observed in the venetoclax arm compared to the control; a subgroup analysis of patients with t(11,14) revealed an ORR of 90% versus 47% in the total treated population, with improved rates of MRD negativity and PFS (Kumar S. *EHA Library*. 2019;273254; LB2601) without excess mortality in that subset of patients.

Another promising agent is isatuximab, a CD38 monoclonal antibody; the ICARIA-MM phase 3 trial evaluated isatuximab-pomalidomide-dexamethasone versus PD in RRMM, resulting in a PFS advantage, with mPFS of 11.5 months in the isatuximab-pomalidomide-dexamethasone group versus 6.5 months in the PD group (HR 0·596, 95% CI 0·44–0·81; p = .001) (*Lancet*. 2019;394(10214):2096–2107).

Other exciting emerging options include therapies targeting B-cell maturation antigen (BCMA); chimeric antigen receptor T-cells (CAR-T) targeting BCMA, such as bb2121 (*N Engl J Med.* 2019;380:1726–1737); antibody-drug conjugates (ADC), such as belantamab mafodotin, a humanized anti-BCMA antibody that is conjugated to monomethyl auristatin-F, a microtubule disrupting agent (*Lancet Oncol.* 2020; 21(2):207–221); and bi-specific T-cell engagers (BiTE), such as CC93269, targeting BCMA and CD3 (ASH. 2019 Dec 7. Abstract #143). Another promising therapeutic includes a novel class of drugs such as peptidase-enhanced compounds including Melflufen that exploits the increased aminopeptidase activity of malignant cells (*Lancet Haematol.* 2020 May;7(5):e395–e407).

▓ REFERENCES FOR SUPPLEMENTAL READING

1. Rajkumar SV, Dimopoulos MA, Palumbo A, et al. International Myeloma Working Group updated criteria for the diagnosis of multiple myeloma. *Lancet Oncol.* 2014;15(12):e538–e548.

2. Palumbo A, Avet-Loiseau H, Oliva S, et al. Revised International Staging System for multiple myeloma: a report from International Myeloma Working Group. *J Clin Oncol.* 2015;33(26):2863–2869.

3. Chang WJ, Dispenzieri A, Chim CS, et al. IMWG consensus on risk stratification in multiple myeloma. *Leukemia.* 2014;28(2):269–277.

4. Rajkumar SV. Multiple myeloma: 2018 update on diagnosis, risk-stratification, and management. *Am J Hematol.* 2018;93(8):1091–1110.

5. Palumbo A, Rajkumar VS, Dimopoulos MA, et al. Prevention of thalidomide and lenalidomide-associated thrombosis in myeloma. *Leukemia.* 2008;22(2):414–423.

30 Waldenström Macroglobulinemia

Ariel Grajales-Cruz and Rachid Baz

▣ INTRODUCTION

Waldenström macroglobulinemia (WM) is an uncommon lymphoproliferative disorder characterized by bone marrow (BM) infiltration with lymphoplasmacytic lymphoma (LPL) cells producing monoclonal immunoglobulin M (IgM). The median age at diagnosis is 70 years, with a Caucasian male predominance (60%). WM is very rare in African Americans (5%). Although the etiology of WM is unknown, an association with autoimmune disorders, infections, and exposures to pesticides has been suggested. Familial predisposition can be seen in about 20% of patients who have a first-degree relative with WM or another clonal B-cell disorder. Familial WM is usually diagnosed at an earlier age, with greater BM involvement. WM is a subtype of LPL; however, the majority of LPL occurs as WM where LPL is characterized as a B-cell neoplasm composed of small lymphocytes, plasmacytoid lymphocytes, and plasma cells involving the BM, with variable involvement of lymph nodes and/or spleen.

▣ DIAGNOSIS

Prior to initiating treatment, patients must undergo studies to confirm the diagnosis and establish the extent of the disease, the presence of associated conditions, and their performance status. Laboratory investigations should include a complete blood count (CBC) with differential, complete metabolic panel (CMP), serum protein electrophoresis (SPEP) with immunofixation, and serum viscosity (usually obtained in patients who have signs and symptoms of hyperviscosity). A contrast-enhanced computed tomography (CT) scan of the chest, abdomen, and pelvis or positron emission tomography/computed tomography (PET/CT) scan should be obtained for staging. In addition, a BM aspiration and biopsy with flow cytometry, cytogenetic analysis, and fluorescence in situ hybridization (FISH) studies should be performed if possible. Molecular analysis (by conventional Sanger or next-generation sequencing) for *MYD88* L265P and *CXCR4* mutations can be performed for diagnostic and prognostic purposes (see the following). Additional testing may be warranted based on the presentation, including evaluation for cryoglobulins, cold agglutinins, myelin-associated glycoprotein (MAG) antibodies, and amyloidosis.

In patients with WM, multiple myeloma, and monoclonal gammopathy of unknown significance (MGUS), the neuropathy is usually demyelinating with sensory involvement. Physical examination and electromyography are helpful in differentiating from other causes, such as amyloidosis and POEMS.

According to the Waldenström Study Group, the diagnostic criteria for WM are:

- IgM monoclonal protein of any concentration
- BM infiltration by small lymphocytes showing plasmacytoid/plasma cell differentiation (usually intertrabecular and >10% involvement)
- Immunophenotype: sIgM+, CD5−/+, CD10−, CD19+, CD20+, CD22+, CD23−, CD25+, CD27+, FMC7+, CD103−, CD138−

Importantly, the presence of B-cells with lymphoplasmacytic differentiation or IgM paraprotein is not diagnostic of WM. The differential diagnosis of WM includes marginal zone lymphoma with plasmacytic differentiation, as some of those patients may present with IgM paraproteinemia, which may be difficult to distinguish from WM (see Chapter 44). IgM-secreting myeloma can be distinguished by IgH translocations (e.g., 11;14 or 4;14) and/or the presence of bone disease. IgM MGUS is associated with <10% BM involvement and absence of end-organ damage (see Chapters 28 and 29). More recently, *MYD88* L265P mutation was found in >90% of patients with WM (91% of LPL patients), a subset of active B-cell (ABC) type-diffuse large B-cell lymphoma, and was rarely present in other mature B-cell neoplasms, such as IgM myeloma or marginal zone lymphoma (*N Engl J Med*. 2012;367:826–833). While the *MYD88* mutation can be noted in some MGUS cases, there are data to suggest a higher likelihood of progression to WM. Symptoms can be related to the lymphoplasmacytic infiltrate or to the production of the IgM paraprotein. The most common presenting symptom is anemia due to BM infiltration. Additional symptoms associated with tumor infiltration include other cytopenias, constitutional symptoms, lymphadenopathy, and organomegaly. IgM paraproteinemia may result in hyperviscocity (up to 30% of patients), cryoglobulinemia, cold agglutinin disease, amyloidosis, or neuropathy. Interestingly, about 20% of WM patients have cryoglobulinemia, but only 5% are symptomatic (Raynaud disease, skin ulcers, necrosis, and cold urticaria). Neuropathy can occur as a result of paraprotein deposition, MAG antibodies, and/or amyloidosis. IgM paraproteins can also deposit in extranodal sites, such as the skin, gastrointestinal tract, and kidney. Large-cell transformation and secondary myelodysplastic syndrome/acute myeloid leukemia occur in a low percentage of patients with WM (approximately 5%) and are associated with nucleoside analogs treatment. Bing–Neel syndrome is an extremely rare neurologic complication of WM and is associated with lymphoplasmacytoid infiltration of the central nervous system (CNS). In these cases, cranial radiation therapy with intrathecal

Table 30.1 ISSWM

ISSWM			
Risk Factors		1. Age >65 Years	
		2. Hemoglobin <11.5 g/dL	
		3. Platelet count <100 × 10⁹/L	
		4. Beta 2 microglobulin >3 mg/L	
		5. M protein >7 g/dL	
Risk Category	**Definition**	**Distribution (%)**	**5-Year Survival (%)**
Low	0–1 Risk factors	27	87
Intermediate	2 Risk factors or age >65	38	68
High	>2 Risk factors	35	36

IPSSWM, International Prognostic Scoring System for Waldenström macroglobulinemia; M protein, monoclonal protein; WM, Waldenström macroglobulinemia.

Source: Morel M, Duhamel A, Gobbi P, et al. International prognostic scoring system for Waldenström macroglobulinemia. *Blood.* 2009;30;113(18):4163–4170.

chemotherapy is more likely to result in sustainable remission (*CLML.* 2009;9:462–466), although a recent report of treatment with ibrutinib by Castillo et al. suggests good efficacy (*Blood.* 2019;133(4):299–305).

▓ PROGNOSIS

Although WM is typically an indolent disease, considerable variability in prognosis can be seen. Median overall survival (OS) ranges between 5 and 10 years, although more contemporary numbers are likely better. The International Prognostic Scoring System for WM (ISSWM) is used to define three risk groups and has been externally validated through independent cohorts (Table 30.1), although it currently does not affect treatment decisions (*Blood.* 2009;30;113(18):4163–4170). Similar to other lymphoid malignancies, serum lactate dehydrogenase (LDH) is associated with higher tumor burden and more aggressive behavior, suggesting that LDH is an adverse prognostic factor for patients with WM (*Leuk Res.* 2010;34(10):1340–1343).

▓ TREATMENT

Few randomized trials have been conducted for WM, and most recommendations are based on small phase 2 studies with variable patient populations as well as some phase 3 studies. Accordingly, there is often limited evidence to support the treatment recommendations that follow. In general, assessment of responses relies on serial measurements of the paraprotein as well as evaluation of the BM biopsy (Table 30.2). WM remains an incurable disease with current therapies, and there is no evidence that treatment of asymptomatic patients provides a survival advantage. Approximately a quarter of patients with

Table 30.2 Updated Response Criteria from the 6th International Workshop on WM

Response Assessment in Patients With WM	
CR	• IgM in normal range and disappearance of monoclonal protein by immunofixation • No histologic evidence of BM involvement • Resolution of any adenopathy/organomegaly (if present at baseline), along with no signs or symptoms attributable to WM • Reconfirmation of the CR status is required by repeat immunofixation studies
VGPR	• A ≥90% reduction in serum IgM and resolution of any adenopathy/organomegaly (if present at baseline) on physical examination or on CT scan • No new symptoms or signs of active disease
PR	• A ≥50% reduction in serum IgM and decrease in adenopathy/organomegaly (if present at baseline) on physical examination or on CT scan • No new symptoms or signs of active disease
MR	• A ≥25% but ≤50% reduction in serum IgM • No new symptoms or signs of active disease
SD	• A <25% reduction and <25% increase in serum IgM without progression of adenopathy/organomegaly, cytopenias, or clinically significant symptoms due to disease and/or signs of WM.
PD	• A ≥25% increase in serum IgM by protein confirmed by a second measurement or progression of clinically significant findings due to disease (i.e., anemia, thrombocytopenia, leukopenia, bulky adenopathy/organomegaly) or symptoms (unexplained recurrent fever ≥38.4°C, drenching night sweats, ≥10% body weight loss, or hyperviscosity, neuropathy, symptomatic cryoglobulinemia, or amyloidosis) attributable to WM

BM, bone marrow; CR, complete response; CT, computed tomography; IgM, immunoglobulin M; MR, minor response; PD, progressive disease; PR, partial response; SD, stable disease; VGPR, very good partial response; WM, Waldenström macroglobulinemia.

Source: Owen RG, Kyle RA, Stone MJ, et al. Response assessment in Waldenström macroglobulinaemia: update from the VIth International Workshop. *Br J Haematol.* 2013;160(2):171:6.

WM fall into the category of smoldering Waldenström macroglobulinemia (SWM) and therefore should not be treated (*Br J Haematol.* 2019:184(6):1014). Independent risk factors, such as BM lymphoplasmacytic infiltration ≥70%, serum IgM ≥4,500 mg/dl, β2-microglogulin ≥4 mg/dl, and albumin ≤3.5 g/dl, were associated with a ≥60% probability of disease progression within 2 years and therefore identified asymptomatic patients who were more likely to require therapy (*J Clin Oncol.* 2019;37(16):1403–1411). Indications for treatment should be based on symptoms and not the absolute IgM levels according to the Eighth International Workshop on WM (IWWM-8) consensus

Table 30.3 Guidelines for Initiation of Therapy in Patients With WM (IWWM-8 Consensus)

Clinical Indications for Initiation of Therapy

- Recurrent fever, night sweats, weight loss, or fatigue
- Lymphadenopathy that is either symptomatic or bulky (≥5 cm in maximum diameter)
- Symptomatic hepatomegaly and/or splenomegaly
- Symptomatic organomegaly and/or organ or tissue infiltration
- Peripheral neuropathy due to WM
- Hyperviscosity

Laboratory Indications for Initiation of Therapy

- Symptomatic dryoglobulinemia
- Cold agglutinin disease
- Immune hemolytic anemia and/or thrombocytopenia
- Neuropathy related to WM
- Amyloidosis related to WM
- Hemoglobin ≤10 g/dL
- Platelet count <100 × 10^9/L

WM, Waldenström macroglobulinemia.

Source: Dimopoulos MA, Kastritis E, Owen RG, et. al. Treatment recommendations for patients with Waldenström macroglobulinemia (WM) and related disorders: IWWM-7 consensus. *Blood.* 2014;124(9):1404–1411.

guidelines. Constitutional symptoms, progressive lymphadenopathy, organomegaly, symptomatic anemia, and certain complications of WM, such as hyperviscosity syndrome, symptomatic sensorimotor peripheral neuropathy, or symptomatic cryoglobulinemia, are all possible indications for therapy (see Table 30.3). First-line agent choice should depend on individual patient considerations, including the need for rapid disease control, comorbidities/age, and presence of cytopenias, hyperviscosity symptoms, or candidacy for future autologous transplant. The intensity of the treatment regimens is dictated by the severity of symptoms. Emergent plasmapheresis in addition to systemic therapy for WM is needed for symptoms of hyperviscosity to provide rapid improvement due to the large size of the IgM molecule. Transplant-eligible patients should not be treated with regimens that could impair stem cell collection. Symptomatic patients are mostly treated with combinations that include rituximab, an anti-CD20 monoclonal antibody, as part of the backbone. For patients with only mild symptoms, single-agent rituximab can be considered, as it is very well tolerated. However, a transient IgM flare can be seen that leads to worsening hyperviscosity (*Blood.* 2015;126(6):721). Rituximab can also be used in combination with alkylators (bendamustine and cyclophosphamide) or proteasome inhibitors (bortezomib and carfilzomib). Nucleoside analogs, such as fludarabine and cladribine, have also demonstrated activity in patients with WM when used in combination with rituximab, but they carry a higher risk of myelosuppression and immunosuppression as well as secondary malignancies, such as myelodysplasia, leukemias, and possible transformation to high-grade lymphoma (*J Clin Oncol.* 2009;27(2):250). Although other regimens have been utilized to treat WM, Ibrutinib, a Bruton's tyrosine kinase (BTK) inhibitor, is the only Food and Drug Administration–approved (FDA-approved) therapy (as single agent or in combination with rituximab). The initial approval of ibrutinib was based on a prospective study of 63 patients with symptomatic WM who had previously received at least one line of therapy. It demonstrated an overall response rate >90%, with the highest being among patients with *MYD88* and *CXCR4* mutations. Moreover, the study also showed durable response and increased progression-free survival (PFS) and OS (*N Engl J Med.* 2015;372:1430–1440).

The INNOVATE trial, a double-blind, placebo-controlled phase 3 study, randomized patients to ibrutinib and rituximab or placebo and rituximab. It demonstrated that ibrutinib in combination with rituximab resulted in significantly higher PFS in treatment-naïve patients as well as those with relapsed/refractory disease. Although generally well tolerated, ibrutinib in combination with rituximab resulted in more frequent rates of hypertension (13% vs. 4%) and atrial fibrillation (12% vs. 1%). There were no fatalities attributed to the use of ibrutinib. Limitations of this study included the fact that rituximab alone may not be appropriate therapy for many patients with WM, and it remains unclear whether adding rituximab to ibrutinib is necessary (*N Engl J Med.* 2018;378(25):2399–2410). While the INNOVATE trial confirmed the activity and safety of ibrutinib, it left several questions unanswered. Because of the need for continuous therapy to prevent disease progression, we generally recommend using ibrutinib as second-line therapy for many patients with WM.

RESISTANCE TO IBRUTINIB

The molecular basis of disease progression during treatment with ibrutinib remains unclear. Ibrutinib binds to the Cysteine 481 residue of BTK. De novo subclonal BTK^{Cys481} mutations were identified in *MYD88*-mutated WM cells from patients who progressed while on ibrutinib. Ibrutinib-resistant WM cell lines that lack BTK^{Cys481} mutation have also been documented; AKT and Bcl-2 associated pathways seem to play a role (*J Blood Med.* 2019;10:291–300). Acalabrutinib, a novel irreversible BTK inhibitor, is active as a single agent for patients with treatment-naïve or relapsed/refractory WM, with overall response rates of 93%. Although the median durations of response, PFS, and OS have not been reached, they seem to be similar to those reported for ibrutinib. Adverse events included atrial fibrillation, hypertension, and bleeding events (*Lancet Haematol.* 2020;7:e112–e121). BCL-2 is highly expressed in WM cells, particularly in patients with *MYD88* mutations. BCL-2 inhibition with venetoclax was well tolerated and resulted in high levels of response (overall response rate of 87%

Table 30.4 Potential Suggested Therapeutic Approaches Based on Clinical Scenarios

Clinical Scenarios	Recommended Potential Treatment Options
• Anemia with low IgM • Comorbidities and cytopenias • Cold agglutinin disease	• Rituximab alone
• Symptomatic anemia • Organomegaly with high IgM level	• DRC
• High IgM level • Hyperviscocity • Renal insufficiency due to IgM/light chain deposition • Cryoglobulinemia	• Bortezomib • Rituximab/dexamethasone • BR
• Transformation to large-cell lymphoma	• R-CHOP (see Chapter 35)
• Sensorimotor neuropathy • Paraprotein-related neuropathy (MAG neuropathy)	• Rituximab alone
• Significant lymphadenopathy • Bulky extramedullary disease • Splenomegaly	• Cyclophosphamide • Bendamustine-based regimens
• Symptomatic cryoglobulinemia	• Rituximab • Thalidomide (based on anecdotal experience)
• Candidate for autologous transplant	• DRC • BR • Avoidance of continuous chlorambucil or nucleoside analogs due to stem cell damage (also, increased risk for transformation)
• IgM flare due to rituximab • Hyperviscosity	• Most patients return to their baseline serum IgM by 12 weeks. • In patients with baseline serum IgM >40 g/dL or serum viscosity >3.5 centipoises, hyperviscosity is a risk, and plasmapheresis should be considered or rituximab should be omitted in the first few cycles until safer IgM levels are achieved (see Chapter 60).
• Intolerance to rituximab	• Ofatumumab is an alternative.

(continued)

Table 30.4 Potential Suggested Therapeutic Approaches Based on Clinical Scenarios (continued)

Clinical Scenarios	Recommended Potential Treatment Options
• Nontransplant candidate with indolent disease • Elderly patients with poor performance status	• Oral fludarabine • Will not offer rapid disease control
• Younger patients	• Avoid nucleoside analogs due to short- and long-term toxicities (prolonged myelosuppression, sustained cytopenias, and secondary malignancies).
• Neuropathy-sparing approach when a proteasome inhibitor is recommended	• CaRD • In patients naïve to bortezomib and rituximab, common toxicities include elevated lipase and decreased IgA and IgG, leading to recurrent infections (potential need for intravenous immunoglobulin therapy).
• Maintenance therapy	• Rituximab for 2 years every 2–3 months • Observation
• Relapsed WM	• Clinical trial • If patient initially had a great response, it is reasonable to reuse the original treatment choice. • If duration of response was short, consider clinical trial, BR, or ibrutinib.
• Intolerance to Ibrutinib	• Consider dose reduction. • Clinical trial of novel BTK inhibitor (acalabrutinib, zanubrutinib, or vecabrutinib)
• Refractory disease	• Clinical trial of novel BTK inhibitor (acalabrutinib, zanubrutinib, vecabrutinib) • Venetoclax • Other compounds

BR, bendamustine and rituximab; CaRD, carfilzomib, rituximab, and dexamethasone; DRC, dexamethasone, rituximab, and cyclophosphamide; IgA, immunoglobulin A; IgG, immunoglobulin G; IgM, immunoglobulin M; MAG, myelin-associated glycoprotein; R-CHOP, Rituximab, cyclophosphamide, dodorubicin, vincristine, prednisone.

and major response rate of 80%) in patients with previously treated WM, including those with prior exposure to BTK inhibitors. Patients with previous exposure to BTK inhibitors or with refractory disease demonstrated lower major response rates than those with relapsed WM. Venetoclax was well tolerated, and no clinical tumor lysis syndrome was observed (*Blood.* 2018;132(Suppl1):2888). A phase 2 trial of the oral mammalian target of rapamycin (mTOR) inhibitor everolimus showed single-agent activity in relapsed/refractory WM, with an overall response rate of 50% and median PFS of 21 months, while carrying manageable toxicities (*Am J Hematol.* 2014;89(3):237). Ixazomib, an oral proteasome inhibitor, was evaluated in combination with dexamethasone and rituximab, and an overall response rate of 96% was seen, though median PFS has not been reached after a median follow-up of 22 months (*Clin Cancer Res.* 2018;24(14):3247). Table 30.4 discusses clinical scenarios with possible therapy choices. As a disclaimer, these recommendations are experience and clinically based, due to the lack of trial data. Evidence for stem cell transplantation in WM is also scant. Table 30.5 includes available therapies for WM based on class of drug. The role of maintenance therapy in WM has limited data, and there are no randomized trials demonstrating

Table 30.5 Available Therapies for Treatment of WM

Type	Examples
Monoclonal antibodies	• Rituximab • Ofatumumab • Alemtuzumab
Alkylators	• Chlorambucil • Cyclophosphamide • Bendamustine
Proteasome inhibitors	• Bortezomib • Carfilzomib • Ixazomib
Nucleoside analogs	• Cladribine • Iudarabine • Bendamustine
Immunomodulators	• Lenalidomide • Thalidomide • Pomalidomide
Signal inhibitors	• Everolimus • Ibrutinib • Panobinostat • Acalabrutinib • Zanubrutinib • Venetoclax

WM, Waldenström Macroglobulinemia.

a clear survival benefit that would justify its clinical and financial toxicity, making observation a reasonable approach. Rituximab, however, has been recommended by the National Comprehensive Cancer Network (NCCN) and the International Workshops on WM (IWWM) for those patients who showed initial response to chemoimmunotherapy. Splenectomy has a palliative role in patients with symptomatic, painful splenomegaly.

▓ POTENTIAL PRACTICE-CHANGING CLINICAL TRIALS

Zanubrutinib is a promising next-generation BTK inhibitor with greater selectivity for BTK than ibrutinib but minimal inhibition of TEC and epidermal growth factor (EGFR) family off-target kinases, resulting in a better toxicity profile. There is an ongoing phase 3 trial comparing zanubrutinib versus ibrutinib (*Future Oncol. 2018;14(22):2229–2237*).

▓ REFERENCES FOR SUPPLEMENTAL READING

1. D'Sa S, Kersten MJ, Castillo JJ, et al. Investigation and management of IgM and Waldenström-associated peripheral neuropathies: recommendations from the IWWM-8 consensus panel. *Br J Haematol*. 2017;176(5):728.

2. Leblond V, Kastritis E, Advani R, et al. Treatment recommendations from the Eighth International Workshop on Waldenström's Macroglobulinemia. *Blood*. 2016;128(10):1321–1328.

3. Buske C, Sadullah S, Kastritis E, et al. Treatment and outcome patterns in European patients with Waldenström's macroglobulinaemia: a large, observational, retrospective chart review. *Lancet Haematol*. 2018;5(7):e299.

4. Treon SP, Hunter ZR, Castillo JJ, et al. Waldenström macroglobulinemia. *Hematol Oncol Clin N Am*. 2014;28:945–970.

5. Oza A, Rajkumar SV. Waldenström macroglobulinemia: prognosis and management. *Blood Can J*. 2015;5:e296.

6. Rossi D. Role of MYD88 in lymphoplasmacytic lymphoma diagnosis and pathogenesis. *Hematology Am Soc Hemtol Educ Program*. 2014(1):113–118.

7. Treon SP, Tripsas CK, Meid K, et al. Ibrutinib in previously treated Waldenström's macroglobulinemia. *N Engl J Med*. 2015;372(15):1430–1440.

8. Treon SP, Gustine J, Meid K, et al. Ibrutinib monotherapy in symptomatic, treatment-naïve patients with Waldenström macroglobulinemia. *J Clin Oncol*. 2018;36(27):2755.

31 Immunoglobulin Light Chain Amyloidosis

Taxiarchis Kourelis and Morie A. Gertz

▓ INTRODUCTION

Immunoglobulin light chain amyloidosis (AL) represents a protein-misfolding disease and is a hematologic malignancy. The production of amyloidogenic immunoglobulins is driven by a plasma-cell clone that is usually more indolent compared to cells in multiple myeloma (MM). These proteins misfold and deposit in organs, causing tissue damage. Although virtually all organs can be involved, cardiac involvement dictates long-term survival in most patients. Eradicating the plasma-cell clone is imperative but is not always enough to halt or reverse further amyloid deposition in organs. Given the rarity of the disease, high-quality data from randomized trials are sparse. The recommendations outlined here reflect how we manage AL in our institution.

▓ DIAGNOSIS

The first step in diagnosis is recognizing the disease. AL is "a great imitator" and presents with nonspecific findings, such as dyspnea in patients with cardiac involvement, proteinuria in patients with renal involvement, and neuropathy in patients with nerve involvement. Furthermore, up to 20% of patients have comorbidities (diabetes and cardiovascular disease) that are severe enough to confound the differential diagnosis. This leads to delays in diagnosis of approximately a year from symptom onset, during which organ function continues to deteriorate. The diagnosis should be suspected in all patients presenting with heart failure with preserved ejection fraction (HFpEF), nephrotic range proteinuria, or peripheral neuropathy. The classic signs of macroglossia and periorbital involvement are not very common (approximately 10%–15%) but are relatively specific in the correct context. When identified, AL should be suspected.

If the diagnosis is suspected, the following tests should be performed:

1. Protein electrophoresis and immunofixation of the serum and urine: Mass spectrometry-based immunofixation techniques have identified an increased incidence of glycosylated light chains in AL compared to other dysproteinemias, which are present in the monoclonal gammopathy of undetermined significance (MGUS) phase and can be detected years before symptom onset. These MGUS patients could be considered for closer follow-up.

2. Serum-free light chain (SFLC) levels.

3. Fat pad and bone marrow (BM) biopsy with Congo red staining.
4. If there is no evidence of amyloid deposition in a fat pad or BM biopsy, an organ should be directly targeted for biopsy.

Absence of a circulating monoclonal protein makes the diagnosis of AL highly unlikely but does not exclude other types of amyloid or localized AL. The sensitivity of a biopsy sample from a symptomatic organ is more than 95%, compared to 75% to 80% for fat pad combined with a BM biopsy and 50% to 65% for either BM biopsy or fat pad alone. However, if the fat/BM biopsy demonstrates amyloid in the correct clinical setting, then no additional organ biopsies are required. Regardless of the clinical presentation, typing should be performed in all cases to identify the nature of the amyloidogenic protein (light chain versus not), because MGUS can frequently coexist in non-AL patients.

▨ STAGING AND PROGNOSIS

Assessing for organ involvement includes a thorough review of systems and a physical examination, including orthostatic vital signs, to assess for autonomic dysfunction. All patients should be evaluated for cardiac involvement with cardiac biomarkers (N-terminal pro b-type natriuretic peptide [NT-proBNP] and troponin) and an echocardiogram. Ejection fraction is usually preserved, but when decreased, it usually denotes advanced cardiac involvement. Renal involvement is suggested by the presence of nephrotic range proteinuria, regardless of renal clearance/GFR. However, renal AL with perivascular amyloid deposits, which is seen in approximately 10% of cases, can present with little/no proteinuria and significantly decreased GFR. Looking for the classic "CRAB" (hypercalcemia, renal failure, anemia and bone lesions) criteria of MM is important. Patients with concurrent CRAB have inferior outcomes; however, their survival is similar to that of AL patients with ≥10% BM plasma cells and no CRAB. This suggests that the bulk of the plasma-cell clone, not the mere presence of CRAB/MM, correlates better with outcomes. In contrast to MM, trisomies predict for inferior survival in AL patients treated with an autologous stem cell transplant (ASCT), while t(11;14)(q13;q32) *CCND1-IgH* predicts for worse survival only in patients not treated with an ASCT.

Several prognostic/staging systems have been developed, and they all seem to perform equally. In our practice, we routinely use the Mayo Clinic 2012 system, which requires NT-proBNP, troponin, and dFLC (the difference between the involved and uninvolved free light chain [FLC] levels) to risk-stratify patients (Figure 31.1; Table 31.1). Median survival can be misleading and underestimate long-term outcomes in some patients, because a third or more of patients die within the first 12 to 18 months (Figure 31.2) as a result of delayed diagnosis and advanced cardiac involvement. Patients who survive longer than 18 months tend to have much better long-term outcomes.

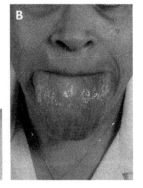
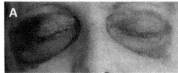

Figure 31.1 Soft tissue involvement in light chain amyloidosis. (A) Periorbital purpura. (B) Macroglossia.

Table 31.1 Mayo Clinic 2012 Prognostic Staging System of AL

Stage	Parameters	Median Survival (Months)	5-Year Survival (%)
I	All below cut-off	Not reached	68
II	One above cut-off	69	60
III	Two above cut-off	17	27
IV	All below cut-off	7	14

Parameters: Troponin T (TnT) <0.025 ng/mL or hs-TnT ≤40, NT-proBNP <1,800 pg/mL, dFLC <18 mg/dL.

▓ TREATMENT

Treatment should be initiated immediately in all patients to prevent further amyloid deposition and progressive organ damage. One exception is patients who have incidentally discovered amyloid deposits in BM biopsies without evidence of organ involvement or myeloma. These patients should be followed closely, with periodic assessment of cardiac biomarkers and 24-hour urine collections to identify evolving cardiac and renal involvement, respectively. Recommendations for the treatment of AL are limited by the paucity of phase 3 data for this rare disease, and clinical trials should always be considered as well as referral for an ASCT. Eligibility criteria for ASCT in AL patients are different from those of MM and include "physiologic age" ≤70, Eastern Cooperative Oncology Group (ECOG) performance score ≤2, systolic blood pressure ≥90 mmHg, and TnT <0.06 ng/mL (or hs-TnT <75 ng/ml). Well-selected

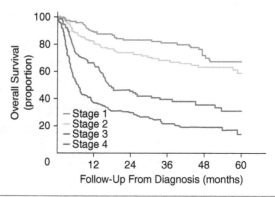

Figure 31.2 Overall survival of patients according to stage.

AL, amyloidosis.

Source: From Kumar S, Dispenzieri A, Lacy MQ, et al. Revised prognostic staging system for light chain amyloidosis incorporating cardiac biomarkers and serum-free light chain measurements. *J Clin Oncol.* 2012;30(9):989–995. Used with permission.

transplant candidates have a transplant-related mortality of <5% in high-volume transplant centers, comparable to that of MM patients. Induction therapy prior to ASCT is not necessary but can be considered especially in patients with >10% BM plasma cells or in patients who for logistical reasons cannot proceed immediately to transplant.

Patients who are not fit or do not wish to proceed with an ASCT are treated with plasma cell–directed therapies similar to those used in MM patients. Combination regimens offer the best chance of a complete response (CR) and are preferred in the first line. Our preferred regimen is CyBorD (Cyclophosphamide, Bortezomib, and Dexamethasone given weekly in 28 day cycles). Preferably with the addition of daratumumab, because it is safe in patients with cardiac involvement and achieves rapid hematologic response. MVP (Melphalan, Bortezomib, and Prednisone) is also a reasonable choice and the only option with randomized data showing a survival benefit versus MP. Lenalidomide and other immunomodulatory drugs are not well tolerated in patients with cardiac involvement and should not be considered first-line options for these patients. Bortezomib should be used cautiously in patients with existing neuropathy. Dexamethasone should be used at a decreased dose (we use 20 mg weekly). If patients have achieved a hematologic very good partial response (VGPR) after 6 to 12 months of therapy, treatment can be interrupted, and patients can be observed or be considered for maintenance therapy. Unlike with MM, treatment should be reinitiated immediately when SFLC levels start rising. Our preferred approach for patients with relapsed disease is to use daratumumab-based regimens.

FRONTLINE TREATMENT

- **Transplant candidates:** ASCT (*J Clin Oncol.* 2018;36(13):1323–1329).
- **Non-transplant candidates:** CyBorD (≥VGPR in 40%–45%, renal and cardiac response in 25% and 17% of patients in recent, "real-life" cohorts; *Blood.* 2015;126(5):612–615; *Blood.* 2019;134(25):2271–2280) or MVP (paper published *J Clin Oncol.* 2020 Oct 1;38(28):3252–3260).

RESPONSE ASSESSMENT

The goals of treatment are (a) to maintain the patient in the deepest possible hematologic response and (b) to achieve organ response. Therefore, both hematologic and organ response parameters should be followed with every visit. Hematologic response criteria in AL are different from those used in MM. A CR is defined as a negative serum and urine immunofixation and a normal SFLC ratio. VGPR is a dFLC level <2 mg/dL, and a partial response (PR) is a dFLC decrease of ≥50%. Recent data suggest that targeting an involved FLC level of <2 mg/dL is associated with improved outcomes. Organ-response criteria have been recently updated (see References for Supplemental Reading), and specific response criteria for heart and kidneys are shown in Table 31.2.

SUPPORTIVE CARE

Of patients who achieve a complete hematologic response or normalization of their SFLC ratios, approximately one third do not achieve organ responses. Of those who do, optimal responses might take several months to occur. Therefore, aggressive supportive treatment should be initiated early. Patients with cardiac involvement require periodic follow-up from cardiologists with expertise in cardiac AL. Beta-blockers should be avoided if possible. Long-acting anti-hypertensives (e.g., angiotensin-converting enzyme [ACE] inhibitors, calcium channel blockers) are not tolerated well and should also be avoided. A nephrologist should be involved early in patients with

Table 31.2 Cardiac and Renal Response Criteria in AL

Response type	Criteria
Cardiac response	• Decrease in NT-proBNP by >30% and 300 pg/mL (if baseline NT-proBNP >650 pg/mL) • ≥2-point decrease in NYHA class (if baseline NYHA class III or IV)
Renal response	• >30% decrease in proteinuria • Drop below 0.5 g/24 h in the absence of renal progression, defined as a >25% decrease in eGFR

AL, amyloidosis; eGFR, estimated glomerular filtration rate; NYHA, New York Heart Association.

impaired renal function at baseline. Finally, nutritional counseling helps patients with AL improve quality of life and maintain weight.

■ POTENTIAL PRACTICE-CHANGING CLINICAL TRIALS

The most promising agents in development are "amyloid-clearing" monoclonal antibodies. After the failure of NEOD001 to demonstrate benefit in randomized clinical trials, another agent, 11-1F4 (CAEL-101), with promising results in early-phase trials, will be tested in randomized clinical trials. Additionally, the combination of daratumumab and CyBorD is being tested in newly diagnosed patients (NCT03201965). Finally, venetoclax remains a promising agent under development for patients harboring t(11;14).

■ REFERENCES FOR SUPPLEMENTAL READING

1. Merlini G, Dispenzieri A, Sanchorawala V, et al. Systemic immunoglobulin light chain amyloidosis. *Nat Rev Dis Primers*. 2018;4(1):38.

2. Palladini G, Dispenzieri A, Gertz MA, et al. New criteria for response to treatment in immunoglobulin light chain amyloidosis based on free light chain measurement and cardiac biomarkers: impact on survival outcomes. *J Clin Oncol*. 2012;30(36):4541–4549.

3. Muchtar E, Kumar SK, Gertz MA, et al. Staging systems use for risk stratification of systemic amyloidosis in the era of high-sensitivity troponin T assay. *Blood*. 2019;133(7):763–766.

4. Muchtar E, Therneau TM, Larson DR, et al. Comparative analysis of staging systems in AL amyloidosis. *Leukemia*. 2019;33(3):811–814.

5. Palladini G, Sachchithanantham S, Milani P, et al. A European collaborative study of cyclophosphamide, bortezomib, and dexamethasone in upfront treatment of systemic AL amyloidosis. *Blood*. 2015;126(5):612–615.

6. Manwani R, Cohen O, Sharpley F, et al. A prospective observational study of 915 patients with systemic AL amyloidosis treated with upfront bortezomib. *Blood*. 2019;134(25):2271–2280.

32   Hodgkin Lymphoma

Anju Nair

With acknowledgments to Dr. Micah Burch for his contribution to the first edition.

▓ INTRODUCTION

Hodgkin lymphoma (HL), formerly known as Hodgkin disease, is a hematologic malignancy derived from germinal-center or post-germinal-center B-cells, with neoplastic "Reed Sternberg" cells in a non-neoplastic inflammatory background. The Surveillance, Epidemiology, and End Results (SEER) data describe the incidence of HL as 0.5% of all new cancers in the United States per year, with a bimodal distribution curve. The median age at diagnosis is 38, with 44% of patients diagnosed at <35 years of age. The percentage of HL-related deaths is highest in people between 75 and 84 years of age.

HL typically presents as painless, localized peripheral lymphadenopathy with variable systemic symptoms, including fever, weight loss, and sweats. HL can be further classified into two major subgroups based on the morphologic and immunophenotypic findings: classical HL (cHL) or nodular lymphocyte predominant HL (NLPHL). All subtypes of cHL share the same tumor cell immunophenotype; however, the various histologic findings, including the nature of the inflammatory background or presence of fibrosis, differ (Table 32.1). On the other hand, NLPHL retains the immunophenotypic features of germinal-center B-cells (Figure 32.1). Treatment and disease outcome are determined by clinical stage and molecular characteristics.

▓ DIAGNOSIS

An excisional lymph node biopsy is the preferred method of diagnosis, but in some cases, a large-core needle biopsy may be adequate. Routine light microscopy findings can provide a diagnosis based on morphology, but confirmatory immunophenotyping with immunohistochemistry can best distinguish between cHL and NLPHL (Table 32.1).

Staging criteria are based on the Ann Arbor staging system, with modifications from Cotswold and Lugano classifications (Table 32.2). Clinical staging includes history, physical examination, complete blood count (CBC) with differential, complete metabolic panel (CMP), and positron emission tomography–computed tomography (PET-CT) scans of the neck, chest, abdomen, and pelvis. Although bone marrow

Table 32.1 Morphologic and Immunophenotypic Features of HL

Subtype	Morphology	Immunophenotypic Features
cHL and NLPHL	**NSHL** (most common) Nodular pattern surrounded by broad bands of fibrosis, thickened capsule, variable numbers of HRS and non-neoplastic inflammatory cells (eosinophils, histiocytes), HRS cells with retraction artifact due to fixative (i.e., "lacunar cells"), "syncytial" variant when abundant large aggregates of HRS cells are present, infrequently associated with EBV	**Positive:** CD15 (85%), CD30 (~100%, membranous with golgi enhancement pattern), and MUM1 **Weakly positive:** PAX-5 (nuclear)
	MCHL Usually diffuse pattern with classic HRS cells, a heterogeneous non-neoplastic inflammatory background (eosinophils, histiocytes, plasma cells, neutrophils, of which one may predominate), normal capsule thickness, no broad fibrotic bands, highest incidence of EBV positivity	**Negative:** CD19, CD20 (small subset can be positive), CD45, CD79a, CD3, CD7
	LRHL More commonly nodular pattern; HRS cells located outside germinal center but within large nodules of small lymphocytes, sparse to absent eosinophils/neutrophils	
	LDHL Heterogenous morphologic spectrum (typical binucleated large HRS cells to pleomorphic, bizarre) but abundant HRS cells that outnumber the background small lymphocytes, hypocellular background (histiocyte rich with few lymphocytes)	
	NLPHL "Popcorn cells" or "LP cells," neutrophils and eosinophils are rarer, associated with PTGC; pathologist should note presence of a diffuse T-cell rich pattern as "THRLBCL-like transformation of NLPHL"	**Positive:** CD20, CD57 "rosette" pattern of T-cells around "popcorn" cells, Oct-2, BOB.1, CD79a, CD45 **Negative:** CD15 and usually CD30

cHL, classical Hodgkin lymphoma; EBV, Epstein–Barr virus; HRS, Hodgkin and Reed/Sternberg; LDHL, lymphocyte-depleted cHL; LP, lymphocyte predominant; LRHL, lymphocyte-rich cHL; MCHL, mixed cellularity cHL; NLPHL, nodular lymphocyte predominant Hodgkin lymphoma; NSHL, nodular sclerosis cHL; PTGC, progressive transformation of germinal centers; THRLBCL, T-cell/histiocyte-rich B-cell lymphoma.

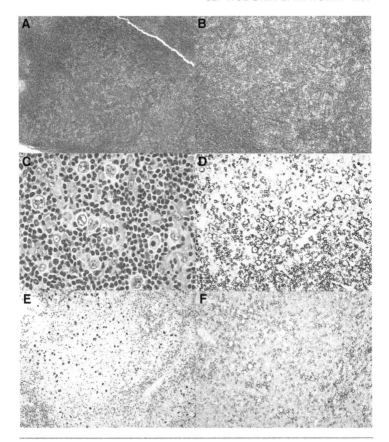

Figure 32.1 A case of nodular lymphocyte predominant Hodgkin lymphoma (NLPHL). Low-power views of the hematoxylin and eosin (H&E) sections showed a vaguely lymphoid nodule embedded with numerous large atypical lymphoid cells, associated with heavy background of small lymphocytes (A and B, ×40 and ×100, respectively). High-power view of these large atypical cells revealed convoluted or lobated nuclei, vesicular chromatin, small but visible nucleoli, and an abundant clear cytoplasm—namely, characteristic "popcorn-cell" or LP cells (C, H&E, ×600). The LP cells were highlighted by B-cell markers— for example, CD20, OCT2 (D and E, immunoperoxidase, ×200 and ×100, respectively), and BOB1 (not shown)— and surrounded by reactive small T-lymphocytes, commonly CD3, CD4, CD57 (not shown), and dendritic cell marker PD1 (F, immunoperoxidase, ×100).

(BM) biopsy was historically required to complete disease staging, it can be avoided with a negative PET-CT scan (negative predictive value of 99.3%; *Am J Hematol.* 2015;90(8):686–690). For treatment purposes, HL is classified as early stage (stage I–II) or advanced stage (stage III–IV), and early-stage HL can further be divided into favorable and unfavorable prognostic categories.

Table 32.2 Ann Arbor Staging System With Cotswold Modifications	
Stage	**Description of Prognostic Group**
I	Involvement of a single lymphatic site (or nodal region) or lymphoid structure (e.g., Waldeyer ring, thymus, or spleen) without nodal involvement
II	Involvement of two or more lymph node regions on the same side of the diaphragm or with involvement of single continuous extra-lymphatic organ or site on the same side of the diaphragm
III	Involvement of lymph node regions or lymphoid structures on both sides of the diaphragm
IV	Diffuse or disseminated involvement of one or more extra-lymphatic organs, with or without associated lymph node involvement
	Includes any involvement of the liver, BM, lungs (other than by direct extension from another site), or cerebrospinal fluid

BM, bone marrow.

Modifiers: B, unexplained fever, weight loss >10% body weight, drenching night sweats; A, no B-symptoms; X, bulky disease (≥10 cm or 1/3 intrathoracic diameter); E, extra-nodal extension (limited involvement of an extra lymphatic organ contiguous with nodal site); S, splenic involvement.

■ PROGNOSIS

Stages I and II HL are stratified into favorable and unfavorable prognosis based on the presence of other clinical features: B-symptoms, erythrocyte sedimentation rate (ESR) >50, number of regions involved, and large mediastinal adenopathy (Table 32.3). The definition of unfavorable may vary slightly, depending on which cooperative group guidelines are used; however, in the United States, the National Comprehensive Cancer Network (NCCN) guidelines are the most commonly used and are listed in Table 32.3.

Table 32.3 Early Stage Unfavorable Prognostic Indicators per NCCN
Early-Stage (Stage I/II) Prognostic Indicators
Large mediastinal adenopathy (>1/3 maximum transverse thoracic diameter) or any lymph node ≥10 cm
Involvement of 4 or more sites
ESR >50 mm/h
B symptoms

ESR, erythrocyte sedimentation rate; NCCN, National Comprehensive Cancer Network.

Table 32.4 IPS and Associated 5-Year Event-Free Survival Rates, FFP Rates, and OS Rates

IPS Cumulative Score	5-Year Event-Free Survival Rate (%)	FFP Rate (%)	Overall Survival Rate (%)
No factors (0 score)	84	88	98
One factor (1 score)	77	84	97
Two factors (2 score)	67	80	91
Three factors (3 score)	60	74	88
Four factors (4 score)	51	67	85
Five or more factors (≥5 score)	42	62	67

FFP, freedom from progression; IPS, International Prognostic Score; OS, overall survival.

Source: Moccia AA, Donaldson J, Chhanabhai M, et al. International Prognostic Score in advanced-stage Hodgkin's lymphoma: altered utility in the modern era. *J Clin Oncol.* 2012;30(27): 3383–3388.

The International Prognostic Score (IPS) is a strong predictor of outcome in HL. It uses prognostic factors to identify the patients at highest risk of relapse and who should be treated initially with intensive therapy. The IPS system is largely used for patients with advanced stage (stage III or IV) HL and is based on the following seven unfavorable features at time of diagnosis:

1. Serum albumin <4 g/dL
2. Hemoglobin <10.5 g/dL
3. Male gender
4. Age >45 years
5. Stage IV disease
6. White blood cell (WBC) count >15,000/mcL
7. Absolute lymphocyte count <600/mcL and/or <8% of total WBC count

Each of these unfavorable features is given 1 point, and the risk of relapse increases with the total score. The 5-year event-free survival rates, freedom from progression (FFP) rates, and overall survival (OS) rates correlated with IPS scores are listed in Table 32.4. The FFP and OS rates documented in the table are from 740 cases of advanced-stage HL treated with doxorubicin, bleomycin, vinblastine, and dacarbazine (ABVD) in a 77-month follow-up study (*J Clin Oncol.* 2012;30:3383).

▦ TREATMENT

Treatment for cHL is based on the clinical stage of the disease and, for stage I or II, further classification as either a favorable or unfavorable prognosis. The widely used regimen for HL is ABVD. Treatment response is determined with repeat PET-CT scans during treatment and after treatment is complete. The Deauville criteria are used for visual interpretation of the PET-CT scans to determine treatment response.

FRONTLINE TREATMENT OF STAGE I AND STAGE II (EARLY) CHL

- **Favorable** (no clinical risk factors; see Table 32.3): Two cycles of ABVD followed by 20 Gray (Gy)-involved field radiation therapy (IFRT), if fewer than 3 sites of disease (*N Engl J Med.* 2010;363:640–652) or 4 cycles of ABVD ± IFRT (*J Clin Oncol.* 2005;23:4634–4642).
- **Unfavorable:** ABVD × 4 cycles plus IFRT of 20 to 30 Gy to involved sites or ABVD × 6 cycles. Number of ABVD cycles determined by PET-CT scan after 2 cycles of chemotherapy. Additional radiation therapy can be considered for bulky disease (*J Clin Oncol.* 2003;21:3601; *N Engl J Med.* 2012;366:399–408).

FRONTLINE TREATMENT OF STAGE III AND STAGE IV (ADVANCED) CHL

- **Nonbulky disease:** ABVD × 6 cycles, then observation (*Cancer.* 1975;36(1):252).
- **Bulky disease:** ABVD × 6 cycles with consolidation-involved site radiation therapy (ISRT) 30 to 36 Gy (*J Clin Oncol.* 2003;21:607) or A + AVD × 6 cycles (brentuximab vedotin, doxorubicin, vinblastine, and dacarbazine) can be used in patients with increased risk of pulmonary toxicity (*N Engl J Med.* 2018;378(4):331), or BEACOPP (standard or escalated—bleomycin, etoposide, doxorubicin, cyclophosphamide, vincristine, procarbazine, and prednisone) can be used if IPS is 4 or greater in patients younger than 50 years (*J Clin Oncol.* 2003;21:607; *N Engl J Med.* 2003;348:2386–2395).
- Treatment response is determined with repeat PET-CT scans after completion of all therapy.

After treatment is complete, surveillance for HL relapse should be continued every 3 to 4 months for the first 2 years and can be widened to every 6 months after. The majority of relapses will occur within the first 3 years of therapy. Once HL relapse is detected, salvage chemotherapy and autologous stem cell transplantation (ASCT) are treatments of choice. Salvage chemotherapy regimens should include different agents due to presumed resistance to prior agents.

TREATMENT FOR RELAPSED CHL

First Relapse or Primary Refractory

- **Relapse at single site of known primary disease:** Radiation therapy alone can be used as salvage therapy.
- **Relapse/progression at more than one site:** Patient should receive salvage chemotherapy with ICE (ifosfamide, carboplatin,

etoposide), DHAP (dexamethasone, cytarabine, cisplatin), or gemcitabine-containing regimen (*Oncologist*. 2009;14(4):425).

- Once the patient obtains a remission, the patient should undergo an ASCT (*Cochrane Database Syst Rev*. 2013; 6:CD009411). Brentuximab maintenance therapy can be used in select patients (primary cHL, relapse within 12 months of initial treatment or extranodal relapse) every 3 weeks × 16 cycles post-ASCT. This nearly doubles progression free survival (PFS) in this patient population (*Lancet*. 2015;385(9980):1853–1862).

Second or Subsequent Relapse

- Brentuximab vedotin once every 3 weeks for a maximum of 16 cycles (*Blood*. 2015;125(8):1236–1243; *J Clin Oncol*. 2012; 30(18):2183–2189).
- ICE, miniBEAM, DHAP, gemcitabine-containing regimen, nivolumab, or bendamustine.
- Nivolumab once every 2 to 4 weeks until disease progresses or reaches unacceptable toxicity (*J Clin Oncol*. 2018;36(14):1428).
- Pembrolizumab every 3 weeks until disease progresses or reaches unacceptable toxicity for 2 years (*J Clin Oncol*. 2017;35(19): 2125).

TREATMENT OF NODULAR LYMPHOCYTE-PREDOMINANT HL

Stage I/II disease: ISRT with 30 to 36 Gy or active surveillance in non-bulky disease. With B-symptoms, treat as stage III/IV disease (*Cancer*. 2005;104(6):1221).

Stage III/IV disease: Combination chemotherapy with ABVD or R-CHOP (rituximab, cyclophosphamide, doxorubicin, vincristine, and prednisone; *J Clin Oncol*. 1999;17(3):776).

Relapsed/refractory disease: Localized disease can be treated with radiation therapy of 30 to 36 Gy. Extensive disease will require combination chemotherapy with or without rituximab (RICE or RDHAP).

▦ POTENTIAL PRACTICE-CHANGING CLINICAL TRIALS

There are multiple well-designed clinical trials available with new drug combinations in attempts to avoid the long-term side effects of the curative therapy used in HL. Prospective studies are evaluating whether substituting brentuximab for bleomycin will provide acceptable treatment results without the potentially fatal pulmonary toxicity (NCT01534078).

There are ongoing studies suggesting that a programmed cell death 1 (PD-1) pathway-blocking antibody, such as pembrolizumab, can be effective as maintenance therapy post-ASCT (NCT02362997) (*Blood*. 2019;134(1):22).

▓ REFERENCES FOR SUPPLEMENTAL READING

1. Johnson P, McKenzie H. How I treat advanced classical Hodgkin lymphoma. *Blood.* 2015;125(11):1717–1723.

2. Meyer RM, Gospodarowicz MK, Connors JM, et al. ABVD alone versus radiation-based therapy in limited-stage Hodgkin's lymphoma. *N Engl J Med.* 2012;366:399–408.

3. Diehl V, Franklin J, Pfreundschuh M. Standard and increased-dose BEACOPP chemotherapy compared with COPP-ABVD for advanced Hodgkin's disease. *N Engl J Med.* 2003;348:2386–2395.

4. Mendler JH, Friedberg JW. Salvage therapy in Hodgkin's lymphoma. *Oncologist.* 2009;14(4):425.

5. Diehl V, Sextro M, Franklin J, et al. Clinical presentation, course, and prognostic factors in lymphocyte-predominant Hodgkin's disease and lymphocyte-rich classical Hodgkin's disease: report from the European Task Force on lymphoma project on lymphocyte-predominant Hodgkin's disease. *J Clin Oncol.* 1999;17(3):776.

6. Moccia AA, Donaldson J, Chhanabhai M, et al. International Prognostic Score in advanced-stage Hodgkin's lymphoma: altered utility in the modern era. *J Clin Oncol.* 2012;30(27): 3383–3388.

33 Diagnosis and Classification of Non-Hodgkin Lymphomas

Johnny Nguyen, Haipeng Shao, and Ling Zhang

■ INTRODUCTION

The current classification of lymphomas originates from the Revised European-American Classification of Lymphoid Neoplasms (REAL) published in 1994 by a group of expert pathologists through the International Lymphoma Study Group (ILSG).[1] Several classification systems have been previously proposed, such as the Rappaport classification initially for follicular lymphoma (FL) in 1956,[2] the Lukes–Collins classification,[3] the Kiel classification,[4] and the Working Formulation of Non-Hodgkin's Lymphoma for Clinical Use.[5,6] In contrast to the aforementioned classifications that heavily emphasized the morphologic features or cellular differentiation, the REAL classification was the first classification system to incorporate immunophenotypic and molecular data.[1] The delineation of the normal development of B-, T-, and natural killer (NK) cells along with the discovery of surface antigen and receptor expression in lymphocytes enabled the classification of specific disease entities.[7–10] Schematic diagrams of the cell origin, differentiation, and corresponding lineage-specific neoplasms are summarized in Figures 33.1 and 33.2. The 4th edition of the World Health Organization (WHO) classification of tumors of hematopoietic and lymphoid tissues published in 2008 utilizes a comprehensive multi-parameter approach for classification by encompassing morphologic, immunophenotypic, cytogenetic, molecular, and clinical data.[11] A large amount of clinical and pathological data has been collected during the last decade, and such molecular technologies as next-generation sequencing (NGS) are increasingly used in routine clinical practice. As a result, the WHO classification is continuously revised to incorporate new information, and the resultant revised 2016 edition of WHO classification provides the latest frameworks and diagnostic criteria for hematopoietic neoplasms, including non-Hodgkin lymphomas.[12]

An accurate diagnosis of lymphoma requires adequate tissue for morphologic evaluation and ancillary studies, such as flow cytometry and cytogenetic and molecular analysis. Morphologic evaluation remains the initial step and most important in the diagnosis and classification of lymphomas. All other analytic methods are secondary in priority and supplement the morphologic diagnosis. When tissue is received in the laboratory, the diagnosis starts with macroscopic

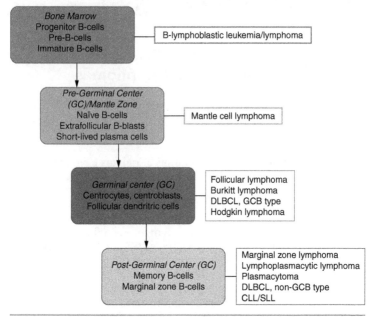

Figure 33.1 Schematic diagram of normal B-cell maturation and differentiation and corresponding cell-of-origin of precursor and mature B-cell neoplasms.

CLL, chronic lymphocytic leukemia; DLBCL, diffuse large B-cell lymphomas; GC, germinal center; GCB, germinal center B-cell; SLL, small lymphocytic lymphoma.

Precursor B-cells (progenitor B-cells, pre-B-cells, and immature B-cells) differentiate into naïve B-cells, an intermediate stage that can give rise to either transient plasma cells or enter the GC of a lymph node. The GC is the site of somatic hypermutation and immunoglobulin class switching. Transformed cells in the GC (centroblasts) can either be removed via apoptosis or differentiate into centrocytes. Follicular dendritic cells are located within primary and secondary follicles and form a stable structural network. Memory B-cells and marginal zone B-cells are post-germinal-center B-cells and can develop into various mature B-cell and plasma-cell neoplasms.

Source: Adapted from Swerdlow SH, Campo E, Harris NL, et al. *WHO Classification of Tumours of Haematopoietic and Lymphoid Tissues* (4th ed.). WHO Press; 2008:159.[11]

evaluation of the lesion. Such properties as single or multiple lesions, the texture of the lesion, and the presence of fibrosis or necrosis should be documented and provide valuable information for the differential diagnosis. Touch preparations should be made whenever possible for the evaluation of the cytologic features of lymphoma cells. Some lymphomas, such as Burkitt lymphoma (BL), have distinctive cytologic features that help narrow down the differential diagnosis and allow adequate tissue to be submitted for ancillary studies early in the process. When processing tissue, pieces of the

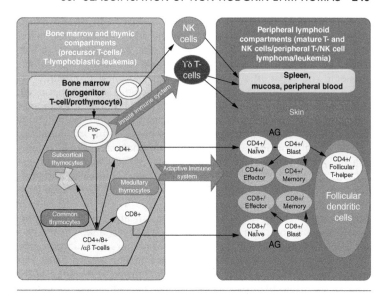

Figure 33.2 Schematic diagram of T-cell differentiation and corresponding T-cell lymphoma/leukemia.

After exiting the bone marrow, progenitor T-cells migrate to the thymus, where differentiation into various naïve T-cells occurs (subcortical, medullary, and common). Pro-T-cells develop into γδ T-cells, which, along with NK and NK-like T-cells in circulation, migrate to specific organs and tissues and form the innate immune system, which lacks the specificity and memory that are characteristic of B-cell maturation. Conversely, the T-cells of the adaptive immune system are more sophisticated and represented by naïve, effector, and memory T-cells. Effector T-cells not only are found in the peripheral regions of lymph node tissue but also reside in the germinal center (GC) as follicular helper T-cells. The clinical presentations of various T-lymphoid neoplasms may reflect the cell of origin from either the innate or adaptive immune system.

Source: Adapted from Swerdlow SH, Campo E, Harris NL, et al. *WHO Classification of Tumours of Haematopoietic and Lymphoid Tissues* (4th ed.). WHO Press;2008:161.[11]

lesion should be allocated to ancillary studies, such as flow cytometry, fluorescence in situ hybridization (FISH), polymerase chain reaction (PCR), or NGS. The microscopic evaluation starts with evaluating the architecture of the lesion followed by examining cytologic features of the lymphoma cells. The architectural features include nodular/follicular, diffuse, interfollicular, and sinusoidal infiltrate pattern. The cytologic features include small, intermediate, or large lymphoid cells; round, irregular, or lobated nuclei; coarse, open, or blastoid chromatin; or presence and prominence of nucleoli. Determination of the phenotypes of the lymphoma cells by immunohistochemistry or flow cytometry is essential for diagnosis. In terms of B-cell non-Hodgkin lymphomas, the difference between low-grade B-cell lymphoma and high-grade B-cell lymphoma is mostly determined by the size and chromatin pattern of the lymphoma cells, with certain exceptions. Low-grade lymphomas are mostly small in size with coarse chromatin, and high-grade B-cell lymphomas are typically large lymphoid cells with open or blastoid chromatin and variably prominent nucleoli. The differential diagnosis of an abnormal proliferation of small mature lymphoid cells commonly includes small lymphocytic lymphoma (SLL), mantle cell lymphoma (MCL), nodal or extranodal marginal zone lymphoma (MZL), low-grade FL, and (rarely) lymphoplasmacytic lymphoma (LPL). Lymphomas with medium-sized lymphoid cells include such aggressive lymphomas as BL; B-lymphoblastic lymphoma (B-ALL); blastoid variant of MCL; high-grade B-cell lymphoma with *MYC, BCL2,* and/or *BCL6* rearrangements; and high-grade B-cell lymphoma, not otherwise specified (NOS). Diffuse large B-cell lymphomas (DLBCL) are characterized by the proliferation of large lymphoid cells. Nonetheless, the classification of B-cell lymphomas frequently requires the incorporation of cytogenetic or molecular features that also have prognostication or therapeutic importance. The revised 4th edition of the WHO classification incorporates several proposed changes that reflect the increasing knowledge of the underlying molecular pathways and clinical outcomes of various entities. For instance, the classification of DLBCL is not only based on Han's algorithm[13] that uses immunohistochemical (IHC) staining for CD10, BCL6, and MUM1 for subtyping (see Chapter 35); it also mandates FISH testing for *MYC, BCL2*, and *BCL6* gene rearrangements to exclude high-grade B-cell lymphoma with *MYC, BCL2,* and/or *BCL6* rearrangements ("double-hit" or "triple-hit" lymphomas) (see Figure 33.3), which are associated with very aggressive clinical behavior and adverse outcomes. Further, it is recommended to assess the presence of "dual expressor" status per IHC results (defined as MYC positivity >40% and BCL2 positivity >50% by IHC stains)—namely, "Double Expressor Lymphoma."[14] These changes were made because these subgroups define patient populations with inferior clinical outcomes as well as patient groups to target with novel therapies. The "Double Expressor Lymphoma" is associated with a poorer clinical outcome than DLBCL, NOS, but it is less aggressive than high-grade B-cell lymphoma with *MYC, BCL2,* and/or *BCL6* rearrangements.[15] Clinical trials are increasingly enrolling patients based on determining cell of origin in DLBCL via multiple techniques and molecular/cytogenetic features. Of note, the revised 4th edition of WHO classification also includes several early B-cell neoplasms (in situ follicular neoplasia, in situ mantle cell neoplasia), an updated definition of Epstein–Barr virus (EBV) positive DLBCL, NOS, and newly proposed entities, such as EBV-positive mucocutaneous ulcer. There are no major changes to the classification of classical Hodgkin lymphomas in the revised 4th edition of WHO classification. In terms of T-cell lymphomas, the diagnosis relies on the incorporation of clinical features, architectural and cytologic changes, as well as phenotypes of the lymphoma cells.

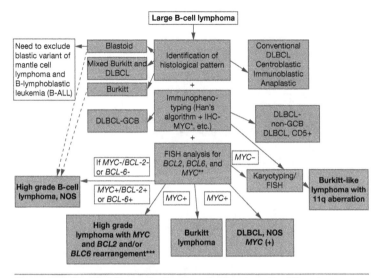

Figure 33.3 Modified diagnostic algorithm of diffuse large B-cell lymphoma.

*Overexpression of *MYC* by immunostaining (>40% of neoplastic B-cells). "Double Expressor lymphoma" (dual MYC +/BCL2+ by IHC) is diagnosed if further FISH is negative for *MYC* gene rearrangement. In addition to CD10, BCL2, BCL6, MUM1, and MYC IHC studies, CD5 and Ki-67 are commonly determined. **FISH study shows *MYC* gene rearrangement by the *MYC* break-apart probe, not including amplification of *MYC* signal. ***The new terminology is to replace "double-" or "triple-hit" "lymphoma." DLBCL, diffuse large B-cell lymphomas; GCB, germinal center B-cell; FISH, fluorescence in situ hybridization; IHC, immunohistochemical; NOS, not otherwise specified.

The determination of small or large lymphoid cells plays a minor role in the classification of T-cell lymphomas. In the updated classification, a modified classification of mature T-cell neoplasms was proposed, including several new categories, such as two indolent T-cell lymphoproliferative disorders, changed type II enteropathy-associated T-cell lymphoma (EATCL) to monomorphic epitheliotropic intestinal T-cell lymphoma (MEITL), and added 4 other rare mature T-cell lymphomas.[12]

■ SUMMARY

Morphologic analysis of tissue is central to rational triaging for ancillary studies that will allow for an accurate diagnosis according to current classification schemes and optimal management of patients. The revised 4th edition of the WHO classification of tumors of hematopoietic and lymphoid tissues has evolved over many years with the increasing understanding of the clinical and molecular cytogenetic features of different lymphomas and will continue to be modified as new biological pathways are discovered.

▓ REFERENCES

1. Harris NL, Jaffe ES, Stein H, et al. A revised European-American classification of lymphoid neoplasms: a proposal from the International Lymphoma Study Group. *Blood.* 1994;84(5):1361–1392.

2. Hicks EB, Rappaport H, Winter WJ. Follicular lymphoma; a re-evaluation of its position in the scheme of malignant lymphoma, based on a survey of 253 cases. *Cancer.* 1956;9(4):792–821.

3. Lukes RJ, Collins RD. Lukes-Collins classification and its significance. *Cancer Treat Rep.* 1977;61(6):971–979.

4. Lennert K, Collins RD, Lukes RJ. Concordance of the Kiel and Lukes-Collins classifications of non-Hodgkin's lymphomas. *Histopathology.* 1983;7(4):549–559.

5. National Cancer Institute sponsored study of classifications of non-Hodgkin's lymphomas: summary and description of a working formulation for clinical usage. The Non-Hodgkin's Lymphoma Pathologic Classification Project. *Cancer.* 1982;49(10):2112–2135.

6. Robb-Smith AH. U.S. National Cancer Institute working formulation of non-Hodgkin's lymphomas for clinical use. *Lancet.* 1982; 2(8295):432–434.

7. Papermaster BW, Good RA. Relative contributions of the thymus and the bursa of Fabricius to the maturation of the lymphoreticur system and immunological potential in the chicken. *Nature.* 1962;196:838–840.

8. Cooper MD, Peterson RD, Good RA. Delineation of the thymic and bursal lymphoid systems in the chicken. *Nature.* 1965;205:143–146.

9. Shevach EM, Jaffe ES, Green I. Receptors for complement and immunoglobulin on human and animal lymphoid cells. *Transplant Rev.* 1973;16:3–28.

10. Jaffe ES, Braylan RC, Nanba K, et al. Functional markers: a new perspective on malignant lymphomas. *Cancer Treat Rep.* 1977;61(6):953–962.

11. Swerdlow SH, Campo E, Harris NL, et al. *WHO Classification of Tumours of Haematopoietic and Lymphoid Tissues* (4th ed.). International Agency for Research on Cancer; 2008:229.

12. Swerdlow SH, Campo E, Harris NL, et al. *WHO Classification of Tumours of Haematopoietic and Lymphoid Tissues.* IARC Press;2017.

13. Hans CP, Weisenburger DD, Greiner TC, et al. Confirmation of the molecular classification of diffuse large B-cell lymphoma by immunohistochemistry using a tissue microarray. *Blood.* 2004;103(1):275–282.

14. Hu S, Xu-Monette ZY, Tzankov A, et al. MYC/BCL2 protein coexpression contributes to the inferior survival of activated B-cell subtype of diffuse large B-cell lymphoma and demonstrates high-risk gene expression signatures: a report from the International DLBCL Rituximab-CHOP Consortium Program. *Blood.* 2013;121(20):4021–4031; quiz 4250.

15. Johnson NA, Slack GW, Savage KJ, et al. Concurrent expression of MYC and BCL2 in diffuse large B-cell lymphoma treated with rituximab plus cyclophosphamide, doxorubicin, vincristine, and prednisone. *J Clin Oncol.* 2012;30(28):3452–3459.

34 Burkitt Lymphoma

Anju Nair

With acknowledgments to Dr. Micah Burch for
his contribution to the first edition.

▮ INTRODUCTION

Burkitt lymphoma (BL) is a highly aggressive form of non-Hodgkin lymphoma, derived from the germinal- or post-germinal-center B-cells and defined by a translocation of the *c-MYC* gene on chromosome 8. There are three distinct clinical forms of BL: endemic, sporadic, and immunodeficiency associated. Although all forms of BL present with a rapidly enlarging tumor, each form has its own epidemiology, clinical signs, and genetic features. The endemic variant is seen in Africa nearly 50 times more frequently than in the United States and accounts for nearly 30% to 50% of all childhood cancer in equatorial Africa. Cases are most commonly seen in children ages 4 to 7 years, with a higher predilection for males than females. Endemic BL presents as a jaw or facial bone tumor in 50% to 60% of cases. Chronic Epstein–Barr virus (EBV) infections are seen in nearly all case of endemic BL but can also be seen in some sporadic and immunodeficiency-associated variants of BL.

Sporadic variants are seen in the United States and make up <1% of adult non-Hodgkin lymphomas in the United States. Cases are typically seen in male patients <35 years of age, with a median age of 30 years at time of diagnosis. The majority of sporadic BL patients present with bulky abdominal adenopathy, and only 25% of cases involve the jaw or facial bones.

Immunodeficiency-associated BL variant is seen largely in patients with human immunodeficiency virus (HIV) infection. The use of antiretroviral therapy (ART) in the HIV population has not decreased the incidence of BL, as patients with cluster of differentiation 4 (CD4) counts >200 cells/mcL develop BL at a similar rate (see Chapter 40).

▮ DIAGNOSIS

BL is diagnosed by using pathologic examination of involved tissue to assess morphology, immunophenotype, and genetic features. Diffuse large B-cell lymphoma, B-lymphoblastic leukemia/lymphoma, and blastoid variant of mantle cell lymphoma must be ruled out, as they can also present as large facial or abdominal masses. With BL, an excisional biopsy of the tumor typically reveals sheets of monotonous, medium-sized, atypical lymphoid cells with extensive necrosis or apoptosis and a high rate of proliferation (Ki-67 ranging from 90% to 100%). The classic "starry sky" pattern is present from multiple benign tingible-body macrophages or histiocytes ("stars") that have ingested apoptotic tumor cells (Figure 34.1). The macrophages contain abundant clear cytoplasm set against a background of basophilic malignant lymphocytes ("sky").

The tumor cells usually express surface immunoglobulins (Ig), B-cell-associated antigens, and germinal center–associated markers, listed in Table 34.1. BL tumor cells do not express CD5, BCL-2, or TdT, and they typically lack CD23 expression. Nearly all endemic BL tumors are EBV positive and express CD21, the EBV C3d receptor (also known as the complement receptor 2 [CR2]).

BL is almost always characterized with a translocation of the *c-YC* oncogene on the long arm of chromosome 8 and one of three locations on Ig genes. The *c-MYC* translocation with the Ig heavy chain

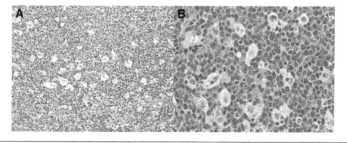

Figure 34.1 Starry sky pattern of BL. Microscopic examination reveals sheets of atypical lymphoid cells associated with increased tingible-body/phagocytizing macrophages in the background forming the "starry sky" pattern (A, hematoxylin and eosin [H&E], ×200). Cytologically, the atypical lymphoid cells are uniformly medium in size with scant cytoplasm, exhibit high nuclear to cytoplasmic ratio, and usually have more than one nucleoli (B, H&E, ×600).

Table 34.1 Tumor Cell Surface Markers	
Surface Markers Expressed in BL	
Ig	IgM and Ig light chains (kappa > lambda)
B-cell-associated antigens	CD19, CD 20, CD22, CD79a
Germinal center–associated markers	CD10 and BCL 6
BL, Burkitt lymphoma; Ig, immunoglobulin; IgM, immunoglobulin M.	

gene on chromosome 14 [t(8;14)] is the most common. However, other variant translocation partners include the kappa light chain gene on chromosome 2 [t(2;8)] and the lambda light chain gene on chromosome 22 [t(8;22)], observed in 15% and 5% of cases, respectively. *c-MYC* gene rearrangements can be detected through routine cytogenetic analysis or fluorescent in situ hybridization (FISH). In the rare 5% of cases that present without a *c-MYC* rearrangement, morphologic and immunophenotypic findings consistent with BL can be used to confirm the diagnosis. Before treatment is initiated, patients with suspected or confirmed BL should undergo pretreatment evaluation with laboratory studies, including complete blood count (CBC) with differential, complete metabolic panel (CMP), lactate dehydrogenase (LDH), and uric acid. Screening for hepatitis B and HIV must be completed. For staging, all patients with BL are recommended to have a bone marrow (BM) biopsy and a lumbar puncture to evaluate for central nervous system (CNS) involvement (cytology and flow cytometry). In addition, patients require a contrast-enhanced computed tomography (CT) scan of the chest, abdomen, and pelvis with IV contrast or positron emission tomography–computed tomography (PET-CT) scan. Furthermore, cardiac function must be assessed by echocardiogram or multigated acquisition (MUGA) scan study prior to anthracycline-based therapy. Fertility preservation must be discussed with patients of child-bearing age. BL is staged based on the Ann Arbor Staging criteria (Table 34.2).

For treatment purposes, BL is further risk stratified as low-risk or high-risk disease. Low-risk patients have nonbulky (<10 cm diameter, extra-abdominal single mass), early-stage (I or II) disease with good performance status and a normal LDH. Patients are classified as high risk if they do not fall into the low-risk category.

Table 34.2 Ann Arbor Staging

Stage	Sites of Involvement
I	Single lymphatic site (or nodal region) or extra-lymphatic structure
II	Involvement of two or more lymph node regions on the same side of the diaphragm
III	Involvement of lymph node regions or lymphoid structures on both sides of the diaphragm
IV	Diffuse or disseminated involvement of one or more extra-lymphatic organs, with or without associated lymph node involvement

Modifiers: A, no B symptoms; B, B symptoms (fevers, sweats, weight loss >10% body weight); X, bulky disease, mass >10 cm.

PROGNOSIS

Overall, BL has a favorable prognosis, with long-term survival ranging from 75% to 90% with current available first-line chemo-immunotherapy. As expected, patients with limited-stage disease have a lower risk of death than patients with advanced stage. A similar correlation between age and survival is also seen with patients younger than 20 years of age having an 87% 5-year survival compared to only a 33% 5-year survival for patients above the age of 60. However, based on a large population study (3,691 cases), patients in the general population have inferior survival rates in comparison to patients treated on clinical trials (3-year overall survival [OS] of 56% vs. 82%–95%), which could be related to selection bias but also to lack of specialized care in a tertiary center.

TREATMENT

In all cases of BL, patients are encouraged to enter an appropriate clinical trial if possible. For patients who are not candidates for clinical trials, an aggressive combination chemotherapy regimen with CNS prophylaxis must be initiated, preferably within 48 hours of encountering a patient with suspected BL. Without appropriate CNS prophylaxis, 30% to 50% of patients will develop CNS relapse, typically within 5 to 12 months of the initial diagnosis. There is no role for radiation therapy or surgery, even in cases of localized disease. Standard treatment is based on a risk-adapted approach modified from the guidelines proposed by the National Cancer Institute (NCI). In HIV-positive patients, ART must be initiated (or continued if the patient has known HIV infection prior to BL diagnosis) in addition to cytotoxic therapy. Appropriate treatment considerations and caution should be given to elderly patients, patients with heart disease, and those with CNS involvement. Due to the disease's aggressive nature and tumor bulk, tumor lysis prophylaxis with intravenous hydration and allopurinol ± rasburicase should be administered (see Chapter 59).

FRONTLINE THERAPY IN LOW-RISK PATIENTS

- R-CODOX-M × 3 cycles (cyclophosphamide, vincristine, doxorubicin, high-dose methotrexate (MTX) with rituximab, and IT MTX and cytarabine) (*Ann Oncol.* 2011;22(8):1859–1864; *J Clin Oncol.* 1996;14(3):925–934)

- HyperCVAD (hyperfractionated cyclophosphamide, vincristine, doxorubicin, dexamethasone alternating with high-dose MTX, cytarabine with rituximab, and IT MTX and cytarabine) (*Cancer.* 2006;106(7):1569–1580)

- DA-EPOCH (etoposide, prednisone, vincristine, cyclophosphamide and doxorubicin) + rituximab, at least 3 cycles, with 1 cycle beyond complete response (*Blood.* 2017;130(Suppl1):188)

FRONTLINE THERAPY IN HIGH-RISK PATIENTS

- R-CODOX-M and IVAC × 2 cycles each, in alternating courses (IVAC: ifosfamide, etoposide, cytarabine with rituximab, and IT MTX and cytarabine) (*Ann Oncol.* 2011;22(8):1859–1864; *J Clin Oncol.* 1996;14(3):925–934)
- HyperCVAD × 6 cycles alternating with high dose methotrexate and cytarabine (*Cancer.* 2006;106(7):1569–1580)
- Dose-adjusted EPOCH with rituximab (DA-EPOCH-R) × 6 cycles (infusional etoposide, prednisone, vincristine, cyclophosphamide, doxorubicin with IT MTX, and rituximab) in patients without CNS disease (*Ann Oncol.* 2008;19(Suppl4):iv83–iv84)

Within 1 month of treatment completion, response should be assessed by using history, physical examination, routine laboratory studies, and CT imaging study, followed by periodic surveillance for possible relapse.

TREATMENT FOR RELAPSED/REFRACTORY DISEASE

Patients with refractory or relapsed disease should be encouraged to participate in clinical trials, as they have extremely poor prognosis outside clinical trials. Limited data are available for second-line therapies.

- CODOX/IVAC × 2 cycles each or DA-EPOCH-R or RICE (rituximab, ifosfamide, carboplatin, etoposide, and IT MTX if not previously received) or RIVAC or RGDP (rituximab, gemcitabine, dexamethasone, cisplatin) or high-dose cytarabine and rituximab (*Pediatr Blood Cancer.* 2009;52:177–181).
- Responders should consider high-dose therapy with stem cell transplant (*J Clin Oncol.* 1996;14(9):2465–2472).

▓ POTENTIAL PRACTICE-CHANGING CLINICAL TRIALS

An open-label, multicenter, single-arm, phase 2 trial of CPI-613 (anti-mitochondrial metabolism agent) monotherapy is currently ongoing in patients with relapsed or refractory BL. In a phase 1 study, CPI-613 showed efficacy in a patient with heavily treated BL (*Clin Cancer Res.* 20(20):5255–5264). An open-label study is planned to assess immunotherapy with CD19 CAR (Chimeric antigen receptor)—T-cells for high-risk children and young adults with high-risk hematologic malignancies, including BL. Furthermore, mutations in genes *TCF3* and *ID3* were found in 70% of sporadic BL patients. Potentially, a less toxic, targeted therapeutic regimen for BL could become available in the future.

▓ REFERENCES FOR SUPPLEMENTAL READING

1. Hill QA, Owen RG. CNS prophylaxis in lymphoma: who to target and what therapy to use. *Blood Rev.* 2006;20:319.

2. Lacasce A, Howard O, Lib S, et al. Modified magrath regimens for adults with Burkitt and Burkitt-like lymphomas: preserved efficacy with decreased toxicity. *Leuk Lymphoma*. 2004;45:761.

3. Barnes JA, Lacasce AS, Feng Y, et al. Evaluation of the addition of rituximab to CODOX-M/IVAC for Burkitt's lymphoma: a retrospective analysis. *Ann Oncol*. 2011;22(8):1859–1864.

4. Thomas DA, Faderl S, O'Brien S, et al. Chemoimmunotherapy with hyper-CVAD plus rituximab for the treatment of adult Burkitt and Burkitt-type lymphoma or acute lymphoblastic leukemia. *Cancer*. 2006;106(7):1569–1580.

5. Dunleavy K, Little RF, Pittaluga S, et al. A prospective study of dose-adjusted EPOCH with rituximab in adult patients with newly diagnosed Burkitt lymphoma: a regimen with high efficacy and low toxicity. *Ann Oncol*. 2008;19(Suppl4):iv83–iv84.

35   Diffuse Large B-Cell Lymphoma

Jose D. Sandoval-Sus and Julio C. Chavez

▤ INTRODUCTION

Diffuse large B-cell lymphoma (DLBCL) is a heterogeneous group of mature B-cell-derived neoplasms characterized by large lymphocytes with a diffuse growth pattern. It is the most common lymphoid neoplasm in the Western world, accounting for approximately 25% to 30% of non-Hodgkin lymphomas (NHL), with an incidence of 7 cases per 100,000 persons/year and a higher prevalence in developing countries (40% of NHL). Even though it is more prevalent in white males and its incidence increases with age (median age at diagnosis is 66 years), it can also occur in children and young adults of all ethnicities. Patients usually present with rapidly enlarging lymphadenopathy/mass and constitutional symptoms. Up to 40% of DLBCL cases have extranodal involvement at diagnosis (e.g., bones, gastrointestinal tract, central nervous system [CNS], etc.). Recognizing that DLBCL is not a single disease but a heterogeneous entity with diverse molecular, pathophysiologic, and prognostic features has improved our ability to make accurate diagnoses and enhance therapeutic effectiveness.

▤ DIAGNOSIS

2016 WORLD HEALTH ORGANIZATION (WHO) DLBCL VARIANTS, SUBGROUPS, AND SUBTYPES

An excisional or incisional biopsy from an enlarged lymph node or from an extranodal mass is the preferred diagnostic method. However, an image-guided core-needle biopsy can be considered when the lymph node/extranodal mass is not easily accessible. A fine-needle aspirate is usually inadequate for diagnosis, which results in higher incidence of sampling error and false negatives (Table 35.1).

Morphology

- Lymph nodes show a diffuse infiltrate of large lymphoid cells that typically efface the nodal architecture. Most common morphologic variants are centroblastic, immunoblastic, anaplastic, and T-cell rich.

Table 35.1 DLBCL Variants, Subgroups, and Subtypes

DLBCL GCB and DLBCL ABC*	EBV-positive DLBCL, NOS
CD5+ DLBCL	PMBL (thymic)
T-cell/histiocyte-rich large B-cell lymphoma	Intravascular large B-cell lymphoma
Primary DLBCL of the CNS	DLBCL associated with chronic inflammation
Primary cutaneous DLBCL, leg type	Lymphomatoid granulomatosis
ALK-positive large B-cell lymphoma	DLBCL with IRF4/MUM1 rearrangement
HHV8+ DLBCL, NOS**	Primary effusion lymphoma
B-cell lymphoma, unclassifiable, with features intermediate between DLBCL and classical HL***	High-grade B-cell lymphoma with *MYC*, *BCL2*, and/or *BCL6* rearrangements****

ABC, activated B-cell; ALK, anaplastic lymphoma kinase; CNS, central nervous system; DLBCL, diffuse large B-cell lymphoma; EBV, Epstein–Barr virus; GCB, germinal-center B-cell; HL, Hodgkin lymphoma; NOS, not otherwise specified; PMBL, primary mediastinal B-cell lymphoma.

*Molecular DLBCL overall response rate (NOS) subgroups.

**Diagnostic category changed from "large B-cell lymphoma arising in HHV8-associated multicentric Castleman disease" in the 2016 WHO updates.

***Previously designated gray-zone lymphomas.

****Known as double-hit or triple-hit lymphoma (see Chapter 36).

Immunophenotype

- Typical immunophenotype by immunohistochemistry (IHC): B-cells markers, such as CD19+, CD20+, CD45+, CD79a+ and CD3–.
- IHC for CD10, BCL-6, and IRF4/MUM1 (per Hans algorithm) should be included as a surrogate tool to determine the cell of origin phenotype (germinal-center B-cell [GCB] vs. non-GCB) a prognostic feature in DLBCL with no proven predicted value at moment (see Figure 35.1).
- The IHC panel should also include *MYC* and *BCL-2* in order to identify "double-expressor" large B-cell NHL lymphoma variants, an aggressive subtype of DLBCL with poor prognosis (see Chapter 36).
- Consider other IHC stains in special circumstances: cyclin D1, CD5, CD30, CD138, EBER-ISH, ALK, and HHV8.
- Flow cytometry to assess cell surface markers: CD45, CD3, CD5, CD19, CD10, CD23, CD20, kappa, and light chain surface immunoglobulin (sIg).

Fluorescence In Situ Hybridization (FISH)

- t(3;v) and t(14;18): most common translocations seen in DLBCL (30% for both).

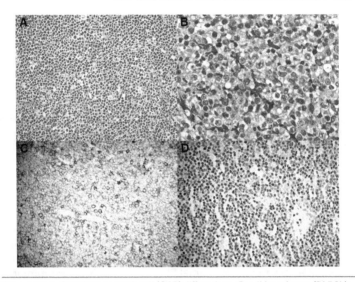

Figure 35.1 Germinal center B-cell (GCB) diffuse large B-cell lymphoma (DLBCL): The section of lymph node shows a complete replacement by large atypical lymphoid cells (A, hematoxylin and eosin [H&E], ×200). A high-power view shows the lymphoma cells displaying large round to overall nuclei, vesicular chromatin, one or more visible nucleoli, and abundant cytoplasm (B, H&E, ×600). They coexpress germinal-center cell markers CD10 (C, ×200) and BCL-6 (D, ×200). The large cells were also CD20+/CD3– (not shown).

- t(8;14): translocation of the *MYC* gene occurs in ≤10% of DLBCL and usually confers a poor prognosis, especially in the presence of other partner translocations (*BCL-2/BCL-6*; see Chapter 36).

Initial laboratory workup must include a complete blood count (CBC) with differential, complete metabolic panel (CMP) with phosphorus levels, lactate dehydrogenase (LDH), and uric acid. Serologic evaluation of hepatitis B/C and human immunodeficiency virus (HIV), and pregnancy testing in women of child-bearing age should be done prior to treatment. Beta-2-microglobulin can also be considered as a baseline prognostic factor. In terms of tumor staging, either a positron emission tomography–computed tomography (PET-CT) scan (preferred) or a chest/abdomen/pelvis computed tomography (CT) scan with contrast and a bone marrow (BM) biopsy should be performed as part of the baseline diagnostic assessment. In patients with neurological deficits at diagnosis or at high risk for CNS involvement, a magnetic resonance image of the brain with/without contrast or CT brain scan with contrast and a lumbar puncture (LP) with cerebrospinal fluid (CSF) analysis are recommended. CNS imaging and/or CSF studies are also recommended in cases with epidural, testicular, or breast involvement; HIV-related DLBCL with 2 or more extranodal sites and/

or elevated LDH levels. The CNS International Prognostic Index (CNS-IPI) (score ≥4) can be used to determine the risk of CNS relapse. Finally, either a 2D-echocardiogram or a multigated acquisition (MUGA) scan is needed before using an anthracycline-based chemoimmunotherapy (CIT) to determine baseline cardiac function.

▓ STAGING

DLBCL is currently staged using the Ann Arbor staging system with Cotswold modifications. In 2014, a Lugano staging system was proposed in which DLBCL is divided into limited (stages I, II, and II bulky) and advanced stages (stages III and IV).

▓ KEY DIAGNOSTIC DILEMMA

B-cell lymphoma, unclassifiable, with features intermediate between DLBCL and classical Hodgkin lymphoma (cHL), commonly known as "gray-zone" lymphoma (GZL), is commonly seen in young men (20–40 years) and usually presents with a bulky mediastinal mass. The morphology of the tumor is characterized by large pleomorphic B-cells in a background of stromal fibrosis. It usually shares immunophenotypic markers present in primary mediastinal B-cell lymphoma (PMBL) and cHL.

▓ PROGNOSIS

DLBCL is considered a curable disease; however, prognosis and individual therapeutic outcomes can vary among patients. The IPI has been typically used to classify patients into four risk groups based on five clinical variables (Table 35.2). However, the IPI was designed in the pre-rituximab era and may overestimate the risk of patients treated with rituximab containing CIT. Redistribution of the IPI factors into a revised IPI (R-IPI) developed in the post-rituximab era identified three distinct prognostic groups that are more clinically relevant in CIT-based treatments (Table 35.2). The most comprehensive prognostic score available is the national comprehensive cancer network (NCCN-IPI), which identifies more accurately patients with very good (5-year overall survival [OS] = 96%) and very poor prognoses (5-year OS = 33%). These prognostic scores are useful, because they separate patients into risk-category groups that can give prognostic information to patients. Nonetheless, there is considerable heterogeneity within those groups. Gene-expression profiling (GEP) studies determined at least three different DLBCL genetic subtypes (GCB, ABC, and PMBL) with clear distinct outcomes among molecular classes that were independent from the IPI score or other prognostic factors (e.g., *MYC/BCL2* dual expression).

▓ TREATMENT

DLBCL is potentially curable with CIT, with more than two-thirds of patients achieving prolonged complete remissions (CR). In preparation for chemotherapy, the risk of tumor lysis syndrome should be

Table 35.2 Revised International Prognostic Index (R-IPI)

IPI Risk Factors Age >60 years, PS ≥ 2, serum LDH > ULN, Extranodal Sites ≥ 2, Stages III to IV

Risk Factors	Risk Groups	5-Year PFS (%)	5-Year OS (%)
0	Very good	94	94
1, 2	Good	80	79
3, 4, 5	Poor	53	55

IPI, International Prognostic Index; LDH, lactate dehydrogenase; OS, overall survival; PFS, progression free survival; PS, performance status; ECOG, eastern cooperative oncology group; R-IPI, revised International Prognostic Index; ULN, upper limit of normal.
Blood. 2007;109(5):1857–1861.

assessed, and prophylaxis with allopurinol or rasburicase should be considered accordingly. Also, in patients with positive hepatitis-B serologies (surface antigen or IgG core antibody), a viral load and initiation of antiviral therapy before using rituximab is recommended. Rituximab, cyclophosphamide, doxorubicin, vincristine, and prednisone every 21 days (RCHOP-21) is currently the standard frontline therapy for newly diagnosed DLBCL patients. However, initial treatment can be individualized based on age, comorbidities, and the disease burden at presentation.

FIRST-LINE THERAPY

Stages I and II Nonbulky (<7.5 cm) DLBCL (Limited Disease)

- RCHOP × 3 cycles + involved site radiation therapy (ISRT; *J Clin Oncol.* 2008;26:2258–2263).
- RCHOP × 4 cycles + 2 cycles of rituximab every 21 days for patients with age-adjusted IPI = 0 (*Lancet.* 2020;394:2271–2281).
- RCHOP × 3 cycles followed by PET-CT. If PET-CT is negative (DS 1–3), 1 more cycle of RCHOP is given without need for ISRT (Persky DO, et al. *J Clin Oncol.* 2020 Sep 10;38(26):3003–3011.
- RCHOP × 6 cycles ± ISRT for residual masses (*Lancet Oncol.* 2011;12:1013–1022).

Stage I or II Bulky (≥7.5 cm) or Stages III and IV DLBCL (Advanced Disease)

- RCHOP × 6 cycles ± ISRT for residual masses or clinical trial (NCCN Category 1; *J Clin Oncol.* 2019;37(21):1790–1799).

When indicated, include CNS prophylaxis with either systemic methotrexate (MTX) (3–3.5 g/m^2 for 2–4 cycles) on day 15 of every other cycle OR intratechal MTX, and/or cytarabine (4–8 doses). Interim restaging imaging with contrasted CT scans after 3 to 4 cycles is recommended to assess response. Although interim PET-CT is controversial, it should be used in disease that is only imaged by PET-CT (e.g., bone lymphoma). Interpretation of interim images should be taken with caution and must be evaluated in conjunction with the clinical response. If there are suspicious lesions in the context of a suboptimal therapeutic response (e.g., patients with less than a partial response [PR]), a new biopsy should always be done before implementing therapeutic changes. On the other hand, if the patient has a favorable response, treatment should be continued without alterations. Posttreatment restaging should be done between 6 and 8 weeks after the last CIT cycle, using PET-CT as the preferred imaging modality based on proven prognostic value.

SURVEILLANCE AFTER CR

Clinical follow-up with full history, physical examination, and laboratory workup is recommended every 3 to 6 months for at least 5 years. A post-remission long-term imaging surveillance has not proven to be beneficial and is currently not recommended on a routine basis. Rituximab maintenance is not recommended in DLBCL, and, to date, consolidation with autologous hematopoietic stem cell transplant (AutoHCT) for aggressive DLBCL (age-adjusted IPI >3) is controversial, and we recommend evaluation in a tertiary cancer center with lymphoma expertise if this consolidation strategy is considered.

RELAPSE/REFRACTORY (R/R) DLBCL

Treatment depends on the patient's performance status (PS), comorbidities, and tumor chemosensitivity. Patients with progressive or stable disease after frontline CIT, with a CR of <12 months after standard CIT, and/or with relapse in ≤12 months after AutoHCT have the poorest survival outcomes. The current approach is to categorize patients as transplant eligible or ineligible. Patients who are eligible for AutoHCT or chimeric antigen receptor T-cell (CAR-T) therapy should be treated with curative intent. Enrollment in clinical trials should always be offered whenever possible.

Patients Eligible for Transplant

- Consider salvage chemotherapy regimens—such as rituximab, ifosfamide, etoposide (RICE); rituximab, dexamethasone, cytarabine, cisplatin (R-DHAP); rituximab, etoposide, dexamethasone, cytarabine, cisplatin (R-ESHAP); or rituximab, gemcitabine, dexamethasone, cisplatin (R-GDP)—followed by consolidation therapy with AutoHCT if evidence of chemosensitive disease.
- R-GDP or gemcitabine plus oxaliplatin (R-GemOx) are options that can be used before AutoHCT in patients with suboptimal response to RICE, R-DHAP, or R-ESHAP.
- Patients who achieve PR after salvage therapy are technically considered to have chemosensitive disease, and AutoHCT is recommended; however, patients have higher risk of relapse, especially

if prior they exhibited short response or no response to initial CIT. Consideration for CAR-T therapy should be discussed and the patient referred to a CAR-T–certified center.

- For patients with stable or progressive disease post-salvage treatments, anti-CD19 CAR-T therapy is recommended. Axicabtagene ciloleucel and tisagenlecleucel are the 2 CAR-T products currently approved for R/R DLBCL after 2 lines of therapy (see Chapter 56).

Patients Ineligible for Transplant

- The choice of therapy will depend on the patient's comorbidities, PS, and previous therapies.
- Some options are GDP ± rituximab; GemOx ± rituximab; lenalidomide ± rituximab (predominantly of non-GCB subtype); ibrutinib (predominantly of non-GCB subtype); PEPC (prednisone, etoposide, procarbazine, cyclophosphamide); and brentuximab vedotin for DLBCL with any level of CD30 expression by IHC (*Blood.* 2015;125(9):1394–1402).
- Polatuzumab vedotin (PV) + bendamustine + rituximab every 21 days for up to 6 cycles is indicated in patients with R/R DLBCL after ≥2 prior therapies (*J Clin Oncol.* 2019;38:155–165).

▓ POTENTIAL PRACTICE-CHANGING CLINICAL TRIALS

In newly diagnosed DLBCL patients, several phase 3 clinical trials have recently reported negative results (Alliance/CALGB 50303, ROBUST, PHOENIX, and REMoDL-B trials); hence, RCHOP remains the standard of care. Nonetheless, this regimen is not curative in ≥35% of patients, with further improvement needed. Due to the single-agent activity of PV in DLBCL, reinforced by its recent approval in R/R disease, this agent was combined with rituximab plus cyclophosphamide, doxorubicin, and prednisone (PV + RCHP) on a phase 1b/2 study. The combination was well tolerated and showed an overall response rate (ORR) and a CR of 89% and 77%, respectively (*Lancet Oncol.* 2019;20(7):998–1010). A phase 3 RCT of PV + RCHP + vincristine placebo versus RCHOP + PV placebo for frontline therapy of DLBCL is ongoing (POLARIX trial; NCT03274492). In DLBCL, one of the goals is to avoid overtreatment by de-escalating therapy when possible, and the recently presented S1001 phase 3 trial showed excellent outcomes in treatment-naïve patients with nonbulky (<10 cm) stage I/II DLBCL treated with 4 cycles of RCHOP ± ISRT based on interim PET-CT scans. Patients who had negative PET after 3 treatment cycles had excellent outcomes without ISRT, showing 5-year PFS and OS of 88% and 91%, respectively. Together with the FLYER trial, this study establishes a new standard of care for patients with limited-stage DLBL. In the R/R setting, the most exciting advance is CAR-T cell therapy, a topic covered in other chapters. For patients not eligible for hematopoietic stem cell transplant (HCT) or CAR-T therapy, several trials are ongoing. A phase 3 trial of PV + R-GemOx versus R-GemOx + placebo in in R/R DLBCL patients (POLARGO trial; NCT04182204) recently started that could be a good option for this population. Multiple cytotoxic chemotherapy-free strategies are being tested in clinical trials, such as the anti-CD19 monoclonal antibody (MOR-209; tafasitamab) that showed single-agent ORR of 26% with minor side effects (*Ann Oncol.* 2018;29(5):1266–1272). When combined with lenalidomide, the ORR was 58%, and the 12-month PFS and OS were 70% and 73%, respectively. A phase 3 trial of tafasitamab + bendamustine versus rituximab + bendamustine in R/R DLBCL is enrolling (B-MIND trial; NCT04182204). The anti-CD47 antibody treatment with magrolimab (Hu5f9-G4) + rituximab has also showed promising activity in heavily treated R/R DLBCL patients. Lastly, bi-specific antibodies, such as mosunetuzumab and REGN1979 (anti-CD20 × anti-CD3 antibodies), recently showed promising safety and efficacy data in heavily pretreated patients, including clinical responses in the post-CAR-T setting (Bennerji R, et al. *Blood.* 2019;134(Suppl1):762; Schuster SJ, et al. *Blood.* 2019;134(Suppl1):6). While these early reports are encouraging, large confirmatory studies are needed.

▣ REFERENCES FOR SUPPLEMENTAL READING

1. Liu Y, Barta SK. Diffuse large B-cell lymphoma: 2019 update on diagnosis, risk stratification, and treatment. *Am J Hematol.* 2019;94:604–616.

2. Poeschel V, Held G, Ziepert M, et al. Four versus six cycles of CHOP chemotherapy in combination with six applications of rituximab in patients with aggressive B-cell lymphoma with favorable prognosis (FLYER): a randomized, phase 3, non-inferiority trial. *Lancet.* 2020;394:2271–2281.

3. Bartlett NL, Wilson WH, Jung SH, et al. Dose adjusted EPOCH-R compared to R-CHOP as frontline therapy for diffuse large B-cell lymphoma: clinical outcomes of the phase III Intergroup trial alliance/CALGB 50303. *J Clin Oncol.* 2019;37(21):1790–1799.

4. Sehn LH, Herrera AF, Flowers CR, et al. Polatuzumab vedotin in relapsed or refractory diffuse large B-cell lymphoma. *J Clin Oncol.* 2019;38:155–165.

5. Younes A, Sehn LH, Johnson P, et al. Randomized phase III trial of Ibrutinib and rituximab plus cyclophosphamide, doxorubicin, vincristine, and prednisone in non-germinal center B-cell diffuse large B-cell lymphoma. *J Clin Oncol.* 2019;37:1285–1295.

36   Double-Hit Lymphoma

Nikhil Mukhi

▒ INTRODUCTION

Double-hit lymphoma (DHL) is a genetically defined subset of diffuse large B-cell lymphomas (DLBCL) that has a significantly poorer prognosis. By definition, it is characterized by the detection of chromosomal breakpoint affecting the *MYC*/8q24 locus in combination with the breakpoint in *BCL2*/18q21, or less commonly *BCL6*/3q27 (Figure 36.1). Rarely, *MYC* gene rearrangement can occur in conjunction with both *BCL2* and *BCL6*, which is known as "triple hit" lymphoma (THL). World Health Organization (WHO) 2016 revised classification of tumors of hematopoietic and lymphoid tissues included a new category, "B-cell lymphoma with MYC and BCL2 and/or BCL6 aberration," in recognition of key differences in tumor biology and treatment. In most studies, it accounts for 2% to 12% of DLBCL, and its incidence increases with patient age.

▒ GENETIC BASIS

Lunenburg Biomarker Consortium conducted a large analysis of DLBCL patients and reported *MYC* translocation in 11% of cases. Isolated *MYC* translocation is associated with worse overall survival (OS) but similar progression-free survival (PFS) when treated with rituximab, cyclophosphamide, doxorubicin, vincristine, and prednisone (R-CHOP) compared with those without translocation. Fifty-five percent of patients with *MYC* translocation have concomitant *BCL6* and/or *BCL2* translocation. Data indicate that the outcomes for DHL with *BCL2/BCL6* translocation and THL are similar, with inferior PFS and OS compared to those of patients without translocation. An example of fluorescence in situ hybridization (FISH) studies for *MYC*, *BCL2*, and *BCL6* rearrangements is demonstrated in Figure 36.1.

▒ DIAGNOSTIC DIFFERENTIATION FROM DOUBLE EXPRESSORS

It is now recognized that high expression of *MYC* and *BCL2* proteins can occur via mechanisms other than gene rearrangements. Tumors with high expression of these proteins detected by immunohistochemistry (IHC) known as "double-expressor" lymphoma (DEL) cases have a poor prognosis. This is not a distinct category in WHO classification and is grouped under DLBCL. Conversely, 20% of patients

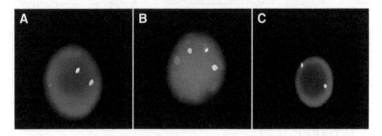

Figure 36.1 Fluorescence in situ hybridization (FISH) representation of double hit lymphoma (DHL) by demonstration of *MYC/BCL2* rearrangement. (A) FISH test using *c-MYC* break-apart probe: one isolated red, one isolated green, and one fusion indicate presence of *c-MYC* gene rearrangement. (B) One red (*BCL2*), one green (*IgH*), and two fusion signals (*IgH/BCL2*/t(14;18)(q32;q21)). (C) FISH test using *BCL6* break-apart probe; two fusion signals indicate no *BCL6* gene rearrangement.

with DHL do not demonstrate overexpression of *MYC* and *BCL2*. In biologic terms, the entity DHL and the prognostic group DEL overlap with cell of origin concept, which subdivides DLBCL into germinal-center B-cell (GCB) lymphoma and non-GCB lymphoma. Eighty to ninety percent of DHL cases occur with GCB DLBCL. DEL has a higher correlation with non-GCB subset (63%) versus GCB subtype (37%).

■ TREATMENT AND OUTCOMES

Over the past two decades, R-CHOP has become the standard initial chemotherapy for large B-cell lymphomas and has led to significant improvement in OS. However, this regimen remains ineffective in DHL, with a median survival of approximately 1.5 years. The majority of data in DHL come from retrospective reviews of patients treated with a variety of regimens (Table 36.1). Current data suggest that more aggressive regimens, such as DA-EPOCH-R and R-Hyper-CVAD, confer higher complete remission (CR) rates, event-free survival (EFS), and OS. In an MD Anderson clinical experience, 2-year EFS rates in patients who received R-CHOP, R-EPOCH, and R-Hyper-CVAD/MA were 25%, 67%, and 32%, respectively. Pooled multivariate analysis from nonrandomized retrospective data suggests that response rates are highest for dose-adjusted R-EPOCH. CNS involvement is seen in 13% of these patients, and 4 cycles of intrathecal methotrexate is recommended for prophylaxis. Patients with documented central nervous system (CNS) disease should be treated with a high methotrexate/cytarabine-based regimen.

Autologous hematopoietic stem cell transplant (HSCT) in first CR does not improve 3-year relapse-free survival or OS rate. Relapsed/refractory disease is treated similar to large B-cell lymphomas with salvage regimens, such as RICE (rituximab, ifosfamide, carboplatin, etoposide) followed by autologous HSCT in responders.

Table 36.1 Retrospective Analyses of Outcomes in DHL Based on Chemotherapy Regimen

Study	Number of Patients	Treatments	Outcomes
Li et al. *Mod Pathol.* 2012;25(1): 145–156	52	19 R-CHOP 30 Hyper-CVAD 3 Others	Median OS: 18.6 months; more intensive therapy ($p = .54$) not associated with better outcome
Oki et al.[4]	129	57 R-CHOP 34 Hyper-CVAD 28 DA-EPOCH-R 10 Other	Median OS: 18 months; CR rates: R-CHOP: 40%. DA-EPOCH-R: 68% ($p = .017$) R-Hyper-CVAD: 68% ($p = .011$) EFS and OS: similar to R-CHOP or R-Hyper-CVAD R-EPOCH better than EFS (HR: .38, $p = .008$) and longer OS at 3 years (76% vs. 35%)
Petrich et al.[3]	311	100 R-CHOP 65 R-Hyper-CVAD 65 DA-EPOCH-R 44 R-CODOX-M/ IVAC 37 Other	PFS 10.9 months OS 21.9 months R-CHOP vs. intensive regimens PFS 7.8 vs. 21.6 months No difference between intensive regimens

CR, complete remission; DA-EPOCH-R, dose adjusted infusional etoposide, prednisone, vincristine, cyclophosphamide, doxorubicin and rituximab; DHL, double-hit lymphoma; EFS, event-free survival; OS, overall survival; PFS, progression-free survival; R-CHOP, rituximab, cyclophosphamide, doxorubicin, vincristine, prednisone; R-CODOX-M/IVAC, cyclophosphamide, vincristine, doxorubicin, high-dose methotrexate [MTX] with rituximab/IVAC: ifosfamide, etoposide, cytarabine with rituximab; R-EPOCH, infusional etoposide, prednisone, vincristine, cyclophosphamide, doxorubicin and rituximab; R-Hyper-CVAD, hyperfractionated cyclophosphamide, vincristine, doxorubicin, dexamethasone alternating with high-dose MTX, cytarabine with rituximab.

CNS prophylaxis not uniform but frequent intrathecal methotrexate ± cytarabine.

Anti-CD19 chimeric antigen receptor (CAR) T-cells have revolutionized the treatment of relapsed refractory diffuse large B-cell lymphoma. Trials involving axicabtagene and tisagenlecleucel have shown significant promise in the treatment of DHL. The Juliet trial had 16 patients with DHL/THL treated with tisagenlecleucel and showed a

3-month CR rate of 60%. Additional data are awaited to further evaluate long-term outcomes.

■ POTENTIAL PRACTICE-CHANGING CLINICAL TRIALS

Thus far, data are clear that DHL represents a patient population group with poor outcomes, and retrospective data suggest that dose intensification improves outcomes. DHL is still an unmet need and poses a treatment challenge. Anti-CD19 CAR T-cells has shown the most promise in this subset of patients and should be considered for young fit patients with relapsed refractory disease.

■ REFERENCES FOR SUPPLEMENTAL READING

1. Friedberg JW. How I treat double-hit lymphoma. *Blood*. 2017;130(5):590–596.
2. Rosenwald A, Bens S, Advani R, et al. Prognostic significance of *MYC* rearrangement and translocation partner in diffuse large B-cell lymphoma: a study by the Lunenburg Lymphoma Biomarker Consortium. *J Clin Oncol*. 2019;37(35):3359–3368.
3. Petrich AM, Gandhi M, Jovanovic B, et al. Impact of induction regimen and stem cell transplantation on outcomes in double-hit lymphoma: a multicentric retrospective analysis. *Blood*. 2014;124(15):2354–2361.
4. Oki Y, Noorani M, Lin P, et al. Double-hit lymphoma: the MD Anderson Cancer Center clinical experience. *Br J Hematol*. 2014;166(6):891–901.
5. Landsburg DJ, Falkiewicz MK, Maly J, et al. Outcomes of patients with double-hit lymphoma who achieve first complete remission. *J Clin Oncol*. 2017;35(20):2260–2267. doi: 10.1200/JCO.2017.72.2157

37   Mantle Cell Lymphoma

Ruchi Desai and Bijal Shah

▓ INTRODUCTION

Mantle cell lymphoma (MCL) is a mature B-cell neoplasm comprising about 8% of adult non-Hodgkin lymphomas (NHLs). The median age at diagnosis for MCL is around 65 years old, and the majority of patients are male, with White people more commonly affected.[1] Clinically, MCL is a heterogeneous disease that shares features of indolent and aggressive NHLs. Currently, MCL is incurable without hematopoietic stem cell transplant. However, new therapies and understanding of genomic and proteomics are changing the treatment landscape and survival of patients with MCL.

▓ PATHOGENESIS

Development and maintenance of MCL are mediated by a complex array of aberrant-cell cycle regulation, DNA damage response, and B-cell receptor (BCR) signaling in addition to molecular and genomic alterations. The hallmark of MCL is overexpression of *cyclin D1* mediated by chromosomal translocation t(11;14)(q13;q32) *IgH/CCND1*. Cyclin D1 activates cyclin-dependent kinases 4 and 6, which deactivate Rb (tumor-suppressor gene) and promote G1 to S phase of the cell cycle, leading to cell proliferation. The majority of patients exhibit *cyclin D1* translocation (<10% are negative). In the small subset of patients who lack *cyclin D1* translocation, *cyclin D2* and *cyclin D3* translocations are frequent. In addition, *SOX-11* overexpression is observed in the majority of MCL patients. SOX-11 is a transcription factor that results in augmentation of BCR signaling, suppression of *BCL-6* to avoid germinal-center transit and *IgHV* mutation, blocking of B-cell maturation to plasma cells, promotion of angiogenesis, and migration and adhesion of MCL to stromal cells. Genomic alterations are noted in DNA repair genes, chromatin remodeling and modifier genes, and tumor-suppressor genes, including *TP53*, *ATM*, *CKDN2A*, *NOTCH 1* and *2*, *CCND1*, *NSD2*, *KMT2D*, *BTK*, and *BIRC3*, among others.[2,3] The World Health Organization (WHO) 2016 lymphoma update[4] recognizes two different MCL subtypes with different clinicopathologic and molecular features. Nodal MCL is characterized by naive B-cells that do not undergo germinal-center reactions and exhibit unmutated *IgHV* gene rearrangement, *SOX-11* overexpression, a higher degree of genomic instability (*ATM*, *CDKN2A*, and chromatin-modifier mutations), and other oncogenic mutations and epigenetic modifications. Leukemic MCL occurs in 10% to 20% of cases and presents with lymphocytosis and splenomegaly. The cell of origin in leukemic MCL is suspected to be a memory B-cell with germinal-center experience, mutated *IgHV*, and lack of *SOX-11* overexpression and has a stable genome with few epigenetic modifications.

▧ DIAGNOSIS

Initial laboratory evaluation includes a complete blood count (CBC) with differential, complete metabolic panel (CMP), lactate dehydrogenase (LDH), and beta 2-microglobulin level. An excisional lymph node (LN) biopsy is preferred for diagnosis if nodal disease is present. A bone marrow (BM) biopsy and a computed tomography (CT) scan of the chest/abdomen/pelvis with contrast or fluorodeoxyglucose–positron emission tomography–computed tomography (FDG-PET-CT) scan are essential to complete clinical staging. Pathologic diagnosis is based upon tissue morphology that typically shows small to medium-sized lymphocytes with irregular nuclear membranes (Figure 37.1). Histologic variants include the blastoid (lymphoblastic-appearing with high proliferative index), pleomorphic (larger cells, many with prominent nucleoli), small cell (resembles chronic lymphocytic leukemia/small lymphocytic lymphoma [CLL/SLL]), and marginal zone–like MCL types. Flow cytometry of involved tissue, BM, or peripheral blood will express MCL immunophenotype: CD20 (bright), CD19, CD5, BCL-1 (cyclin D1), and FMC7 (Figure 37.1). MCL is negative for CD10, CD23 (or weakly positive), and BCL6 and also shows lambda light chain restriction in up to 80% of cases. Conventional karyotype or fluorescence in situ hybridization (FISH) testing should be performed to evaluate for t(11;14)(q13;q32) *IgH/CCND1*. Lack of this translocation should prompt clinicians to also consider alternative lymphoma diagnoses. *SOX-11* overexpression by immunohistochemistry can be a diagnostic marker for MCL and is helpful in cases that lack cyclin D1. However, indolent MCL may fail to show expression of SOX-11. In such cases, alternative cyclin abnormalities (e.g., cyclin D2 or D3) may be aberrantly overexpressed. Blastoid/pleomorphic MCL may show phenotypic aberrancies, including absence of CD5 and/or expression of CD10, in which case performing cyclin D1 immunohistochemistry is important. It is worth noting that pleomorphic and blastoid variants of MCL harbor a higher rate of chromosomal abnormalities, including gains of 3q26, 7p21, 8q24, and tetraploidy. An attempt should be made to characterize the proliferative rate (using Ki-67 immunohistochemistry) for prognostic purposes. Targeted DNA sequencing for *TP53* mutation and *IgHV* mutational status should be performed, as aberrancy could affect the prognosis and choice of therapy. If available to clinicians, expanded DNA sequencing could be performed to identify other genomic alterations that may influence outcomes, but currently it is not routinely recommended. Human immunodeficiency virus (HIV) testing and hepatitis-B evaluation (if rituximab is planned) should be completed prior to treatment initiation. Evaluation of the cerebrospinal fluid (CSF) is not routinely performed, unless neurological symptoms are present (which is rare),

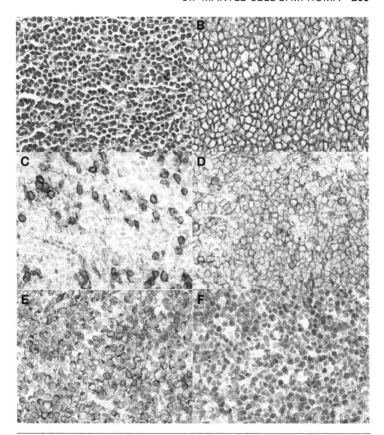

Figure 37.1 Classic morphology of mantle cell lymphoma (MCL) sections show a lymph node with complete effacement of the normal lymph node architecture by a monotonous population of atypical small to medium-sized lymphoid cells with round to oval nuclei, condensed chromatin, occasional small visible nucleoli, and scant cytoplasm, in a background of increased vasculature (A, hematoxylin and eosin [H&E] ×600). By immunohistochemical staining, the atypical cells are positive for CD20 and negative for CD3 (B and C, Immunoperoxidase, ×600). The neoplastic B-cells also coexpress CD5, BCL-1, and BCL-2 (D, E, and F, immunoperoxidase, ×600, respectively).

the proliferative index by Ki-67 is increased, or a blastoid/pleomorphic variant is noted. In the latter instance, the rate of central nervous system (CNS) involvement is approximately 20% to 25%, and, thus, CSF evaluation is often performed in the context of CNS prophylaxis.

▓ KEY DIAGNOSTIC DILEMMA

CLL/SLL is another small B-cell lymphoma that shows expression of CD5; however, it also coexpresses CD23, CD20 is often dim, and uniform cyclin D1 expression is not seen. The loss of CD5 may also pose a challenge in distinguishing blastoid/pleomorphic MCL from diffuse large

B-cell lymphoma. In such cases, the absence of SOX11 and expression of BCL6 in DLBCL may be useful in distinguishing between the two.

▦ PROGNOSIS

The natural history of MCL is variable. Patients with nodal MCL generally have a more aggressive course and typically present with Stage III or IV disease. Patients with leukemic MCL usually have an indolent course with lymphocytosis and splenomegaly. Currently used prognostic models are the Mantle Cell International Prognostic Index (MIPI) and the simplified MIPI (sMIPI), which is concordant with the MIPI (Table 37.1).[5] The MIPI identifies three risk groups: low (5-year overall survival [OS] 60%), intermediate (5-year OS 35%), and high (5-year OS 20%). The prognostic value of the sMIPI is improved with the addition of Ki-67 (biologic MIPI). Ki-67 >30% is considered to be high risk. Notably, there are not enough data to inform of the utility of beta-2 microglobulin or high-risk genomic losses (e.g., *TP53*) within the MIPI models. In addition, for patients with leukemic MCL who present with leukocytosis at baseline but follow a more indolent course, the MIPI may overestimate disease risk. Other factors commonly identified that correlate with poor prognosis are blastoid and pleomorphic histology, presence of complex karyotype, unmutated *IgHV*, *MYC* overexpression, and genomic alterations in *TP53*. Genomic mutations in *ATM, CKDN2A (locus 9p21), NOTCH 1 and 2, NSD2, CCND1, SMARCA4, BIRC3, KMT2D/MLL2, BTK, MAP3K14,* and *CARD 11* have also been associated with poor prognosis in the literature.

▦ TREATMENT

Currently, there is no absolute standard of care in MCL due to a paucity of randomized clinical trial data in MCL patients. The treatment approach should be tailored to the aggressiveness of the disease and the patient's age and comorbidities. Until recently, treatment options in MCL were limited to chemoimmunotherapy followed by consolidation (most often with autologous stem cell transplantation) and/or maintenance strategies (most commonly with rituximab). While this approach remains a good choice for some patients, the recent

Table 37.1 Simplified MCL International Prognostic Index[5]

Points	Age (Years)	ECOG Performance Status	LDH:ULN Ratio	WBC (k/mcL)
0	<50	0–1	<0.67	<6.7
1	50–59	–	0.67–0.99	6.7–9.9
2	60–69	2–4	1.00–1.49	10.0–14.9
3	>70	–	>1.50	>15.00

ECOG, Eastern Cooperative Oncology Group; LDH, lactate dehydrogenase; ULN, upper limit of normal; WBC, white blood cell. Patients with 0 to 3 points in summary were classified as low risk, patients with 4 to 5 points as intermediate risk, and patients with 6 to 11 points as high risk.

advances in chemotherapy-free regimens have become important for the treatment of others, with overall fewer toxicities.

INDOLENT MCL

Similar to other low-grade lymphomas, a subset of MCL patients (good performance status, asymptomatic disease, non-bulky disease, low Ki-67, normal LDH, non-aggressive cytomorphology, mostly leukemic MCL) does not need immediate systemic treatment. Given the incurable nature of MCL, close observation is a reasonable approach. As with most indolent lymphomas, progression to symptomatic and/ or high-volume disease occurs in most patients, albeit at variable rates, such that some continue on observation for many years. When patients develop symptomatic disease, options for treatment include aggressive induction therapy followed by autologous transplantation or less aggressive regimens. Optimal management of patients with *TP53* mutations is not known, though. Recommended less aggressive regimens are Rituximab, cyclophosphamide, doxorubicin, vincristine, prednisone (R-CHOP) (*JCO*. 2005;23:1984–1992; *N Engl J Med*. 2012;367:520–531), R-bendamustine (BR) (*Lancet*. 2013;381:1203–1210; *Blood*. 2014;123:2944–2952), VR-CAP (bortezomib substituted for vincristine from CHOP; *Lancet Oncol*. 2018;19;1449–1458), R-lenalidomide (*N Engl J Med*. 2015;373(19):1835–1844), R-bendamustine and cytarabine (R-BAC) 500 (*Lancet Haematol*. 2017;4:e15–e23), or a clinical trial.

YOUNG (<65 YEAR)/AGGRESSIVE MCL

Although this subset reflects only 20% to 30% of all MCL patients, it has been the subject of considerable study. Clinical trials have documented improvements in remission rates and remission depth by increasing treatment intensity, most commonly via the inclusion of high-dose cytarabine into the therapeutic regimen. Relevant examples include Rituximab, hyperfractionated cylcophosphomide, vincristine, doxorubicin, dexamethasone (R-Hyper-CVAD) (*J Clin Oncol*. 2006;24(4):724), R-CHOP or R-dexamethasone, high dose cytarabine, cisplatin (DHAP) (*Blood*. 2013;121:48–53), or maximum strength rituximab, cyclophosphamide, doxorubicin, vincristine, prednisone alternating with rituximab, high dose cytarabine (R-MaxiCHOP) (*Blood*. 2008;112:2687–2693). Consolidation with autologous stem cell transplantation in first remission can be performed, as it has improved progression-free survival (PFS) (*Blood*. 2005;105:2677–2684). However, rituximab maintenance has shown comparable remission duration in at least one large study (*N Engl J Med*. 2012;367:520–531). Presence of *TP53* mutations has been associated with poor prognosis in patients treated with conventional therapy, and participation in clinical trial should be considered for this poor-risk subset.

ELDERLY/AGGRESSIVE MCL

Treatment of elderly patients with aggressive MCL is challenging, as comorbid medical conditions often limit treatment intensity, and patients may not be transplant candidates. In this cohort, less aggressive chemotherapy regimens, such as those proposed for progressive indolent MCL, can be used with maintenance rituximab to improve survival. New approaches that bundle low- to intermediate-intensity chemotherapy with novel targeted agents (lenalidomide, ibrutinib) will likely also play a role in this subset of patients.

RELAPSED/REFRACTORY MCL

Previously, the most common method of treatment for recurrent MCL was an aggressive salvage regimen of chemoimmunotherapy (akin to diffuse large B cell lymphoma) followed by consolidation with allogeneic stem cell transplantion. The advent of novel targeted therapies has fundamentally changed this paradigm, and it is likely that the treatment of MCL may more closely resemble myeloma, with chemotherapy reserved for those with highly aggressive or otherwise refractory disease. Targeted therapies currently available with or without immunotherapy for MCL include bortezomib (*Ann Oncol*. 2009;20:5200–5225; *Cancer*. 2011;117:2442–2451); lenalidomide (*BR J Haematol*. 2009;145:344–349); Bruton's Tyrosine Kinase (BTK) inhibitors, including ibrutinib (*N Engl J Med*. 2013;369:507–516; *Blood*. 2015;126:739–745); acalabrutinib (*Lancet Oncol*. 2018;391:659–667); and zanubrutinib ([abstract] *Hemat. Oncol.* 2019;37:45–46; [abstract] *Hemat. Oncol.* 2019;37:245–247). In addition, the *BCL-2* inhibitor venetoclax has shown promise as both a single agent and in combination with ibrutinib in early-phase studies, with responses seen even among patients who had progressed on BTK inhibitors (*J Clin Oncol*. 2017;35:826–833; *NEJM*. 2018;378:1211–1233; *Haematologica*. 2019;104:68–71).

▨ POTENTIAL PRACTICE-CHANGING CLINICAL TRIAL

Treatment regimens are rapidly changing in MCL, and many trials are garnering attention. Currently, these trials include frontline use of ibrutinib in combination with BR (NCT01776840); a phase 3 study evaluating venetoclax and ibrutinib combined in the relapsed setting (NCT03112174); multiple CD19-directed chimeric antigen receptor T-cell (CART-19) studies, most notably axicabtagene ciloleucel (NCT0201313); and multiple new BTK inhibitors.

▨ REFERENCES FOR SUPPLEMENTAL READING

1. Fu S, Wang M, Lairson DR, et al. Trends and variations in mantle cell lymphoma incidence from 1995 to 2013: a comparative study between Texas and National SEER areas. *Oncotarget*. 2017;8(68):112516–112529.

2. Bertoni F, Rinaldi A, Zucca E, et al. Update on the molecular biology of mantle cell lymphoma. *Hemat. Oncol.* 2006;24(1):22–27.

3. Jain P, Wang M. Mantle cell lymphoma: 2019 update on the diagnosis, pathogenesis, prognostication, and management. *Am J Hemat*. 2019;94(6):710–725.

4. Swerdlow SH, Campo E, Pileri SA, et al. The 2016 revision of the World Health Organization classification of lymphoid neoplasms. *Blood*. 2016;127(20):2375–2390.

5. Hoster E, Dreyling M, Klapper W, et al. A new prognostic index (MIPI) for patients with advanced-stage mantle cell lymphoma. *Blood*. 2008; 111(2):558–565.

38 Primary Mediastinal Large B-Cell Lymphoma

Vania Phuoc, Andreas Saltos, and Julio C. Chavez

▧ INTRODUCTION

Primary mediastinal large B-cell lymphoma (PMBCL) is a relatively uncommon subtype of non-Hodgkin lymphoma (NHL) that is distinct from diffuse large B-cell lymphoma (DLBCL). It is generally thought to arise from thymic medullary B-cells. PMBCL is characterized by a pathologic and molecular profile that is between that of DLBCL and nodular sclerosis classical Hodgkin lymphoma (HL) (see Chapters 32 and 35). It is a clinically aggressive lymphoma and most frequently occurs in adolescents and young adults, with a slight female predominance. The typical presentation involves an isolated large mediastinal mass with initial locoregional spread to the supraclavicular, cervical, and hilar lymph nodes as well as into the mediastinum and lung, but distant disease can occur in approximately one-quarter of patients at diagnosis.

▧ DIAGNOSIS

Common presenting symptoms include chest pain, cough, dyspnea, and B-symptoms (e.g., fever, night sweats, or weight loss). Patients may also present with oncologic emergencies, including superior vena cava (SVC) syndrome, tumor lysis syndrome (TLS), or airway compression (see Chapter 59). Pleural or pericardial effusions are common, and pericardial tamponade may occur. Adequate tissue biopsy, frequently performed by image-guided core needle biopsy or mediastinoscopy, is imperative prior to starting treatment to confirm the correct diagnosis and to guide therapy. The histologic features are common to both DLBCL and HL, consisting of large cells with pale cytoplasm as well as delicate strands of background sclerosis, which often compartmentalize tumor cells (Figure 38.1). Lobulated or multinucleated cells resembling the Reed–Sternberg cells of HL may be present. PMBCL cells stain positive for pan-B-cell antigens (cluster of differentiation 19 [CD19], CD20, CD22, and CD79a) and CD30, and are typically negative for CD10, CD15, CD21, and surface immunoglobulin (Ig). Rearrangements or mutations in the *CIITA* gene, a class II major histocompatibility complex transactivator, occur in 30% to 50% of PMBCL patients and are also found in classical HL patients. *CIITA* translocations also occur with *CD274* and *PDCD1LG2*, or programmed death ligand 1 (PD-L1) and PD-L2, respectively, and gains in chromosome 9p24 involving JAK2 in 50% to 75% of patients can lead to overexpression of PD-L1. Other cytogenetic abnormalities in

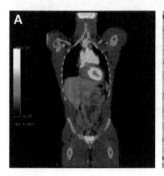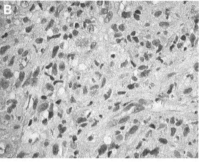

Figure 38.1 PET/CT and histologic findings in primary mediastinal large B-cell lymphoma. (A) High-metabolic activity of mediastinal mass/adenopathy, as well as significant pericardial effusion, without distant involvement outside the mediastinum. (B) Large cells with pale cytoplasm divided by strands of background sclerosis, or "compartmentalizing alveolar fibrosis."

PMBCL involve chromosome 2p15 involving *c-REL* and loss in chromosomes 1p, 3p, 13q, 15q, and 17p. Rearrangements of *BCL2*, *BCL6*, and *MYC* are absent or rare in PMBCL. Laboratory evaluation includes complete blood count (CBC) with differential, complete metabolic panel (CMP), uric acid, lactate dehydrogenase (LDH), and beta-2 microglobulin. Hepatitis B serology should be obtained due to possible reactivation with rituximab therapy, and other viral serology, including human immunodeficiency virus (HIV) and hepatitis C virus, should be considered. Pregnancy testing and fertility counseling are recommended for appropriate patients in this generally younger population. Positron emission tomography/computed tomography (PET/CT) scans are recommended for staging. An echocardiogram or multigated acquisition (MUGA) scan should be obtained prior to anthracycline-based therapy. The incidence of central nervous system (CNS) involvement is low, and CNS prophylaxis is generally not indicated, although it can be considered in patients presenting with extensive extranodal or nasopharyngeal, sinus, or testicular involvement. Staging is classified using the Ann Arbor staging system.

■ KEY DIAGNOSTIC DILEMMA

Systemic DLBCL with mediastinal involvement can be mistaken for PMBCL, but DLBCL is more likely to have distant lymphadenopathy, CNS, and/or bone-marrow involvement. Nodular sclerosing classical Hodgkin lymphoma (cHL) may have similar clinical and histologic features but is usually negative for CD20 (see Chapter 32). PMBCL is typically positive for pan-B-cell antigens and weak CD30 as well as frequent expression of MAL-1, CD200, and, rarely, CD15. Mediastinal "gray-zone" lymphoma is a rare and distinct entity from PMBCL and shares many features, but tumors generally stain positive for CD15 (see Chapter 33).

PROGNOSIS

The International Prognostic Index (IPI) is generally used in PMBCL similarly to other types of NHL. The presence of pleural or pericardial effusions has been proposed as a negative prognostic indicator. Response to initial therapy is a strong predictive marker for progression-free survival. Patients who obtain a complete response (CR) and minimal to no residual uptake by Deauville criteria in the mediastinum have a low risk of relapse. Reported 5-year progression-free survival (PFS) was 98% for those achieving complete metabolic response (CMR), compared to 82% for those with residual uptake after chemoimmunotherapy, and 5-year overall survival (OS) was 100% for CMR, versus 91% for residual uptake (*J Clin Oncol*. 2014;32(17):1769–1775). Response rates and OS are generally favorable, with up to 85% to 90% long-term survival reported in prior studies, but approximately 10% to 20% of patients can develop relapsed/refractory (R/R) disease after first-line treatment. Relapses typically occur in the first few months after treatment, and late relapses (>2 years) are rare.

TREATMENT

Because PMBCL is relatively uncommon, prospective data to guide treatment remain limited. Therefore, some uncertainty exists regarding the optimal treatment approach. Chemoimmunotherapy with rituximab-containing regimens are recommended and have produced generally favorable results.

FRONTLINE TREATMENT

The following first-line regimens are referenced in 2020 National Comprehensive Cancer Network (NCCN) guidelines:

- Dose-adjusted etoposide, doxorubicin, cyclophosphamide, vincristine, and prednisone, plus rituximab (da-EPOCH-R) for 6 to 8 cycles (5-year event-free survival [EFS] 93%, OS 97%; *N Engl J Med*. 2013;368(15):1408–1416).
- Rituximab plus cyclophosphamide, doxorubicin, vincristine, and prednisone (R-CHOP) for 6 cycles, followed by consolidative radiation therapy (5-year EFS 80%, OS 89%; *Oncologist*. 2012;17(2):239–249).
- Dose-dense R-CHOP (every 14 days) for 4 cycles, followed by consolidation with ifosfamide, carboplatin, and etoposide (ICE) for 3 cycles (44-month PFS 79%, OS 90%; *J Clin Oncol*. 2010;28(11):1896–1903).

ROLE FOR RADIATION THERAPY

Consolidation with mediastinal radiation therapy after chemotherapy has been shown to significantly improve both response rates and PFS, most notably with early regimens before the introduction of rituximab. However, emerging data suggest that patients who achieve a CR to initial therapy (as demonstrated on post-treatment PET/CT scans) have equally good outcomes without the need for radiotherapy (*Am J Hematol.* 2015;90(11):1052–1054).

R/R DISEASE

If residual disease is suspected on a post-treatment PET/CT scan, a biopsy should be obtained to confirm refractory PMBCL and distinguish it from post-treatment inflammation. Salvage chemotherapy regimens, similar to those used to treat DLBCL, have not resulted in significant benefit in the PMBCL R/R setting. There is no consensus on optimal therapy, and patients should consider a clinical trial if possible. Alternatively, high-dose therapy (e.g., R-ICE) followed by autologous stem cell transplantation has shown to improve survival in some patients (*Leuk Lymphoma.* 2008;49(7):1329–1336). Pembrolizumab, a checkpoint inhibitor against programmed cell death protein 1 (PD-1), was approved by the Food and Drug Administration (FDA) in June 2018 for patients who have progressed after two or more prior lines of therapy. The phase 2 KEYNOTE-170 trial with pembrolizumab showed an overall response rate (ORR) of 45%, as defined by International Working Group 2007 criteria, and median duration of response was not reached after median follow-up of 12.5 months (*J Clin Oncol.* 2019;37(34):3291–3299). Nivolumab, an anti-PD-1 immune checkpoint inhibitor, combined with brentuximab vedotin, an anti-CD30 antibody-drug conjugate, can also be considered based on the phase 2 CheckMate 436 study, showing ORR up to 73% and CR rate up to 43% by Lugano 2014 criteria. Median PFS and OS were not reached at median follow-up of 11.1 months (*J Clin Oncol.* 2019;37(33):3081–3089). The chimeric antigen receptor T-cell therapy (CAR T) axicabtagene ciloleucel is currently FDA-approved for patients who progressed after two or more prior lines of therapy (*N Engl J Med.* 2017;377(26):2531–2544).

■ POTENTIAL PRACTICE-CHANGING CLINICAL TRIALS

Multiple ongoing studies are investigating new treatment strategies for PMBCL. A phase 1/2 multicenter, single-arm, non-randomized trial is evaluating brentuximab vedotin in combination with rituximab, cyclophosphamide, doxorubicin, and prednisone as a frontline treatment in patients with CD30-positive PMBCL (NCT01994850). Initial results from 22 patients reported ORR 100% and CR 82%, with median PFS not reached. Another ongoing phase 2 prospective study is evaluating the pan-PI3K inhibitor copanlisib in combination with nivolumab for R/R PMBCL and DLBCL (NCT03484819). Finally, the anti-CD19 CAR T-cell product lisocabtagene maraleucel (JCAR017) is being studied in R/R DLBCL and PMBCL as second-line therapy in the ongoing randomized phase 3 TRANSFORM study, which is comparing CAR T to standard salvage chemotherapy and autologous hematopoietic stem cell transplant (NCT03575351).

▓ REFERENCES FOR SUPPLEMENTAL READING

1. Cheson BD, Richard IF, Sally FB, et al. Recommendations for initial evaluation, staging, and response assessment of Hodgkin and non-Hodgkin lymphoma: the Lugano classification. *J Clin Oncol.* 2014; 32(27):3059–3068. doi: 10.1200/JCO.2013.54.8800

2. Dunleavy K, Pittaluga S, Maeda LS, et al. Dose-adjusted EPOCH-rituximab therapy in primary mediastinal B-cell lymphoma. *N Engl J Med.* 2013;368(15):1408–1416. doi: 10.1056/NEJMoa1214561

3. Locke FL, Ghobadi A, Jacobson CA, et al. Long-term safety and activity of axicabtagene ciloleucel in refractory large B-cell lymphoma (ZUMA-1): a single-arm, multicenter, phase 1–2 trial. *Lancet Oncol.* 2019;20(1):31–42. doi: 10.1016/S1470-2045(18)30864-7

4. Armand P, Rodig S, Melnichenko V, et al. Pembrolizumab in relapsed or refractory primary mediastinal large B-cell lymphoma. *J Clin Oncol.* 2019;37(34):3291–3299. doi: 10.1200/JCO.19.01389

5. Zinzani PL, Santoro A, Gritti G, et al. Nivolumab combined with brentuximab vedotin for relapsed/refractory primary mediastinal large B-cell lymphoma: Efficacy and safety from the phase II CheckMate 436 study. *J Clin Oncol.* 2019;37(33):3081–3089. doi: 10.1200/JCO.19.01492

Primary Central Nervous System Lymphoma

Tony Kurian, Liliana Bustamante,
Peter Forsyth, and Solmaz Sahebjam

▣ INTRODUCTION

Primary central nervous system lymphoma (PCNSL) is an aggressive malignancy arising exclusively in the central nervous system (CNS), involving the brain, leptomeninges, eyes, or spinal cord yet without evidence of systemic disease. This is a rare disorder, representing 4% of newly diagnosed primary CNS tumors and 1% of non-Hodgkin lymphomas (NHL). Risk factors for CNS lymphomas include acquired and/or congenital immunodeficiency states. PCNSL is an acquired immunodeficiency syndrome–defining (AIDS-defining) illness associated with a CD4 cell count of <50 cells/L. With improvements in highly active anti-retroviral therapy (HAART) for human immunodeficiency virus (HIV) patients, the incidence of PCNSL has decreased in this population. Conversely, recent registry studies demonstrate increased overall incidence, particularly in patients >60 years old. Median age of diagnosis is 60 years, with a slight male predominance. Common symptoms at presentation include focal neurological deficits (70%), personality changes (43%), seizures (14%), ocular symptoms (4%), and other symptoms related to an increase in intracranial pressure (33%). Ninety-five percent of PCNSLs are diffuse large B-cell lymphomas (DLBCL), with T-cell lymphomas accounting for only 2% of cases. Prognosis is poor, but PCNSL is highly sensitive to chemotherapy and radiation. Therefore, surgery has a limited role in management of the disease. Historically, treatment had been whole brain radiation therapy (WBRT) alone, with a median survival of only 12 months. However, incorporation of a high-dose methotrexate–based (HD-MTX–based) chemotherapy regimen and consolidation strategies has significantly improved outcomes and obviated the need for high-dose WBRT, which carries significant toxicity, in most cases.

▣ DIAGNOSIS AND INITIAL EVALUATION

Ninety-five percent of PCNSLs are DLBCL and as such have almost constant expression of pan-B-cell markers (CD20, CD19, CD22, and CD79a); the majority are of activated B-cell (ABC) phenotype (i.e., near universal expression of late-germinal-center marker MUM-1 but CD10–). Notably, BCL6 expression is observed in 60% to 80% of cases, although with conflicting data regarding its prognostic impact. A distinguishing histologic feature of PCNSL is angiocentricity or angiotropism—the accumulation of lymphoma cells around small and medium-sized blood vessels as demonstrated in Figure 39.1—a property that likely contributes to the disruption of the blood-brain barrier (BBB). High MYC expression has been identified as a potential mediator of disease pathogenesis. In addition, constitutive activation of the nuclear factor-κB (NF-κB) pathway appears central to the pathogenesis of this disease. Specifically, activating mutations of *MYD88*, an essential adaptor protein of innate immunity, occur in 38% to 50% of cases, and CD79B, a component of B-cell receptor signaling, occurs in 20% to 30% of cases, respectively, leading to activation of NF-κB. The workup for PCNSL is shown in Table 39.1.

■ KEY DIAGNOSTIC DILEMMA

PCNSL usually presents as periventricular-enhancing masses that markedly restrict diffusion on diffusion-weighted magnetic resonance imaging (DW-MRI). Patients who are immunocompromised have increased frequency of multiple lesions. Differential diagnoses include gliomas, metastasis, toxoplasmosis, sarcoidosis, and progressive multifocal leukoencephalopathy and require stereotactic biopsy for differentiation. Notably, patients often present with CNS symptoms and are started on glucocorticoids empirically, which typically induce rapid improvement of symptoms and radiographic responses. However, steroid use may induce significant diagnostic delays by decreasing biopsy yield and may postpone the ability to make a definitive diagnosis for months. Ideally, steroids should be avoided until a definitive diagnosis is established or tapered rapidly if started.

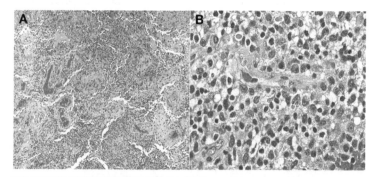

Figure 39.1 Classic histopathologic findings of primary central nervous system lymphoma. (A) Biopsy shows atypical lymphoid infiltrate associated with vascular proliferation, dilatation, congestion, and focal necrosis (left panel, hematoxylin and eosin [H&E], ×100). (B) The atypical lymphoid infiltrate consists of angiocentrically-distributed medium to large-size cells with dispersed to vesicular chromatin, small but distinct nucleoli, and abundant eosinophilic cytoplasm (right panel, H&E, ×600).

Table 39.1 Workup of Patients With PCNSL

Diagnostic Tests	Details
Contrast-enhanced MRI with gadolinium	Brain ± spine
Contrast-enhanced CT scan	If MRI is contraindicated
CSF examination	Flow cytometry and cytology analysis is needed if there is no concern for mass effect. This should be done before or at least 1 week after surgical biopsy to avoid false-positive results.
Stereotactic-guided biopsy	
Ophthalmologic evaluation with slit lamp	Evaluate for ocular involvement.
Contrast CT scan of chest/abdomen/pelvis and BM biopsy or whole-body PET/CT scan	Evaluate for systemic lymphoma (~4%–12% of patients with presumptive PCNSL manifest with extra-CNS disease).
Testicular ultrasonography or PET scan	It may be useful in selected cases to rule out concomitant testicular involvement or systemic disease.
Routine blood studies: CBC with differential, CMP, HIV, hepatitis C/B, LDH	

BM, bone marrow; CBC, complete blood count; CMP, complete metabolic panel; CNS, central nervous system; CSF, cerebrospinal fluid; CT, computed tomography; HIV, human immunodeficiency virus; LDH, lactate dehydrogenase; MRI, magnetic resonance imaging; PCNSL, primary central nervous system lymphoma; PET/CT, positron emission tomography/computed tomography.

PROGNOSIS

PCNSL has a rapidly fatal course if untreated, with a survival rate of approximately 1.5 months from the time of diagnosis in untreated patients. Several positive prognostic factors have been identified and used in the International Extranodal Lymphoma Study Group (IELSG) risk assessment tool (Table 39.2). The most important of these include age and performance status (PS).

TREATMENT
INITIAL TREATMENT IN ADULTS <70 YEARS OF AGE

Most regimens use rituximab and HD-MTX–based ($3.5-8$ mg/m^2) induction chemotherapy (for patients with adequate renal function) and are outlined in Table 39.3. Importantly, survival data may be equivalent among these regimens, as they have not been directly compared. Batchelor et al. demonstrated that patients treated

Table 39.2 The IELSG Risk Assessment

Prognostic Factor	Point
• Age >60	1
• ECOG PS >1	1
• Elevated serum LDH	1
• Elevated CSF protein concentration	1
• Involvement of deep brain regions (periventricular, basal ganglia, brainstem, and/or cerebellum)	1
Risk Category	**2-Year Survival Rate (%)**
Low risk (0–1)	80
Intermediate risk (2–3)	48
High risk (4–5)	15

CSF, cerebrospinal fluid; ECOG, Eastern Cooperative Oncology Group; IELSG, International Extranodal Lymphoma Study Group; LDH, lactate dehydrogenase; PS, performance status. *J Clin Oncol.* 2003;21(2):266–272.

with HD-MTX experienced 52% complete response (CR) and 12.8-month median progression-free survival (PFS) rate. Median overall survival (OS) had not been reached at the 22.8-month follow-up. Patients treated with the MATrix regimen (methotrexate, cytarabine, thiotepa, and rituximab) experienced 49% CR and 67% OS at the 2-year follow-up. Patients treated with R-MPV (methotrexate, procarbazine, vincristine, and rituximab) experienced 66% CR and 81% OS at 2 years. Patients treated with HD-MTX and cytarabine experienced 46% CR and 46% OS at 3 years. Nonmethotrexate-based chemotherapy is only used in patients with severe renal insufficiency (creatinine clearance <30 mL/min) or for patients unable to tolerate HD-MTX due to worsening renal function. Alternative chemotherapy options include temozolomide and rituximab, high-dose cytarabine (with some dose reduction if indicated for severe renal insufficiency), or an anti-folate agent other than methotrexate (MTX).

INITIAL TREATMENT IN OLDER ADULTS (>70 YEARS OF AGE)
Treatment of elderly patients must be individualized according to their comorbidities and PS. In a large meta-analysis, PS was a much stronger predictor for overall survival than age alone in patients >60 years old with PCNSL. HD-MTX–based therapy is still the treatment of choice for elderly patients with good PS and appropriate renal function. This can be combined with high-dose cytarabine or oral alkylating agents, such as temozolomide or procarbazine. Further studies are needed in this population to establish the role of consolidation

Table 39.3 Current Frontline Induction Regimens Used in PCNSL

Chemotherapy Agent(s) ± WBRT	Response (%)	OS
Induction: MTX	CR 52	Median OS not reached at 22.8+ months
Consolidation: MTX[A]		
Induction: MATRix regimen	CR 49	67% at 2 years
Consolidation: ASCT or WBRT[B]		
Induction: R-MPV	CR/CRu 66	81% at 2 years
Consolidation: thiotepa, busulfan, and cyclophosphamide[C]		
Induction: MTX + cytarabine[D]	CR 46	46% at 3 years
Consolidation: WBRT		
Induction: MTX + temozolomide + rituximab[E]	CR 66	65% at 4 years
Consolidation: Etoposide + cytarabine		
Induction: R-MPV[F]	CR 60	87% at 3 years
Consolidation: Reduced-dose WBRT + cytarabine		

The OS could be equivalent, because these regimens have not been directly compared.

ASCT, autologous stem cell transplant; CR, complete response; MATRix regimen, methotrexate, cytarabine, thiotepa, and rituximab; MTX, methotrexate; OS, overall survival; PCB, procarbazine; PCNSL, primary central nervous system lymphoma; R-MPV, methotrexate, procarbazine, vincristine, and rituximab; WBRT, whole brain radiotherapy.

[A]*J Clin Oncol.* 2003;21(6):1044–9. [B]*Lancet Haematol.* 2016;3(5):e217–e227. [C]*Blood.* 2015;125(9):1403–1410. [D]*Lancet.* 2009;374(9700):1512–20. [E]*J Clin Oncol.* 2013; 31(25):3061–8. [F]*J Clin Oncol.* 2013;31(31):3971–9.

therapy. Currently, elderly patients who achieve CR are not routinely treated with consolidation therapy, given the increased toxicity from further chemotherapy and WBRT.

SUPPORTIVE CARE
Glucocorticoids should be avoided if possible prior to biopsy for diagnosis. Once diagnosis has been made, steroids may be initiated as needed for focal neurologic deficits. There is no role for prophylactic

anticonvulsants, but these agents are appropriate for patients with seizures.

CONSOLIDATION

At least 50% of patients who achieve CR with induction chemotherapy will relapse within 5 years, increasing interest in improving outcomes by adding consolidation therapy. There are three main approaches to consolidation: nonmyeloablative chemotherapy, high-dose chemotherapy followed by autologous hematopoietic cell transplantation (HCT), and dose-reduced radiation therapy (3,000 cGy whole brain radiotherapy [WBRT]). Chemotherapy approaches are favored in younger patients in order to avoid the potential decrease in neurocognitive function seen with WBRT, but this remains an alternative for patients unable to tolerate further chemotherapy. The recent IELSG-32 trial compared three different forms of MTX-based induction chemotherapy followed by a second randomization to consolidation with either myeloablative chemotherapy followed by autologous stem cell transplant (ASCT) or WBRT. It demonstrated that both strategies are feasible, effective, and safe. Impairment in attention and executive function was seen in patients who received WBRT, and hematologic toxicity was noted in patients who underwent ASCT (*Lancet Haematol.* 2017; 4(11):e510–e523).

TREATMENT OF RECURRENT CNS LYMPHOMA

It is important to identify patients who have MTX-sensitive recurrent disease (i.e., relapse >6 to 12 months from treatment). In these cases, salvage regimens with dose-intensive HD-MTX–based chemotherapy in combination with other CNS-penetrant agents (e.g., ifosfamide, thiotepa, cytarabine, intrathecal liposomal cytarabine) followed by myeloablative therapy and stem cell transplant have yielded a 2-year PFS rate of 49% (*Haematologica.* 2013;98:364–370). For patients who progressed within 6 to 12 months of consolidation, high-dose salvage may not be a reasonable option, and investigational agents should be considered. These may include high-dose cytarabine, lenalidomide, ibrutinib, pemetrexed, or temozolomide with rituximab, although data are limited, and clinical trial enrollment is encouraged if possible.

TREATMENT OF INTRAOCULAR LYMPHOMA

Ocular PCNSL affects between 15% and 25% of patients with PCNSL. Therapies can be divided into local approaches, such as intravitreal therapy versus ocular radiation and systemic chemotherapy. Systemic administration of MTX and cytarabine yields therapeutic drug levels in the intraocular fluids with well-documented clinical response. However, concentrations of the drug in vitreous humor are unpredictable, and intraocular relapse is common. The usual approach includes intensive systemic chemotherapy and consolidation followed by binocular radiation if there is persistence and/or recurrence of intraocular lymphoma (IOL).

Table 39.4 Potential Practice-Changing Trials in PCNSL

Trial	Identifier	Regimen	Status
CAR-T	NCT04134117	Tisagenlecleucel	Recruiting
Alliance 51101	NCT01511562	Intensive vs. myeloablative consolidation	Active
PRECIS	NCT00863460	Myeloablative vs. WBRT consolidation	Accrual complete
FVD	NCT01960192	Induction: FVD vs. HD-MTX + Ara-C	Active
Ibrutinib for relapse/ refractory	NCT02315326	Ibrutinib	Active

CAR-T, chimeric antigen receptor T cells; FVD, fotemustine, teniposide and dexamethasone; HD-MTX, high-dose methotrexate; PCNSL, primary central nervous system lymphoma; WBRT, whole brain radiation therapy.

▓ POTENTIAL PRACTICE-CHANGING CLINICAL TRIALS

Clinical trials have recently been focusing on evaluating different induction and consolidation strategies in treating PCNSL. Frigault et al. recently published promising results of CAR-T cell therapy with commercial tisagenlecleucel in eight patients with secondary CNS lymphoma, suggesting minimal neurotoxicity and disease response (*Blood*. 2019;134(11):860–866). This is prompting further investigation with an ongoing pilot trial of tisagenlecleucel in primary CNS lymphoma (Table 39.4).

▓ REFERENCES FOR SUPPLEMENTAL READING

1. Schmitt AM, Herbrand AK, Fox CP, et al. Rituximab in primary central nervous system lymphoma—a systematic review and meta-analysis. *Hematol Oncol*. 2019;37(5):548–557.

2. Kasena B, Ferreri AJ, Marturano E, et al. First-line treatment and outcome of elderly patients with primary central nervous system lymphoma—a systematic review and individual patient data meta-analysis. *Ann Oncol*. 2015;26(7):1305–1313.

3. Illerhaus G, Schorb E, Kasenda B. Novel agents for primary central nervous system lymphoma: evidence and perspectives. *Blood*. 2018;132(7):681–688.

4. Kluin PM, Deckert M, Ferry JA. Primary diffuse large B-cell lymphoma of the CNS. In: Swerdlow SH, Campo E, Harris NL, et al. (eds.). *WHO Classification of Tumours of Haematopoietic and Lymphoid Tissues*. IARC WHO Classification of Tum; 2017:300–302.

40 HIV-Related Lymphomas

Danny Nguyen, Nishan Tchekmedyian,
and Jeremy S. Abramson

▓ INTRODUCTION

The World Health Organization (WHO) estimated that by the end of 2018, 37.9 million people in the world were living with human immunodeficiency virus (HIV), with 770,000 people dying from HIV-related illnesses that year. Before the introduction of highly active antiretroviral therapy (HAART), malignancies caused approximately 10% of HIV-related deaths. With the advent of HAART, patients with HIV are living longer and approaching normal life spans. Consequently, the incidence of solid and hematologic malignancy is increasing, with as many as 40% of HIV-infected patients being diagnosed with a malignancy at some point during their lifetimes, and accounting for approximately 30% of deaths in HIV patients. Only three categories of malignancies are recognized as acquired immunodeficiency syndrome (AIDS) defining: (a) Kaposi sarcoma; (b) invasive cervical carcinoma; and (c) high-grade non-Hodgkin lymphomas (NHLs) of B-cell or unknown immunologic phenotype (Table 40.1). Additional malignancies are increased in the setting of HIV infection but not considered AIDS defining, including classical Hodgkin lymphoma.

▓ DIAGNOSIS

Diagnosis is with adequate tissue biopsy, and thus excisional lymph node biopsy is preferred. Fine needle aspiration (FNA) alone is generally insufficient for initial diagnosis (Table 40.2). Laboratory evaluation includes a complete blood count (CBC) with differential, complete metabolic panel (CMP) with special consideration to screen for risk of tumor lysis, phosphate, lactate dehydrogenase (LDH), uric acid, CD4 count, HIV viral load, and hepatitis B and C testing. Primary-effusion lymphoma (PEL) is unique and almost exclusively associated with HIV- and immunodeficiency-related states (Figure 40.1). In Epstein–Barr virus (EBV+) diseases, an EBV viral load can be obtained. Quantitative immunoglobulins and serum protein electrophoresis should be checked at baseline in plasmablastic lymphoma. Radiological evaluation includes a whole-body positron emission tomography–computed tomography (PET-CT) scan (preferred) or computed tomography (CT) scan of the chest, abdomen, and pelvis.

Table 40.1 HIV-Related NHL Based on Severity of Immunodeficiency and Associated Viral Pathogen

Lymphoma	Frequency	Degree of HIV Severity (cells/ mcL)	Associated Viral Pathogen
Burkitt lymphoma	25%–30%	All CD4 ranges, but often >200	EBV in 30%–40%
DLBCL	30%–75%		
—Centroblastic	20%–30%	CD4 <100	EBV in 30%–40%
—Immunoblastic	10%–30%	CD4 <100	EBV in 90%–100%
—Primary DLBCL of the CNS (usually immunoblastic type)	<10%	CD4 <50	EBV 100% (*Note:* nearly absent in immunocompetent patients)
Plasmablastic lymphoma	<5%	CD4 <200	EBV in 50%
PEL	<5%	CD4 <200	HHV-8 in 100%, EBV in 90%

CNS, central nervous system; DLBCL, diffuse large B-cell lymphoma; EBV, Epstein–Barr virus; HHV, human herpes virus; HIV, human immunodeficiency virus; NHL, non-Hodgkin lymphoma; PEL, primary-effusion lymphoma.

Source: Adapted from Chen YB, Rahemtullah A, Hochberg E. Primary effusion lymphoma. *Oncologist.* 2007;12:5569–5576. doi: 10.1634/theoncologist.12-5-569.

Table 40.2 Diagnostic Assays in the Workup of HIV-Related Lymphomas

Diagnostic Assay	Useful Markers
Immunohistochemistry panel	CD3, CD5, CD10, CD20, CD30, CD45, CD138, BCL2, BCL6, MYC, MUM-1, PAX-5, CD15
	Ki-67, kappa/lambda light chain, HHV-8, EBER-ISH preferred
Flow cytometry	CD3, CD5, CD10, CD19, CD20, CD45, surface Ig, CD38, CD138, cytoplasmic Ig, CD56
Cytogenetics/FISH	Consider *BCL2, BCL6, MYC* FISH probes

EBER-ISH, Epstein–Barr virus in situ hybridization; FISH, fluorescence in situ hybridization; HHV, human herpes virus; HIV, human immunodeficiency virus; Ig, immunoglobulin.

Staging evaluation may also include a bone marrow (BM) aspiration and biopsy in selected cases. Cardiac function is assessed via an echocardiogram or multigated acquisition (MUGA) scan prior to anthracycline-containing therapy. Women of child-bearing age should have pregnancy testing. Men and women should be

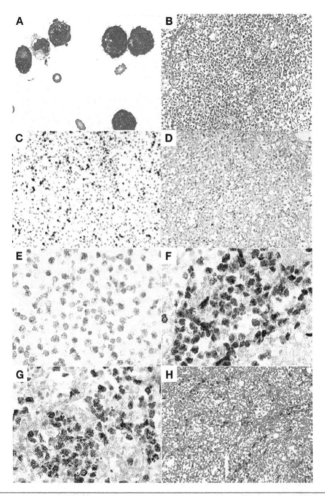

Figure 40.1 Histologic case of primary effusion lymphoma in an HIV patient. (A) Cytospin preparation of a specimen of thoracentesis from a patient with pleural effusion revealed many large atypical lymphoid cells, large in size in contrast to adjacent monocyte/histiocyte, with markedly irregular nuclear contour, one to multiple prominent nucleoli, and deep basophilic cytoplasm (Wright–Giemsa, ×1,000). (B) The cell clot showed a collection of large atypical lymphoid cells with hyperchromatic nuclei, similar to those present in image A, intermingled with fibrins and many histiocytes (oval nuclear, smooth nuclear contour, low in nuclear-to-cytoplasmic ratio, and containing foamy or vacuolated cytoplasm) in the background (H&E, ×200). (C–G) Immunohistochemical stains highlighting the neoplastic cells were negative for CD3 (C, immunoperoxidase ×200), CD20 (D, immunoperoxidase ×200), and PAX5 (E, immunoperoxidase ×600) and positive for MUM1 (F, immunoperoxidase ×600) and HHV-8 (G, in situ hybridization [ISH] ×600). (H) A subset of the neoplastic cells was positive for EBV, highlighted by ISH with EBV-encoded RNA probe (EBER) (×200).

counseled on fertility issues, and men should be offered sperm banking, depending on the regimen. A lumbar puncture should be performed in all HIV patients with Burkitt lymphoma or diffuse large B-cell lymphoma (DLBCL) in the setting of neurologic signs or symptoms or with high-risk central nervous system (CNS) International Prognostic Index (IPI) scores. A high-risk CNS-IPI score is defined as 4 or more of the following adverse risk factors: age >60, advanced-stage disease, poor performance status, elevated LDH, renal or adrenal involvement, and involvement of 2 or more extranodal sites.

▓ PROGNOSIS

With the introduction of HAART, HIV patients with NHL with CD4 counts greater than 100 cells/mcL can be expected to have prognoses close to those of immunocompetent patients. Although the IPI (unchanged from immunocompetent patients) is still prognostic, an AIDS-related lymphoma IPI was developed and validated to be superior to the IPI in prognostic discrimination and prediction of death (Table 40.3). Persistent and/or prolonged high viral load nadir (>100,000 copies/mL) also appears to be a poor prognostic factor. Plasmablastic lymphoma, PEL, and primary central nervous system lymphoma (PCNSL) have inferior prognoses relative to other histologic subtypes.

The AIDS-related lymphoma IPI score consists of (a) points from the age-adjusted IPI, which includes LDH, stage greater than 2, ECOG greater than 1 multiplied by 2 (IPI score given more weight) and then added to (b) the number of extranodal sites and then added to (c) the HIV score. The score ranges from 0 to 15.

▓ TREATMENT

In the modern era, HIV-associated lymphomas are treated similarly to their HIV-negative counterparts, but with increased attention to supportive care, prevention of infection, and drug interactions. HAART can be safely given with chemotherapy and is recommended for all patients. Zidovudine (AZT) and pharmacologic boosters (such as ritonavir and cobicistat) should be avoided due to synergistic risk of myelosuppression with chemotherapy. Preference should be given for a nonprotease inhibitor–based regimen to avoid affecting chemotherapy metabolism. Consultation with an HIV specialist or pharmacist is always recommended. All patients should receive white blood cell growth factor support with chemotherapy. CNS prophylaxis is recommended in patients with Burkitt lymphoma or with high-risk CNS-IPI scores. *Pneumocystis jiroveci* infection (PJP) prophylaxis should be used in all patients irrespective of baseline CD4 count and continued post-chemotherapy until the CD4 is more than 200 cells/mcL. Mycobacterium avium complex (MAC) prophylaxis should be considered if the CD4 is <50 cells/mcL. Gram-negative prophylaxis may

Table 40.3 AIDS-Related Lymphoma International Prognostic Score Index

Risk Factor	Points	Risk Factor	Points
I. Age-adjusted IPI		III. HIV score	
a. LDH		a. CD4 count	
Abnormal	2	CD4 count <50 cells/mcL	3
Normal	0	CD4 count 50–199 cells/mcL	2
b. Stage		CD4 count 200–499 cells/mcL	1
Stage 0–2	0	CD4 count >500 cells/mcL	0
Stage >2	2	b. Viral load (copies/mL)	
c. ECOG PS		<400	0
0–1	0	400–9,999	1
>2	2	≥10,000	2
II. Extranodal sites		c. Prior history of AIDS	
0	0	Yes	1
1	1	No	0
2	2		
≥3	3		

Risk Group	5-year Overall Survival
Low: 0–6	83%
Intermediate: 7–10	64%
High: 11–15	53%

AIDS, acquired immunodeficiency syndrome; ECOG, Eastern Cooperative Oncology Group; IPI, International Prognostic Index; LDH, lactate dehydrogenase; PS, Performance Status.
Source: Data from Barta SK, Xue X, Wang D, et al. A new prognostic score for AIDS-related lymphomas in the rituximab-era. *Haematologica.* 2014;99(11):1731–1737. doi: 10.3324/haematol.2014.111112.

be given during periods of neutropenia, particularly in patients who have had prior episodes of neutropenic fever disease growth factor support. Varicella-zoster virus/herpes simplex virus (VZV/HSV) prophylaxis is given unless contraindicated.

BURKITT LYMPHOMA
Frontline Therapy

- Dose adjusted infusional etoposide, prednisone, vincristine, cyclophosphamide, doxorubicin and rituximab (DA-EPOCH-R) or short-course EPOCH and dose-dense rituximab (SC-EPOCH-RR) (strongly recommended if no evidence of CNS disease; consider other regimens [see the following] if CNS disease): 3 to 6 cycles (1 cycle past complete response [CR]). Overall survival (OS) 90% at 6 years (*N Engl J Med.* 2013;369(20):1915).

- Cyclophosphamide, vincristine, doxorubicin, high-dose MTX with rituximab/IVAC: ifosfamide, etoposide, cytarabine with rituximab (R-CODOX-M/IVAC) (modified): 1-year progression-free survival (PFS) 69%, OS 72%, 2-year OS 69% (*Blood*. 2015;126(2):160–166).

DIFFUSE LARGE B-CELL LYMPHOMA
Frontline Therapy

- DA-EPOCH-R: CR 74%. At 53 months, disease-free survival (DFS) 92%, OS 60% (*Blood*. 2003;101:4653–4659; *Cancer*. 2012;118(16):3977–3983).
- Rituximab, cyclophosphamide, doxorubicin, vincristine, prednisone (R-CHOP): CR 77%, 2-year OS 75% (*J Clin Oncol*. 2006;24(25):4123–4128).

A meta-analysis suggested improved outcome with R-EPOCH relative to R-CHOP in HIV-associated lymphomas, with patients who received R-EPOCH having a 60% lower likelihood of death or progressive disease compared with patients who received R-CHOP (*Cancer*. 2012;118(16):3977–3983).

PRIMARY CNS LYMPHOMA
Frontline Therapy

- Good PS: Treatment similar to PCNSL in immunocompetent patients with high-dose methotrexate-based therapy (see Chapter 39).
- Poor PS: Consider whole-brain radiation therapy alone or best supportive care.

PLASMABLASTIC LYMPHOMA
Frontline Therapy (Note: No prospective data)

- DA-EPOCH: *Oncologist*. 2010;15(3):293.
- CODOX-M/IVAC: *Ann Oncol*. 2004;15(11):1673.
- CHOP: 30-month OS approximately 37%. This should be reserved for patients not considered candidates for more intensive therapies.

PRIMARY EFFUSION LYMPHOMA
Frontline Therapy

Clinical trial if available. Historically, OS 3 months with no treatment. Median OS 6.2 months with intensive chemotherapy and HAART. Regimen options listed under treatment for DLBCL. Methotrexate should be avoided, given that the effusion acts as a reservoir for the drug and increases toxicity (*J Clin Oncol*. 2005;23(19):4372).

THERAPY FOR RELAPSED HIV-RELATED LYMPHOMA

Poor prognosis, median OS generally <1 year. In the era of HAART, given improvement in HIV treatment and consequently immune function, consideration of second and further lines of chemotherapy should

Table 40.4 Chemotherapy Regimens Used in the Treatment of HIV-Related Lymphomas

Chemotherapy Regimen Acronyms/Abbreviations	
DA-EPOCH (dose-adjusted EPOCH)	See Balis et al. *Blood*. 2002;99(8):2685–2693
R-CHOP	Rituximab, cyclophosphamide, doxorubicin, vincristine, prednisone
R-CODOX-M	Dose-adjusted Rituximab, cyclophosphamide, vincristine, doxorubicin, methotrexate (IV and IT), cytarabine (IT)
IVAC	Ifosfamide (with mesna), etoposide, cytarabine
DA-EPOCH-R	Dose-adjusted Rituximab, etoposide, prednisone, vincristine, cyclophosphamide, doxorubicin
SC-EPOCH-RR (short course)	Short course rituximab (RR = 2 doses per cycle), etoposide, prednisone, vincrisitine, cyclophosphamide, doxorubicin

EPOCH, Infusional etoposide, prednisone, vincristine, cyclophosphamide, doxorubicin and rituximab.

be approached similarly to their HIV-negative counterparts. To this degree, a prospective study was conducted with 50 HIV patients with relapse/refractory NHL who were treated with high-dose therapy (HDT) and peripheral blood stem cell transplantation (PBSCT). Of those able to receive transplant ($n = 27$) with a median follow-up of 44 months, OS was 74.6% with PFS 75.9% (*Blood*. 2009;114(7):1306–1313). The anti-CD30 antibody-drug conjugate is an option for relapsed PEL, which is always CD30+, and other CD30-positive DLBCL, which express CD30 (usually positive in EBV+ lymphomas). Chimeric antigen receptor modified T-cells (CAR T-cells) induce durable remissions in HIV+ DLBCL, which have been relapsed/refractory to at least 2 prior lines of chemotherapy and can be considered.

HODGKIN LYMPHOMA

Treatment is similar to that for HIV-negative counterparts, with ABVD-based (Adriamycin, bleomycin, vinblastine, and dacarbazine–based) therapies. Limited-stage patients may be treated with PET-adapted approaches, while advanced-stage patients can be considered for the brentuximab vedotin plus AVD regimen. All patients receive concurrent HAART, increased supportive care to prevent infection, and attention to drug interactions (see Chapter 32) (Table 40.4).

▓ REFERENCES FOR SUPPLEMENTAL READING

1. Barta S, Xue X, Wang D, et al. Treatment factors affecting outcomes in HIV-associated non-Hodgkin lymphomas: a pooled analysis of 1546 patients. *Blood*. 2013;122(19):3251–3262.

2. Dunleavy K, Wilson WH. How I treat HIV-associated lymphoma. *Blood*. 2012;119(14):3245–3255.

3. Hutter G, Nowak D, Mossner M, et al. Long-term control of HIV by CCR5 d32/d32 stem-cell transplantation. *N Engl J Med*. 2009;360:692–698.

4. Ratner L, Lee J, Tang S, et al. Chemotherapy for human immunodeficiency virus-associated non-Hodgkin's lymphoma in combination with highly active antiretroviral therapy. *J Clin Oncol*. 2001;19(8):2171–2178.

5. Scripture CD, Figg WD. Drug interactions in cancer therapy. *Nat Rev Cancer*. 2006;6(7):546–558.

41 Follicular Lymphoma

Jori Kaplan and Celeste Bello

▓ INTRODUCTION

Follicular lymphoma (FL) is the second-most-common subtype of non-Hodgkin lymphoma (NHL), accounting for 35% of NHL in the United States and 20% in South/Central America. FL arises from germinal-center B-cells of lymphoid follicles, both the centrocytes and the centroblasts. It is classically considered an indolent lymphoma, with a characteristic relapsing and remitting pattern primarily involving lymph nodes and the bone marrow. The most common clinical presentation of FL is painless waxing and waning peripheral lymphadenopathy, with only 20% of cases exhibiting B-symptoms (e.g., fevers, night sweats, weight loss) at diagnosis. Large mediastinal masses are rare, though hilar and mediastinal lymph nodes can still be involved. Anemia and thrombocytopenia may be present if there is bone marrow (BM) infiltration (approximately 50% of cases) and <25% present with an elevated lactate dehydrogenase (LDH). The median age at diagnosis is 65 years, with disease rarely occurring in patients <20 years. Pediatric FL does occur, though the majority appear to be biologically distinct from typical adult FL cases. Heterogeneity exists among the various grades of FL, and thus clinical presentations, treatment, and prognosis are highly individualized.

▓ DIAGNOSIS

Diagnosis can be made by histopathologic review of tissue biopsy with morphologic and immunohistochemical examination. FL histology is characterized by uniform, densely packed follicles that efface nodal architecture with poorly defined mantle zones, lack of normal polarization of follicles, and infrequent tingible-body macrophages (Figure 41.1). Histologic grade is determined by the number of centroblasts (cleaved follicle center cells) per high-power field (Table 41.1). Initial laboratory studies include complete blood count (CBC) with differential, complete metabolic panel (CMP), LDH, and beta-2 microglobulin. Hepatitis B/C and human immunodeficiency virus (HIV) serology should be obtained prior to treatment. Baseline BM biopsy with aspirate; computed tomography (CT) scan of neck, chest, abdomen, and pelvis; and/or positron emission tomography–computed tomography (PET-CT) scan is necessary for staging. Immunohistochemistry typically shows neoplastic cells to be

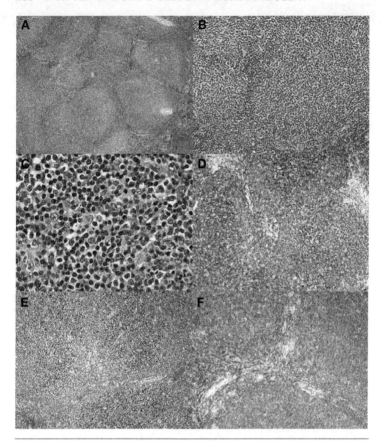

Figure 41.1 Hematoxylin and eosin (H&E) sections (A–F) show abnormal proliferation of follicles arranged in a back-to-back pattern with diminished mantle and marginal zones, devoid of tingible-body macrophages, and loss of normal polarity (A, ×40). The atypical follicles consist of medium-sized centrocytes with cleaved nuclei (B, ×100) and large centroblasts containing vesicular chromatin, often one to two peripherally located nucleoli, and moderate amounts of cytoplasm (C, ×200). Immunohistochemical stains show positivity for CD10 and *BCL6* (D and E, ×200), indicating germinal-center cell origin, and aberrant C-expression of *BCL2* (F, ×200).

CD20+, CD23±, CD10+, CD43–, BCL2+, BCL6+, CD5–, and cyclin D1–, with a low Ki-67 proliferative index. The translocation of chromosome 14 with chromosome 18 (t(14;18)) resulting in the *IgH/BCL2* fusion gene is present in 85% of FL cases, as identified by fluorescence in situ hybridization (FISH) or polymerase chain reaction (PCR) techniques.

Table 41.1 WHO FL Tumor Grading System (2016)

Grade	Histology
Grade 1–2 (low grade)	0–15 centroblasts/hpf
1	0–5 centroblasts/hpf
2	6–15 centroblasts/hpf
Grade 3	>15 centroblasts/hpf
3a	>15 centroblasts/hpf with centrocytes present
3b	Solid sheets of centroblasts

FL, follicular lymphoma; hpf, high-power field; WHO, World Health Organization.

◼ KEY DIAGNOSTIC DILEMMA

2016 WORLD HEALTH ORGANIZATION (WHO) VARIANTS

1. **Pediatric-type FL:** This variant of FL is seen in children and young adults. Localized lymphadenopathy with the absence of *BCL2*, *BCL6*, or *MYC* rearrangements is characteristic of this disease type. Histologically, this subtype is described as large, highly proliferative, expansile follicles with prominent blastoid follicular cells. The most commonly seen genetic mutations are *MAP2K1* and *TNFRSF14*. This variant is indolent, with very good clinical outcomes.

2. **In situ follicular neoplasia (iSFN):** This variant is characterized by follicles with high content of *BCL2* rearrangement-positive B-cells within a lymph node that lacks any other diagnostic criteria for FL. Only a small percentage of these patients have disseminated FL on further workup, which seems to correlate with higher levels of t(14;18) lymphocytes.

3. **Duodenal-type FL:** This variant of FL is confined to the intestines, usually the duodenum. It often presents as multiple small polyps incidentally noted on a colonoscopy in an asymptomatic patient. It is notable for being confined to the mucosa, with partial follicular growth pattern and grade 1 or 2 cytologic features. Patients with duodenal type lack transmural infiltration of the intestine wall, regional lymph node involvement, or large intestine involvement. This variant has a very good outcome.

4. **Large B-cell lymphoma with *IRF4* rearrangement:** This variant of FL is most commonly seen in children and young adults. It is characterized by follicular growth pattern in the Waldeyer's ring and cervical lymph nodes. This variant is notable for strong *IRF4/MUM1* expression and *BCL6+/MUM1+* with variable *CD10* and *BCL2* expression. There are no *BCL2* translocations. This type is considered more aggressive than the pediatric-type FL, but patients do well when treated with chemotherapy +/– radiation.

■ PROGNOSIS

According to Surveillance, Epidemiology, and End Results (SEER) data, overall median survival is 8 to 15 years, with 25% to 30% of FL transforming to diffuse large B-cell lymphoma (DLBCL) (see Chapter 35). The FL International Prognostic Index (FLIPI) was developed in 2004 to categorize patients into risk groups that correlate with overall survival (OS) (Table 41.2). FLIPI2, developed in 2009, includes other variables, such as BM involvement, elevated serum beta-2 microglobulin, and size of largest lymph node; however, this scoring system is not widely used in clinical practice (Table 41.3). WHO tumor grades (Table 41.1) and the Lugano classification for staging (Table 41.4) also have prognostic value. Grades 1, 2, and 3a FL are typically clinically indolent, whereas Grade 3b is considered more aggressive and treated as DLBCL. More recently, progression of disease at 24 months (POD24) has been validated as a predictor of poor OS. Certain genetic mutations have also been correlated with prognosis. Patients with *TP53* mutations, although rare, had inferior OS

Table 41.2 FLIPI Score and Overall Survival

Poor Prognostic Factors	FLIPI Score (Number of Factors)	5-Year OS (%)	10-Year OS (%)
Age ≥60 years	0–1 = Low risk	91	71
LDH above normal hemoglobin <12 g/dL	2 = Intermediate risk	78	51
Ann Arbor stage III or IV nodal sites >4	≥3 = High risk	53	36

FLIPI, Follicular Lymphoma International Prognostic Index; LDH, lactate dehydrogenase; OS, overall survival.

Source: Data from *Blood.* 2004;104(5):1258–1265.

Table 41.3 FLIPI2 Score and Overall Survival

Poor Prognostic Factors	FLIPI Score (Number of Factors)	3-Year PFS (%)	5-Year PFS (%)
Age ≥60 years	0 = Low risk	90.9	79.5
BM involvement Hemoglobin <12 g/dL	1–2 = Intermediate risk	69.3	51.2
Greatest diameter of involved LN >6 cm Serum beta-2 micro-globulin > ULN	3–5 = High risk	51.3	18.8

BM, bone marrow; FLIPI2, Follicular Lymphoma International Prognostic Index 2; LN, lymph node; PFS, progression-free survival; ULN, upper limit of normal.

Source: Data from *J Clin Oncol.* 2009;27(27):4555.

Table 41.4 Revised Staging System for Primary Nodal Lymphomas (Lugano Classification)

Stage		Involvement	Extranodal Status
Limited	I	One node or a group of adjacent nodes	Single extranodal lesions without nodal involvement
	II	≥2 Nodal groups on same side of diaphragm	Stage I or II by nodal extent with limited contiguous extranodal involvement
	II bulky*	≥2 Nodal groups on same side of diaphragm with "bulky" disease	Not applicable
Advanced	III	Nodes on both sides of diaphragm; nodes above the diaphragm with spleen involvement	Not applicable
	IV	Additional noncontiguous extralymphatic involvement	Not applicable

Extent of disease determined by PET-CT. Tonsils, Waldeyer's ring, and spleen are considered nodal tissue.

*Whether stage II bulky disease is treated as limited or advanced disease may be determined by histology and a number of prognostic factors.

Source: Data from *J Clin Oncol.* 2014;32(27):3059–3067.

and progression-free survival (PFS) compared with patients with wild-type *TP53*. Single nucleotide polymorphisms in chromosome 6p have been correlated with a higher risk of transformation to more aggressive lymphoma. Prognostic factors have also been identified involving gene expression and immunohistochemistry patterns of nonlymphoma cells in the surrounding microenvironment.

■ TREATMENT

The decision to initiate treatment is highly individualized and may be based on the histologic grade, presence of symptoms, bulky disease, and cytopenias that can be attributed to FL. Asymptomatic and low-risk patients may be observed clinically. The Groupe d-Etude des Lymphomes Folliculaires (GELF) criteria are often used to determine when patients should be started on therapy (Table 41.5). The presence of any variable on this list indicates a high tumor burden. For patients with localized disease (stage I or contiguous stage II), involved-site

Table 41.5 GELF Criteria

Involvement of ≥3 nodal sites, each with diameter ≥3 cm
Any nodal or extranodal tumor mass with diameter ≥7 cm
B symptoms
Splenomegaly
Pleural effusions or peritoneal ascites
Cytopenias (leukocytosis <1.0 × 10⁹/L or and/or platelets <100 × 10⁹/L
Leukemia (>5.0 × 10⁹/L malignant cells)

radiation therapy (ISRT) is the preferred method of treatment and may be curative in some patients. In contrast, the goal for patients with advanced disease (stage III or IV) is not curative and focuses mainly on controlling symptoms and bulky disease. Grade 3b FL is treated as DLBCL (see Chapter 35).

Treatment Options

- Clinical observation
- ISRT (*J Clin Oncol.* 2003;21:2474–2480).
- Anti-CD20 monoclonal antibody* + bendamustine (*Lancet.* 2013; 381:1203–1210; *Blood.* 2014;123:2944–2952; *NEJM.* 2017;377: 1331–1344).
- Anti-CD20 monoclonal antibody* + CHOP (cyclophosphamide, doxorubicin, vincristine, prednisone). (*Blood.* 2014;123:2944–2952; *N Engl J Med.* 2017;377:1331–1344).
- Anti-CD20 monoclonal antibody* + CVP (rituximab, cyclophosphamide, vincristine, prednisone) (*J Clin Oncol.* 2008;26:4579–4586; *N Engl J Med.* 2017;377:1331–1344).
- Rituximab (375 mg/m² weekly for four doses) (*J Clin Oncol.* 2002; 20:4261–4267; *Blood.* 2001;97:101–106; *J Clin Oncol.* 2010;28: 4480–4484; *Lancet Oncol.* 2014;15:424–435). Consider in elderly or unfit patients.
- Lenalidomide ± Rituximab (*Ann Oncol.* 2017;28:2806–2812. *Lancet Oncol.* 2014;15:1311–1318.). Consider in elderly or unfit patients.
- Single-agent alkylators (e.g., chlorambucil or cyclophosphamide) ± rituximab (*J Clin Oncol.* 2003;21:5–15). Consider in elderly or unfit patients.
- Ibritumomab tiuxetan (*J Clin Oncol.* 2013;31:308–313). Consider in elderly or unfit patients.
- *Anti-CD20 monoclonal antibody = rituximab or obinutuzumab.

Consolidation/Maintenance

- Can be considered after any treatment for any stage.

- Rituximab 375 mg/m^2 1 dose every 8 weeks for 12 doses (*Blood.* 2004;103:4416–4423).
- Chemoimmunotherapy followed by rituximab or obinutuzumab maintenance (*Blood.* 2017;130(Suppl1):486; *N Engl J Med.* 2017;377:1331–1344).
- Ibritumomab tiuxetan (*J Clin Oncol.* 2013;31:1977–1983).

TREATMENT FOR RELAPSED/REFRACTORY DISEASE

Consider re-challenging with frontline therapy if patient achieved a durable remission (i.e., >1 year) or an alternative frontline therapy. Treatment with phosphatidylinositol 3-kinase (PI3K) inhibitors idelisib, copanlisib, and duvelisib is approved in FL after failure of 2 lines of treatment (*N Engl J Med.* 2014:370:1008–1018; *Blood.* 2018;132:1595; *J Clin Oncol.* 2019;37:912–922). Autologous transplantation can be considered as consolidation therapy in patients in their second or third remissions with improved OS and PFS in those with relapsed/ refractory disease. Allogenic transplantation is another option that is associated with lower relapse rates but increased transplant-related mortality. In patients with documented transformation to DLBCL, treat as DLBCL. Consider clinical trial if available.

▓ POTENTIAL PRACTICE-TRAINING CLINICAL TRIALS

Several ongoing clinical trials are underway, with promising results for the management of relapse/refractory FL. A phase 2 trial of taze-metostat, an EZH2 inhibitory, has shown an Overall Response Rate (ORR) in both EZH2 mutant and wild-type (WT) FL patients who have been treated with 2+ lines of treatment (ORR mutant 69%, ORR WT 35%) (NCT01897571). Polatuzumab is a CD79b drug antibody conjugate that has been studied in combination with obinutuzumab and lenalidomide in a phase 1/2 clinical trial that has shown high rates of complete response in the relapsed/refractory patient population (78% CR, 11% PR) (NCT02600897). CD19-directed chimeric antigen receptor modified t cells (CAR-T) has been examined in a phase 1/2 clinical trial in patients with relapsed/refractory FL, with 88% CR with a median duration of response of 10.2 months (NCT01865617). Mosunetuzumab, a CD20/CD3 bi-specific antibody, has shown a 64% ORR and 42% CR in patients with relapsed/refractory disease, including patients who have progressed after CAR-T (NCT02500407).

▓ REFERENCES FOR SUPPLEMENTAL READING

1. Solal-Céligny P, Roy P, Colombat P, et al. Follicular lymphoma international prognostic index. *Blood.* 2004;104(5):1258–1265.
2. Federico M, Bellei M, Marcheselli L, et al. Follicular lymphoma international prognostic index 2: a new prognostic index for follicular lymphoma developed by the international follicular lymphoma prognostic factor project. *J Clin Oncol.* 2009;27(27):4555.

3. Hiddemann W, Cheson BD. How we manage follicular lymphoma. *Leukemia.* 2014;28:1388–1395.

4. Casulo C, Barr P. How I treat early relapsing follicular lymphoma. *Blood.* 2019;133(14):1540–1547.

5. Cheson BD, Fisher RI, Barrington SF, et al. Recommendations for initial evaluation, staging, and response assessment of Hodgkin and non-Hodgkin lymphomas: the Lugano classification. *J Clin Oncol.* 2014;32(27):3059–3067.

42 Chronic Lymphocytic Leukemia/ Small Lymphocytic Lymphoma

Emilie Wang, Ateefa Chaudhury,

and Javier Pinilla-Ibarz

▓ INTRODUCTION

Chronic lymphocytic leukemia/small lymphocytic lymphoma (CLL/SLL) is the most common adult leukemia in Western countries, comprising 25% to 30% of all leukemias. The Surveillance, Epidemiology, and End Results (SEER) data have shown that the incidence of CLL/SLL in the United States has been steadily rising on average by 0.2% each year. The median age at diagnosis is 72 years, with 10% of patients diagnosed at <55 years of age. There is a higher incidence in Caucasians compared to Asian/Pacific Islanders or African Americans. The classic features of CLL include a circulating monoclonal B lymphocyte population (≥5,000 cells/mcL) with varying degrees of cytopenias and hepatosplenomegaly. Although there exists significant heterogeneity regarding disease outcomes, the combination of clinical and molecular tools has refined prognostication. In addition, the treatment landscape has changed dramatically with the addition of B-cell lymphoma-2 (BCL-2) protein inhibition to other targeted therapy.

▓ DIAGNOSIS

2018 INTERNATIONAL WORKSHOP ON CLL (IWCLL) GUIDELINES ON DIAGNOSIS

1. Absolute clonal B lymphocyte count in the peripheral blood (PB) ≥5,000 cells/mcL sustained for at least 3 months.
2. Flow cytometry: Monoclonal B-cells (lambda or kappa light chain restriction) expressing B-cell-associated antigens (CD19, dim CD20, and CD23), CD5 with low levels of membrane-bound immunoglobulin.
3. Morphologically appearing as small, mature lymphocytes with abnormally condensed ("fractured" or "earth-baked") chromatin pattern.

Laboratory evaluation includes complete blood count (CBC) with differential, complete metabolic panel (CMP), serum immunoglobulin, direct antiglobulin test, and lactate dehydrogenase (LDH). Serologic evaluation of hepatitis B and C, cytomegalovirus (CMV), and human immunodeficiency virus (HIV) should be done prior to treatment. Diagnostic workup should also include fluorescence in situ hybridization (FISH) for del(17p), del(11q), trisomy 12, and del(13q). Testing for

immunoglobulin heavy chain variable (IGHV) and *TP53* mutation status should be performed to assist with prognosis and is an important
factor in the treatment decision. Bone marrow (BM) biopsy is recommended for all patients who have cytopenias of unknown cause or
prior to therapy initiation in order to determine the BM cellularity and
degree of CLL infiltration. A chest radiograph should be obtained if a
computed tomography (CT) scan has not been performed. CLL and
SLL are considered the same entity by the World Health Organization
(WHO) based on the commonality of immunophenotypic and pathologic features. If patients have lymphadenopathy, predominately
nodal disease with an absolute PB B-lymphocyte count ≤5,000 cells/
mcL, and no cytopenias due to CLL infiltration, they are diagnosed
with SLL rather than CLL. Patients with an absolute lymphocyte
count <5,000 cells/mcL who are asymptomatic are diagnosed with a
monoclonal B-cell lymphocytosis (MBL). MBL has an annual risk of
transformation to CLL of 1% to 2% per year. Patients with MBL share
an increased risk of secondary malignancy with CLL patients, and
both groups should undergo appropriate cancer screening. Physical
examination of the lymph nodes, liver, and spleen and determination
of the performance status are also essential baseline assessments.

■ KEY DIAGNOSTIC DILEMMA

Mantle cell lymphoma (MCL) expresses CD5 and is usually negative for
CD23 (see Chapter 37). MCL should be ruled out by negative cyclin D1
immunostaining and/or negative FISH for t(11;14).

■ PROGNOSIS

There is great variability in the natural history of CLL, with some
patients presenting with a highly aggressive and treatment refractory disease and others with a very indolent course that never
requires treatment. Prognostic evaluation includes clinical staging
and genetic/laboratory characterization. Commonly utilized clinical
prognostic models include Rai staging (Table 42.1) and Binet staging (Table 42.2). In addition, further prognostic discrimination can be
determined with FISH, IGHV mutation status, and overexpression of
CD38/Zap70 (Table 42.3). The mutational spectrum of CLL has been
well characterized and includes such genes as *ATM*, *BIRC3*, *NOTCH1*,
SF3B1, and *TP53*. In the largest prognostic evaluation to date, a
novel comprehensive scoring system called the CLL International
Prognostic Index (CLL-IPI) was created and validated from analysis of
26 prognostic factors, with only *TP53* mutation and/or del(17p) being
the most predictive (Table 42.4).

■ TREATMENT

The decision to treat should be based on symptomatic disease per
IWCLL active-disease criteria, which includes constitutional symptoms, Rai stage III/IV disease, massive or symptomatic splenomegaly,

Table 42.1 Rai Clinical Staging for CLL/SLL

Rai Staging	Risk	Description	Median OS (Months)
0	Low	Lymphocytosis in PB or BM (>5,000/mcL)	>120
I	Intermediate	Enlarged lymph nodes and lymphocytosis	95
II	Intermediate	Enlarged liver/spleen ± lymphadenopathy and lymphocytosis	72
III	High	Anemia (Hgb <11 g/dL) ± enlarged liver, spleen, or lymph nodes and lymphocytosis	30
IV	High	Thrombocytopenia (platelet count <100,000/mcL) ± enlarged liver, spleen, or lymph nodes and lymphocytosis	30

BM, bone marrow; CLL/SLL, chronic lymphocytic leukemia/small lymphocytic lymphoma; Hgb, hemoglobin; OS, overall survival; PB, peripheral blood.

Table 42.2 Binet Clinical Staging

Binet Staging	Risk	Description	Median OS (Months)
A	Low	Hgb ≥10 g/dL, platelets ≥100,000/mm³, and <3 enlarged areas	>120
B	Intermediate	Hgb ≥10 g/dL, platelets ≥100,000/mm³, and ≥3 enlarged areas	84
C	High	Hgb <10 g/dL, platelets <100,000/mm³, and any number of enlarged areas	24

Hgb, hemoglobin; OS, overall survival.

progressive lymphocytosis with an increase of >50% over a 2-month period or a lymphocyte doubling time <6 months, bulky lymphadenopathy, extranodal involvement, and/or autoimmune cytopenias.

There are many options for the upfront treatment of CLL/SLL. Low-, intermediate-, and high-risk patients who are asymptomatic can be clinically observed with CBC, CMP, and LDH every 3 to 6 months, as median survival can be >10 years without treatment. Treatment is

Table 42.3 FISH/Molecular Markers and OS in CLL

Prognostic Study	Prognosis	Median OS (Years)
CLL-specific FISH		
Del(13q14.3)	Favorable	17
Trisomy 12	Intermediate	11
Del(11q23)	Poor	9
Del(17p)	Very poor	7
IGHV status		
Hypermutated	Favorable	20–25
Unmutated	Poor	8–10
ZAP70		
Positive*	Poor	6–10
Negative	Favorable	15
CD38		
Positive*	Poor	9
Negative	Favorable	20–25

*Overexpression on CLL cell level defined in accordance with individual laboratory validation.

CLL, chronic lymphocytic leukemia; del, deletion; FISH, fluorescence in situ hybridization; IGHV, immunoglobulin heavy chain variable; OS, overall survival.

Table 42.4 CLL-IPI Scoring System

Variables	Points	Risk Group Based on Total Points	Survival After 5 Years (%)
Del(17p)/*TP53* mutation	4	Low = 0–1	93.2
IGHV unmutated	2	Intermediate = 2–3	79.4
β2M, mg/L >3.5	2	High = 4–6	63.6
Binet B/C or Rai stages I–IV	1	Very high = 7–10	23.3
Age >65	1		

β2M, β2 microglobulin; CLL-IPI, CLL International Prognostic Index; del, deletion; IGHV, immunoglobulin heavy chain variable.

indicated in patients who meet the IWCLL criteria to alleviate symptoms and improve progression-free survival (PFS) and overall survival (OS) rates. Several novel drugs have been approved for CLL in the past few years that have significantly influenced survival, but no standard first-line therapy has been established. High-risk patients

Table 42.5 Frontline Therapy

Targeted Regimen	Del (17p)/ *TP53*	Response Data	Clinical Trials
Ibrutinib (Category 1 by NCCN)	Negative	5yr PFS 70%	RESONATE-2 (*N Eng J Med.* 2015;373:2425–2437; *Leukemia.* 2020;34(3):787–798)
		5-yr OS 83%	
	Positive	5-yr estimated PFS 74%	Phase 2 trial 5-year follow-up
		5-yr estimated OS 85%	(*Blood* 2018; 131:2357–2366)
Acalabrutinib	Negative	30-mo estimated PFS 82%	ELEVATE TN (*Blood.* 2019; 134(Suppl1):31)
	Positive	30 mo estimated OS 94%	
Acalabrutinib + Obinutuzumab	Negative	30-mo estimated PFS 90%	
	Positive	30-mo estimated OS 94%	
Venetoclax + Obinutuzumab	Negative	24-mo estimated PFS 88.2%	CLL14 (*N Engl J Med.* 2019;380:2225–2236)
	Positive	24-mo estimated OS 91.8%	
		12 mo undetectable minimal residual disease (uMRD) rate is 81%	

mo, month; NCCN, National Comprehensive Cancer Network; OS, overall survival; PFS, progression-free survival; uMRD, undetectable minimal residual disease; yr, year.

(del(17p) and/or *TP53* mutation) should be considered for clinical trial or allogenic stem cell transplant, given inferior outcomes. Preferred first-line regimens are similar for younger and older patients with or without del(17p) and/or *TP53* mutation.

No head-to-head comparison has been performed between the 3 preferred first-line regimens (Table 42.5). Ibrutinib, a Bruton's tyrosine kinase (BTK) inhibitor, has been shown to improve PFS and OS. It is generally well tolerated but has an increased risk of bleeding and cardiac arrhythmias. Acalabrutinib, a BTK inhibitor, with or without obinutuzumab, an anti-CD20 monoclonal antibody, is another targeted therapy that has improved PFS compared to chlorambucil, an alkylating chemotherapy, plus obinutuzumab. Venetoclax, a BCL-2 inhibitor, with obinutuzumab also improved PFS, but it can cause tumor lysis syndrome in those with rapid disease progression and high tumor burden. Other preferred therapies in younger and older individuals without del(17p) and/or *TP53* mutation are chemoimmunotherapy-based regimens that can include fludarabine or pentostatin with cyclophosphamide and rituximab.

For patients with relapsed/refractory CLL, treatment includes acalabrutinib, ibrutinib, and venetoclax. Phosphoinositide 3-kinase (PI3K) inhibitors, such as idelalisib with rituximab and duvelisib, also can be utilized in patients with relapsed/ refractory disease, which has been associated with increased risk of opportunistic infections, CMV reactivation, colitis, pneumonitis, and hepatitis (Table 42.6). Please refer to National Comprehensive Cancer Network (NCCN) guidelines for additional regimen information. Autoimmune hemolytic anemia and idiopathic thrombocytopenic purpura can occur irrespective of symptomatic disease and should be treated accordingly. Hypogammaglobinemia also occurs in CLL, for which intravenous immunoglobulin (IVIG) can be considered if a patient has a history of recurrent infections and IgG <600 mg/dL. Patients with CLL/SLL can also undergo Richter's transformation into more aggressive diffuse large B-cell lymphoma (see Chapter 35).

▨ POTENTIAL PRACTICE-CHANGING CLINICAL TRIALS

Many clinical trials are evaluating the efficacy of novel agent combinations, most notably in treatment-naïve CLL patients. The phase 2 multicenter CAPTIVATE trial (NCT02910583) assessing frontline ibrutinib and venetoclax demonstrated a high rate of undetectable minimal residual disease (uMRD) in PB and BM, 75% and 72% respectively. The rates of uMRD were sustained even in patients with adverse characteristics, such as del(17p)/*TP53* mutation, unmutated IGHV, and complex karyotype (*Blood*. 2019;134(Suppl1):35). A single-arm open-label phase 2 study combining acalabrutinib, venetoclax, and obinutuzumab resulted in an overall response rate (ORR) of 100%, complete response (CR) of 25%, and partial response (PR) of 75%. uMRD on PB and BM was 68% and 48%, respectively (*Blood*. 2019;134(Suppl1):32). Another triplet combination of venetoclax, obinutuzumab, and ibrutinib (NCT02427451) showed an ORR of 93%, with CR of 42%.

Additional trials are evaluating the efficacy and safety of novel agents in relapsed/refractory disease. LOXO-305, a new BTK inhibitor (NCT03740529), showed a promising 77% ORR in a phase 1 study of 16 CLL patients (*Blood*. 2019;134(Suppl1):501). DTRM-12, another new BTK inhibitor, when combined with everolimus and pomalidomide (NCT02900716), exhibited an acceptable safety profile, with 48% of patients showing >50% reduction in the sum of lymph-node diameters (*Blood*. 2019;134(Suppl1):810). Chimeric antigen receptor

Table 42.6 Preferred Targeted Regimens for Relapsed Refractory Patients

Regimen	Best Response	Trial
Acalabrutinib (*Category 1 by NCCN*)	All ages with/without comorbidities positive or negative for del (17p)/ TP53: 12-mo PFS 88%, 12-mo OS 94%	ASCEND (*Eur Hematol Assoc Congr.* 2019;LB2606)
Ibrutinib (*Category 1 by NCCN*)	All ages with/without comorbidities positive or negative for del (17p)/TP53: Median PFS 44.1 mo at 74-mo follow-up, median OS 67.7 mo at 6-yr follow-up	RESONATE (*N Engl J Med.* 2014;371:213–223; *Am J Hematol.* 2019;94(12): 1353–1363)
Venetoclax + Rituximab (*Category 1 by NCCN*)	All ages with/without comorbidities negative for del (17p)/ TP53: 2-yr PFS 85.9%, 2-yr OS 91.9%	MURANO (*N Engl J Med.* 2018;378:1107–1120)
	Positive for del (17p)/TP53: 2-yr PFS 81.5%, 2-yr OS 91.9%	
Duvelisib	All ages with/without co-morbidities negative for del (17p)/TP53: 12-mo estimated PFS 60%, 12-mo estimated OS 86%	DUO (*Blood.* 2018;132(23): 2446–2455)
	Positive for del (17p)/TP53: 12-mo estimated PFS 55%, 12-mo estimated OS 86%	
Idelalisib + Rituximab	All ages with/without comorbidities negative for del (17p)/ TP53: Median PFS 20.8 mo at 18-mo follow-up, median OS 40.6 mo at 18-mo follow-up	Phase 3 Study (*N Eng J Med.* 2014;370:997–1007; *J Clin Oncol.* 2019;37:1391–1402)
	Positive for del (17p)/ TP53: Median PFS 18.7 mo and median OS 40.6 mo at 18-mo follow-up	
Venetoclax	Positive for del (17p)/ TP53: 24-mo PFS 54%, 24-mo OS 73%	Phase 2 Study (*J Clin Oncol.* 2018;36:1973–1980)

del, deletion; mo, month; NCCN, National Comprehensive Cancer Network; OS, overall survival; PFS, progression-free survival; yr, year.

(CAR)-T-cell therapy targeting CD19 in relapsed/refractory CLL is currently under investigation. One study of 14 heavily pretreated CLL patients achieved an ORR of 57%, CR of 28%, and PR of 28%. MRD was not detected in those who achieved CR (*Sci Transl Med.*

2015;7(303):303ra139). Another study of 19 patients with CLL who were not in CR despite 6 months of ibrutinib had 3-month ORR and CR of 71% and 43%, respectively. Seventy-eight percent of patients had uMRD on PB, and 94% had morphologic CR on BM (*Blood.* 2018;132(Suppl1):298). While still in early phases of clinical trials, these studies show the feasibility of CAR-T in relapsed/refractory CLL and that it may be a viable future treatment option.

▓ REFERENCES FOR SUPPLEMENTAL READING

1. Molica S, Giannarelli D, Mirabelli R, et al. Chronic lymphocytic leukemia international prognostic index (CLL-IPI): a systemic review and meta-analysis. *Blood.* 2018;131(3):365–368.

2. National Cancer Institute. *PDQ® Chronic Lymphocytic Leukemia Treatment.* National Cancer Institute. http://www.cancer.gov/types/leukemia/hp/cll-treatment-pdq

3. Hallek M, Cheson BD, Catovsky D, et al. IWCLL guidelines for diagnosis, indications for treatment, response assessment, and supportive management of CLL. *Blood.* 2018;131(25):2745–2760.

4. Grever MR, Lucas DM, Dewald GW, et al. Comprehensive assessment of genetic and molecular features predicting outcome in patients with chronic lymphocytic leukemia: results from the US intergroup Phase III Trial E2997. *J Clin Oncol.* 2007;25(7):799–804.

5. National Comprehensive Cancer Network. *Chronic Lymphocytic Leukemia/Small Lymphocytic Lymphoma* (Version 4.2020). 2020. https://www.nccn.org/professionals/physician_gls/pdf/cll.pdf

43 Hairy Cell Leukemia

Justin Taylor and Omar Abdel-Wahab

■ INTRODUCTION

Hairy cell leukemia (HCL) is a lymphoproliferative disorder with an estimated 600 to 800 new cases each year in the United States. The characteristic abnormal cell, named after its hairlike cytoplasmic projections, has several features of a mature B-cell, such as expression of surface CD20 and monoclonal surface immunoglobulin. While the instigating factor(s) is unclear, studies have showed that nearly all cases of classic HCL (HCLc) are associated with a *BRAF* V600E mutation.[2] Furthermore, next-generation sequencing efforts have found the *BRAF* V600E mutation in hematopoietic stem cells of patients with HCL, linking the pathogenesis to an earlier cell of origin. The clinical features result from accumulation of the abnormal hairy cells within the blood, bone marrow (BM), and spleen. Thus, most patients present with symptoms related to cytopenias and/or splenomegaly. Monocytopenia is typically seen with HCLc. The median age of onset is 50 to 55 years, with a strong male predominance of 4:1 and three times increased incidence in Caucasians compared to African Americans. While the disease can occur in young adults, it is almost never seen in childhood. Since the advent of the potent purine analogs cladribine and pentostatin, responses to such initial treatment are seen in almost all patients with HCL. However, deeper molecular understanding and characterization of this disease are reshaping the treatment landscape for relapsed and refractory patients.

■ DIAGNOSIS

The diagnosis of HCL previously relied on demonstrating tartrate-resistant acid phosphatase (TRAP) activity using cytochemical method in atypical B-cells in the peripheral blood or marrow (Figure 43.1). However, it is not as specific as flow cytometry or Annexin A1 immunohistochemical (IHC) staining, which has made the use of TRAP staining obsolete. Annexin A1 IHC will stain only HCL cells but not other B-cell neoplasms; however, it is not recommended for minimal residual disease (MRD) analysis due to nonspecific staining with myeloid and T-cells. HCL cells are also stained positive for TRAP (immunoperoxidase), DBA44, and cyclin D1 (subset, without t(11;14)). Currently, flow cytometry and IHC staining are used in conjunction with BM biopsy and aspiration.

- Diagnostic flow cytometric phenotype includes expression of pan-B cell antigens (e.g., surface CD20, CD22) with FMC-7, bright CD11c, CD25, and CD103.

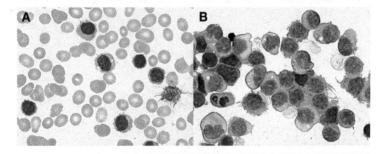

Figure 43.1 The peripheral blood smear includes several atypical lymphoid cells with oval to "kidney bean-shaped" nuclei, condensed chromatin, and clear cytoplasm with visible, radiated cytoplasmic projections—hence the term "hairy cell leukemia." Included also are two small and mature forms of naive lymphocytes (A, Wright, ×1,000). The hairy cells (in cytospin preparation) are stained positive for TRAP (cytochemical method) (B, TRAP, ×1,000).

- Molecular testing for *BRAF* V600E mutation was incorporated into the diagnostic criteria for HCL in the 2016 update to the 2008 World Health Organization (WHO) classification.

■ KEY DIAGNOSTIC DILEMMA

Hairy cell leukemia variant (HCLv) is a disorder that was previously thought to be a subtype of HCL but is now considered to be a distinct biological entity. HCLv appears to have some morphologic similarities to HCLc but is often associated with extreme leukocytosis, presence of monocytes, and neoplastic cells containing prominent nuclei not found in HCLc (Figure 43.2); it also has limited response to purine analog therapy. HCLv can be differentiated from HCLc by immunophenotyping, because, unlike HCL, HCLv cells lack CD25 and are usually negative for Annexin A1 and TRAP (Figure 43.3). Moreover, molecular genotyping for *BRAF* V600E can also be used, because most cases of HCLc harbor the mutation, while HCLv does not and instead is frequently associated with mutation of *MAP2K1* (Table 43.1). Interestingly, it was shown that 40% of HCLv samples and 10% of HCLc samples expressed the IGHV4-34 immunoglobulin variable heavy chain rearrangement (IGHV4-34+). Independent of the variant/classic diagnosis, IGHV4-34 expression is associated with adverse clinical features, including higher disease burden at the time of diagnosis, poor response to single-agent cladribine, and shorter overall survival (OS) (*Leuk Lymphoma*. 2011;52(Suppl2):99–102).

■ PROGNOSIS

The prognosis of HCL has improved with the introduction of purine analog agents that show high levels of sustained remissions with even a single treatment. Even after relapse, patients are usually responsive to

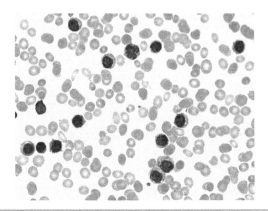

Figure 43.2 Hairy cell leukemia variant. The peripheral blood film shows atypical lymphocytosis composed of predominantly large-sized lymphoid cells with oval to irregular nuclei, prominent nucleoli, and abundant light bluish cytoplasm with hairy projection.

Table 43.1 Diagnostic Value of Somatic Mutations in HCL and HCLv

Classification	Mutation	Percentage of Reported Cases
HCLc	*BRAF* V600E	79%–100% of HCL
		0% HCLv
		0% HCLc IGHV4-34+
*HCLv	*MAP2K1*	50% HCLv
*HCLc IGHV4-34		50% HCLc IGHV4-34+
		0% HCLc

*IGHV4-34 is expressed in 40% of HCLv and 10% of HCLc.

HCL, hairy cell leukemia; HCLc, classic hairy cell leukemia; HCLv, hairy cell leukemia variant.

Source: Data from *Blood.* 2012;119(14):3330–3332; *Nat Genet.* 2014;46(1):8–10.

repeated use of the same initial treatment. The overall 10-year survival rate exceeds 90%. Despite poorer responses to initial therapy, patients with HCLv can have similar survival rates to those with classical HCL. Long-term survivors have a higher incidence of secondary malignancies, and patients should be encouraged to follow up with dermatology and continue other routine cancer screening. There are conflicting data on how much of this increased cancer risk is associated with treatment.

■ TREATMENT

HCL behaves like a chronic indolent leukemia and thus can be observed for some time before treatment is required. The decision to treat should be based upon symptomatic disease, including constitutional

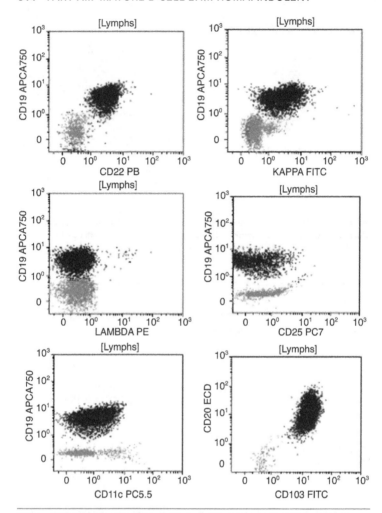

Figure 43.3 Immunophenotyping of hairy cell leukemia variant. Flow cytometry analysis reveals a population of atypical lymphoid cells, phenotypically positive for CD19, CD22, dim CD11c, bright CD103, and negative for CD25 with kappa light-chain restriction.

symptoms, significant cytopenias (absolute neutrophil count <1,000 cells/mcL, hemoglobin <11 g/dL, or platelet count <100,000 k/mcL), or symptomatic splenomegaly.

FRONTLINE TREATMENT

- The treatment options for initial therapy of HCL include splenectomy, interferon, or cytotoxic chemotherapy.

- The purine analog agents cladribine and pentostatin are most commonly used, with cladribine preferred due to ease of administration.
- Cladribine can be given in a single cycle via 7-day continuous infusion, while pentostatin is administered every 2 weeks until maximal response.
- Both produce prolonged immunosuppression as the major side effect, with some evidence that immune recovery is faster after cladribine compared to pentostatin.

RELAPSED/REFRACTORY PATIENTS

- Retreatment with a second cycle of the same purine analog used in initial therapy can result in a second complete remission in up to 70% of patients with relapsed HCL.
- The rates of complete remission as well as disease-free survival time decrease with subsequent lines of treatment.
- Moxetumomab pasudotox is an immunotoxin drug consisting of a CD22 antibody conjugated to pseudomonas toxin and is Food and Drug Administration–approved (FDA-approved) for patients with relapsed/refractory HCL, who have received ≥2 prior systemic therapies, including ≥1 purine nucleoside analog (NCT01829711). Serious treatment-related adverse events included hemolytic uremic syndrome (7.5%) and capillary leak syndrome (5%).
- Researchers in two phase 2 studies published their results together on the targeting of mutant *braf* with vemurafenib in relapsed/refractory HCL,[5] and results indicated a 98% overall response rate (ORR) and that most toxicities were mild (grade 1 or 2). Dabrafenib, another potent *braf* inhibitor, has also been utilized in this previously treated setting, with a mixed response.

▨ POTENTIAL PRACTICE-CHANGING CLINICAL TRIALS

Vemurafenib and the anti-CD20 antibody obinutuzumab are being tested in combination as an upfront treatment for HCL, given their low-toxicity profile in an ongoing phase 2 trial (NCT03410875). The BTK inhibitor ibrutinib is also being tested for relapsed/refractory HCLc and HCLv, with promising preliminary results. The phase 2 trial of ibrutinib (NCT01841723) showed an ORR in this difficult to treat population of 50% and a progression-free survival (PFS) rate at 3 years of nearly 75%.

▨ REFERENCES FOR SUPPLEMENTAL READING

1. Morton LM, Wang SS, Devesa SS, et al. Lymphoma incidence patterns by WHO subtype in the United States, 1992–2001. *Blood.* 2006; 107(1):265–276.
2. Tiacci E, Trifonov V, Schiavoni G, et al. BRAF mutations in hairy cell leukemia. *N Engl J Med.* 2011;364(24):2305–2315.

3. Chung SS, Kim E, Park JH, et al. Hematopoietic stem cell origin of BRAFV600E mutations in hairy cell leukemia. *Sci Transl Med*. 2014; 6(238):238ra71.

4. Swerdlow S, Campo E, Pileri S, et al. The 2016 revision of the World Health Organization (WHO) classification of lymphoid neoplasms. *Blood*. 2016;127(20):2375–2390.

5. Tiacci E, Park JH, De Carolis L, et al. Targeting mutant BRAF in relapsed or refractory hairy-cell leukemia. *N Engl J Med*. 2015;373(18):1733–1747.

6. Kreitman RJ, Dearden C, Zinzani PL, et al. Moxetumomab pasudotox in relapsed/refractory hairy cell leukemia. *Leukemia*. 2018;32:1768–1777. doi: 10.1038/s41375-018-0210-1

44 Marginal Zone Lymphoma

Nishan Tchekmedyian, Danny Nguyen,
Hayder Saeed, and Celeste Bello

▓ INTRODUCTION

The 2016 World Health Organization (WHO) classification divides marginal zone lymphoma (MZL) into three subtypes: (a) extranodal MZL of mucosa-associated lymphoid tissue (MALT); (b) nodal MZL (NMZL); and (c) splenic MZL (SMZL) (*Blood.* 2016;pii:blood-2016-01-643569). MALT lymphoma, NMZL, and SMZL comprise 7% to 8%, 1.5% to 1.8%, and <2% of all B-cell lymphomas, respectively. MZL is often associated with either infection or autoimmune conditions, which cause antigenic stimulation of lymphoid tissues (see Chapter 45). Specifically, hepatitis C seropositivity has been associated with up to 35% of cases of NMZL, SMZL, and nongastric MALT (*Ann Oncol.* 2007;18(2):346–350; *Cancer.* 2004;100(1):107–115). The classic features of MZL include an infiltrate of centrocyte-like small cleaved cells, monocytoid B-cells, or small lymphocytes, sometimes with expanded marginal zones. The cells express B-cell markers, such as CD20 and CD19, but do not express CD5, CD10, and CD23, and they lack cyclin D1 positivity, which helps in distinguishing MZL from most cases of chronic lymphocytic leukemia/small lymphocytic lymphoma (CLL/SLL), mantle cell lymphoma (MCL), and follicular lymphoma (FL) (see Chapters 42, 37, and 41, respectively).

▓ DIAGNOSIS

2008 INTERNATIONAL WORKSHOP GUIDELINES ON THE DIAGNOSIS OF NMZL

- The growth pattern and architecture of NMZL encompasses a spectrum of morphologies, including nodular, diffuse, marginal zone–like/perifollicular, "inverse follicular," interfollicular, perisinusoidal, or follicular colonization of reactive follicles (infiltration of neoplastic lymphocytes into reactive follicles). NMZL cells morphologically are heterogeneous, small- to medium-sized monocytoid B-cells that compose the marginal zone, including centrocyte-like monocytoid B-cells (up to three times the size of normal lymphocytes, round to irregular nuclei with clumped chromatin, with abundant pale cytoplasm), small lymphocytes, and scattered larger, transformed B-cells.
- Clonality can be established, and tumor cells typically express IgM.

- Phenotype: Pan B-cell marker positive (e.g., CD20, CD19, and CD79a) and negative for CD5, CD10, CD23, and cyclin D1.
- Plasmacytic differentiation is common, and a serum paraproteinemia is detected in one-third of cases.
- Localized or generalized lymphadenopathy; one-third of cases represent nodal dissemination of MALT lymphoma.
- BCL2-positive in most cases. CD43 (pan T-cell marker) is reported in approximately half of all cases of NMZL.
- Translocations of MALT are not detected (see Chapter 45).

2008 INTERNATIONAL WORKSHOP GUIDELINES ON THE DIAGNOSIS OF SMZL

- Small B lymphocytes replace the splenic white pulp germinal centers, efface the follicle mantle, and merge with the marginal zone and invade the red pulp.
- The spleen, splenic hilar nodes, and bone marrow (BM) are often involved.
- The peripheral blood may also contain characteristic circulating lymphoma cells, termed "villous lymphocytes" (named for their bipolar villous cytoplasmic projections).
- Splenomegaly and often autoimmune thrombocytopenia or anemia.

Laboratory evaluation includes complete blood count (CBC) with differential, complete metabolic panel (CMP), and lactate dehydrogenase (LDH). Serologic evaluation of hepatitis B/C and human immunodeficiency virus (HIV) should be done prior to treatment with rituximab. Excisional lymph node biopsy is preferred in the diagnosis of NMZL. BM biopsy and aspirate are recommended in NMZL to document stages I to II disease and also in SMZL, given the high frequency of BM involvement. Staging scans with either diagnostic computed tomography (CT) scans of the chest, abdomen, or pelvis with contrast or positron emission tomography–computed tomography (PET-CT) scans should be performed.

■ KEY DIAGNOSTIC DILEMMA

MZL is a small/medium B-cell lymphoma that expresses pan B-cell markers, such as CD20. MCL and SLL, which both express CD5, should be ruled out by showing lack of expression of CD5. In rare cases, MZL can be CD5-positive, but absence of cyclin-D1 positivity distinguishes it from MCL. FL should generally be excluded by lack of CD10 expression. The neoplastic hairy cells in hairy cell leukemia (HCL) may mimic the villous lymphocytes seen in cases of SMZL; however, the absence of annexin A1 expression and other markers, such as the combination of CD11c, CD25, and CD103, essentially excludes HCL (Figure 44.1).

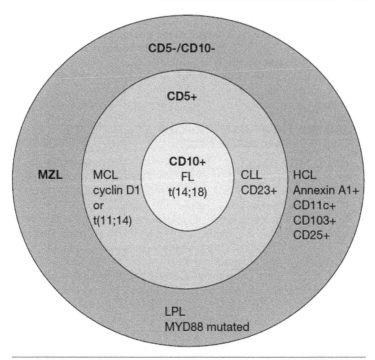

Figure 44.1 Simplified bull's-eye diagram to distinguish the immunophenotypes of low-grade B-cell lymphomas. CLL/SLL, chronic lymphocytic leukemia/small lymphocytic lymphoma; FL, follicular lymphoma; HCL, hairy cell leukemia; LPL, lymphoplasmacytic lymphoma; MCL, mantle cell lymphoma; MZL, marginal zone lymphoma.

▓ PROGNOSIS

Clinically, extranodal MZLs are indolent lymphomas, with 10-year overall survival (OS) rates of 90%. In contrast, the 5-year OS of NMZL is 60% to 70%. Arcaini et al. published the Intergruppo Italiano Linfomi (IIL) prognostic model for SMZL by using hemoglobin <12 g/dL, elevated LDH, and albumin <3.5 g/dL, which classified three prognostic risk groups. Five-year OS rates were 88%, 73%, and 50% for patients with 0, 1, or 2 to 3 risk factors, respectively.[1] Patients with MZL can undergo histologic transformation into more aggressive diffuse large B-cell lymphoma (DLBCL; see Chapter 35).

▓ TREATMENT

FRONTLINE TREATMENT: ASYMPTOMATIC PATIENTS

Asymptomatic and low-risk patients can be clinically observed with CBC, CMP, and LDH every 3 to 6 months.

TREATMENT OF NMZL

The treatment for NMZL is similar to the treatment of FL, as prospective trials isolated to MZL patients are sparse (see Chapter 41). There is no general consensus regarding treatment.

A post-treatment PET-CT scan that shows either a partial response (PR) or a complete response (CR) should prompt consideration for maintenance rituximab for 2 years (*Lancet*. 2011;377(9759):42–51).

FRONTLINE TREATMENT: SYMPTOMATIC PATIENTS OR LOCALIZED DISEASE, NMZL

- Patients with stage I or II NMZL should receive radiation to the involved lymphoid region; if extrapolated from FL, about half of these patients may be cured (*J Clin Oncol*. 1996; 14(4):1282–1290).
- Patients with symptomatic stage III/IV NMZL or with disease that is threatening organ function, causing cytopenias, or becoming bulky disease (>7 cm) can be treated with 6 to 8 cycles of alkylator-based therapy, including bendamustine and rituximab (BR); rituximab, cyclophosphamide, doxorubicin, vincristine, and prednisone (RCHOP); or rituximab, cyclophosphamide, vincristine, and prednisone (RCVP) (*Blood*. 2014;123(19):2944–2952. *Blood*. 2005;106(12):3725–3732. *Lancet*. 2013;381(9873):1203–1210).

SECOND-LINE TREATMENT OF NMZL

- If there is adequate BM reserve, treatment with radioimmunotherapy (Yttrium-90—ibritumomab tiuxetan) can be considered versus an alternative first-line regimen (*Leuk Lymphoma*. 2015;56(6):1750–1755; *J Clin Oncol*. 2002;20(10):2453–2463; *Br J Haematol*. 2014;167(2):207–213).
- Ibrutinib (Bruton's tyrosine kinase [BTK] inhibitor) has an overall response rate (ORR) of 48% and progression-free survival (PFS) rate of 14.2 months in refractory cases; caution should be used in patients who are anticoagulated (*Blood*. 2017;129(16):2224–2232. doi: 10.1182/blood-2016-10-747345).
  - Phosphatidylinositol 3-kinase (PI3K) inhibitors: Idelalisib (inhibits PI3K-δ/delta isoform) has a RR of 57% with PFS of 11 months in heavily pre-treated patients with indolent B-cell lymphomas, including MZL (*N Engl J Med*. 2014;370:1008–1018. doi: 10.1056/NEJMoa1314583).
  - Copanlisib (inhibits P13K-α/alpha and P13K-δ/delta isoforms) demonstrated ORR of 78% with PFS of 24.1 months upon subset analysis (*Blood*. 2019;134(Suppl1):1531).
  - Duvelisib (inhibits PI3K-δ/delta and PI3K-γ/gamma isoforms) showed ORR of 38.9% in the MZL subgroup and PFS of 9.5 months in refractory cases (*J Clin Oncol*. 2019;37(11):912–922. doi: 10.1200/JCO.18.00915).

- Rituxan and lenalidomide demonstrated ORR of 75% in a subset of patients with previously treated MZL (*Haematologica.* 2016;101(5):e196–e199).

FRONTLINE AND SECOND-LINE CONSOLIDATION OR EXTENDED THERAPY, NMZL

Consider rituximab as first-line maintenance therapy or obinutuzumab extended therapy in rituximab refractory disease for an extended period of up to 2 years (*Br J Haematol.* 2016;173(6):867–875. doi: 10.1111/bjh.14007. Epub 2016 Mar 11; *Lancet Oncol.* 2016;17(8):1081–1093. doi: 10.1016/S1470-2045(16)30097-3).

TRANSFORMATION TO DLBCL

Consider anti-CD19 chimeric antigen receptor-T (CAR-T) cell therapy (axicabtagene ciloleucel or tisagenlecleucel) if the patient has already received an anthracycline-containing regimen. Refer to Chapter 35, Diffuse Large B-Cell Lymphoma, and Chapter 56, CD19 CAR T-Cell Therapy, for details and references.

FRONTLINE TREATMENT: SYMPTOMATIC PATIENTS, SMZL

Hepatitis C–negative patients: Splenectomy or rituximab alone[5] (*Clin Lymphoma.* 2002;3(1):41–47; *Leuk Lymphoma.* 2014;55(8):1854–1860). Hepatitis C–positive patients: Treatment of hepatitis C infection with the addition of splenectomy or rituximab in recalcitrant cases.[3]

SECOND-LINE TREATMENT OPTIONS, SMZL

Second-line options for SMZL include chemoimmunotherapy typically used for FL or NMZL (see Chapter 41).

▨ SURVEILLANCE

In general, all patients can undergo clinical follow-up every 3 to 6 months with CBC, CMP, and LDH and with imaging no more than every 6 months for the first 2 years and no more than yearly after 2 years, as indicated by symptoms. Remember to consider transformation to DLBCL if LDH is rising, there are new sites of disease growing disproportionately, or the patient develops B symptoms. Fluorodeoxyglucose positron emission tomography (FDG-PET) can help identify appropriate biopsy sites of the most FDG-avid disease to rule out transformation to DLBCL.

▨ POTENTIAL PRACTICE-CHANGING CLINICAL TRIALS

Targeting of the B-cell receptor signaling has led to a paradigm shift in the treatment of multiple B-cell lymphomas. Ibrutinib, a BTK inhibitor that impedes downstream signaling and inhibits B-cell proliferation, is being tested in a phase 2, open-label study for patients with relapsed/refractory MZL (NCT01980628). Another targeted agent, idelalisib, which is a PI3-kinase delta inhibitor, has shown promising results in patients with FL refractory to rituximab and alkylating agents. In this pivotal study leading to approval in FL (n = 125), 15 patients had MZL (*N Engl J Med.* 2014;370(11):1008–1018). Subset analysis by tumor type is not currently available, but there is interest in this drug for treatment of MZL (NCT01282424). Duvelisib is a small molecule inhibitor of both PI3-kinase delta and PI3-kinase gamma and is being combined with BR in a phase 3 study of patients with indolent NHL, including MZL (NCT02576275 "BRAVURA"). A phase 3 study (NCT01938001) is randomizing patients with relapsed/refractory indolent NHL, including MZL, to rituximab plus placebo versus rituximab plus lenalidomide; a separate phase 3B study is randomizing patients to lenalidomide versus rituximab maintenance after treatment with lenalidomide plus rituximab (NCT01996865 "MAGNIFY"). A phase 2 study is investigating radioimmunotherapy with ^{131}I-rituximab in patients with relapsed, refractory MZL (NCT01678404). Immune checkpoint inhibition is being studied in NHL, including MZL; for example, a phase 2 study is combining pembrolizumab (anti-PD-1) with idelalisib or ibrutinib in patients with relapsed, refractory disease (NCT02332980).

■ REFERENCES FOR SUPPLEMENTAL READING

1. Arcaini L, Lazzarino M, Colombo N, et al. Splenic marginal zone lymphoma: a prognostic model for clinical use. *Blood.* 2006; 107(12):4643–4649.

2. Franco V, Florena AM, Iannitto E. Splenic marginal zone lymphoma. *Blood.* 2003;101(7):2464–2472.

3. Hermine O, Lefrère F, Bronowicki J-P, et al. Regression of splenic lymphoma with villous lymphocytes after treatment of hepatitis C virus infection. *N Engl J Med.* 2002;347(2):89–94.

4. Thieblemont C, Felman P, Callet-Bauchu E, et al. Splenic marginal-zone lymphoma: a distinct clinical and pathological entity. *Lancet Oncol.* 2003;4(2):95–103.

5. Tsimberidou AM, Catovsky D, Schlette E, et al. Outcomes in patients with splenic marginal zone lymphoma and marginal zone lymphoma treated with rituximab with or without chemotherapy or chemotherapy alone. *Cancer.* 2006;107(1):125–135.

45 Mucosa-Associated Lymphoid Tissue Lymphoma

Nishan Tchekmedyian, Danny Nguyen,
and Hayder Saeed

▨ INTRODUCTION

Extranodal marginal zone lymphoma (MZL) of mucosa-associated lymphoid tissue (MALT) lymphoma is the most common of the three subtypes of MZL (see Chapter 44), occurring in 7% to 8% of all non-Hodgkin lymphoma (NHL) cases. It is believed that the increased incidence seen over the past two decades is related to improved diagnostics, given the decline in Helicobacter pylori-associated MALT. Compared to other types of MZL, MALT lymphoma has a more favorable survival outcome, with a 5-year survival rate of 88.7% (*Cancer.* 2013;119(3):629–638). MALT lymphoma has been described in virtually all tissues. The most common involved site is the gastrointestinal (GI) tract (50%), particularly the stomach. Other non-GI sites that are less common are the lung, ocular adnexa, skin, endocrine, and salivary glands. There is no age predilection, but there is a slight female predominance reported. These tumors are usually indolent, and their pathogenesis is postulated to be secondary to clonal-memory B-cell expansion secondary to chronic systemic inflammation and antigen stimulation complicated by oncogenic events, leading to their subsequent independence of the antigenic drive (*Brit J Haematol.* 2011;155(3):362–365). MALT lymphoma at specific sites has shown association with infectious agents or autoimmune conditions (Table 45.1).

▨ DIAGNOSIS

Clinical presentation is indolent, although it depends on the organ of origin. Gastric MALT lymphoma presents with symptoms of dyspepsia, esophageal reflux, nausea, abdominal pain, and/or weight loss. Ocular adnexal MALT lymphoma may present with conjunctival symptoms or with intraocular lesions. MALT lymphoma usually remains localized within the tissue of origin, but one-third of patients may present with more advanced disease. Nongastric MALT can have disseminated disease in up to 50% of patients. Bone marrow (BM) involvement may be present in 15% to 20% of cases.

WORKUP

- **Basic lab studies:** Complete blood count (CBC) with differential, complete metabolic panel (CMP), and lactate dehydrogenase (LDH).

Table 45.1 MALT Subtype Based on Antigenic Stimulus

MZL Subtype	Antigenic Stimulus
Gastric MALT	*Helicobacter pylori*
Cutaneous MALT	*Borrelia burgdorferi*[*]
Ocular adnexal MALT	*Chlamydophila psittaci*[†]
Nodal MZL	Hepatitis C
SMZL	Hepatitis C
Parotid MALT	Sjögren's syndrome
Thyroid MALT	Hashimoto thyroiditis
IPSID	*Campylobacter jejuni*

IPSID, immune proliferative small intestinal disease; MALT, mucosal-associated lymphoid tissue; MZL, marginal zone lymphoma; SMZL, splenic marginal zone lymphoma.

[*]Exclusively in Europe.

[†]50%–80% in Italy, Austria, Germany, and Korea.

- **Specific lab studies:** *Helicobacter pylori* testing (stool antigen, serum antibody, urea breath test); hepatitis B serology testing (hepatitis B surface antigen and core antibody; prior to use of rituximab); hepatitis C virus (HCV) antibody testing, BM aspirate and/or biopsy in case of multifocal disease; pregnancy test (if chemotherapy is planned for younger women); serum protein electrophoresis and immunofixation.
- **Imaging:** Computed tomography (CT) scan with contrast of chest, abdomen, and pelvis or associated organ of origin.
- **Upper GI endoscopy and endoscopic ultrasound (EUS):** Required for diagnosis of gastric MALT for guided biopsies. Fine needle aspiration (FNA) is not ideal. EUS helps in staging and is helpful in predicting efficacy of the treatment for *H. pylori* eradication (associated with depth of tumor invasion).[2]
- **Multigated acquisition (MUGA) scan/echocardiogram:** Prior to treatment with anthracycline-based chemotherapy.

2008 INTERNATIONAL WORKSHOP GUIDELINES ON THE DIAGNOSIS OF EXTRANODAL MZL OR MALT

- Extranodal lymphoma composed of morphologically heterogeneous small B cells, including marginal zone (centrocyte-like) cells, monocytoid cells, small lymphocytes, and scattered immunoblasts, and centroblast-like cells.
- Plasmacytic differentiation is common, and a serum paraprotein is detected in 30% to 50% of cases (usually immunoglobulin M [IgM]).
- Typically, there is infiltration of epithelium with lymphoepithelial lesions.

Table 45.2 Translocations Associated With MALT Lymphoma

Translocation [Frequency]	Genes Involved	Associated Locations
t(11;18)(q21;q21) [15%–40%]	*BIRC3-MALT1*	Lung and stomach
t(1;14)(p22;q32) [<5%]	*BCL10-IgHV*	Lung and stomach
t(14;18)(q32;q21) [15%–20%]	*MALT1-IgHV*	Liver, skin, parotid gland, and ocular adnexa
t(3;14)(p13;q32) [<5%]	*FOXP1-IgHV*	Thyroid, ocular adnexa, and skin

API2, apoptosis 2; *BCL10*, B-cell lymphoma/leukemia 10; *FOXP1*, Forkhead box protein P1; *IgHV*, Immunoglobulin heavy chain; MALT, mucosa-associated lymphoid tissue; MALT1, mucosa-associated lymphoid tissue1.

- Clonality: Tumor cells typically express IgM with light-chain restriction. Cluster of differentiation 20 (CD20) is positive; CD5, CD10, CD23, and cyclin D1 are negative.
- CD43 is aberrantly expressed in approximately 50% of cases.

CYTOGENETICS

Multiple chromosomal translocations have been described, as shown in Table 45.2. The frequencies of the translocations vary with the site of disease and are mutually exclusive. The t(11;18), resulting in fusion protein *API2-MLT*, is the most common chromosomal translocation (6%–26% in gastric MALT), and generally these lymphomas are not driven by *H. pylori*. Trisomies, including trisomy 3 (seen in 40% of cases), 8, 12, and 18, are also seen but are not site-specific.

▒ PROGNOSIS

MALT lymphomas follow an indolent course and are slow to disseminate. They have a good prognosis regardless of the stage. Recurrences may occur after many years and may involve other extranodal sites. Exceptions include gastric MALT lymphomas with t(11;18) and *BCL10* overexpression, which are associated with disseminated disease and resistance to treatment with antibiotics. Staging is not standardized for MALT lymphoma and is based on the organ of origin. The Lugano modification of the Ann Arbor or Paris staging system can be used for gastric MALT (Table 45.3).

▒ TREATMENT

Management is very heterogeneous, and no specific guidelines exist. Treatment differs based on whether the patient has gastric or nongastric MALT lymphoma, the disease stage, and whether the patient is symptomatic (Table 45.4). Main treatment modalities are locoregional radiation therapy (RT) and *H. pylori* eradication by using antibiotics. If either is ineffective or contraindicated, rituximab

Table 45.3 Comparison of Different Staging Systems Used for GI MALT

Stage	Tumor Involvement	Lugano Modification of Ann Arbor Staging	Paris Staging
I	Confined to the GI tract: mucosa, submucosa, muscularis propria, serosa	Based on involvement—	T1-3 N0 M0
		I1: Mucosa or sub-mucosa	
		I2: Muscularis propria or serosa	
II	Extending into the abdomen OR penetration of serosa by tumor to involve adjacent organs or nodes	II1: Local LN involvement	T1-3 N 1-2 M0
		II2: Distant nodal involvement	T4 N0-2 M0
		IIE: Invasion of adjacent structures	
IV	Disseminated extranodal involvement OR concomitant su-pra-diaphragmatic nodal involvement	Involvement of LN on both sides of the diaphragm OR distant metastasis (bone marrow)	AnyT N3 M0
			AnyT Any N M1-2

GI, gastrointestinal; LN, lymph node; MALT, mucosa-associated lymphoid tissue.

or chemo-immunotherapy is used, and, in rare cases, surgical excision is required (Table 45.5).

GASTRIC MALT LYMPHOMA

This is most commonly associated with *H. pylori*, and so testing for *H. pylori* is essentially the first step. In approximately 5% to 10% of cases, which are *H. pylori* negative, t(11;18) has been found with high frequency and is associated with disseminated disease and resistance to antibiotic therapy.

Localized Disease—Stage I (1/2) and Stage IIE

Advanced Disease

Though uncommon, advanced gastric malt lymphoma is believed to be incurable, and treatment should be considered if the patient is symptomatic; has bulky disease, end-organ damage, or GI bleeding;

Table 45.4 Treatment of Localized MALT Lymphoma

Stage of Gastric MALT Lymphoma	H. pylori Positive	H. pylori Negative	Follow-Up
Stage I1, I2, and IIE	Antibiotic treatment for eradication[*]	RT[†] (preferred) or rituximab if RT is contraindicated	Restage with EGD and biopsy and check H. pylori status (if HP+ at start) in 3 months or sooner if patient is symptomatic.
Stage I1, I2, and IIE, and t(11;18) positive	Upfront RT[†] or rituximab if RT is contra-indicated	Upfront RT[†] or rituximab if RT is contraindicated	Follow up with EGD and biopsy in 3 months.

EGD, esophagogastroduodenoscopy; HP, *Helicobacter pylori*; MALT, mucosal-associated lymphoid tissue; RT, radiation therapy.

[*]Antibiotic regimen—Proton pump inhibitor (PPI) + clarithromycin + amoxicillin (metronidazole if PCN allergy).

[†]Maximal benefit from RT: limited disease that can be incorporated in one radiation field, failed antibiotics treatment. Long-term remissions are seen. Average dose is 30 Gy to 36 Gy.

Table 45.5 Management Based on Re staging EGD Evaluation

Lymphoma status	H. pylori (+) at Restaging Biopsy	H. pylori (−) at Restaging Biopsy
Negative	Second-line antibiotic treatment	Observe
Positive	**Stable disease:** Second-line antibiotic treatment	**Asymptomatic:** Observe and follow up in 3 months or RT
	PD or symptomatic: RT + second-line antibiotic treatment	**Symptomatic:** RT

EGD, esophagogastroduodenoscopy; PD, progressive disease; RT, radiation therapy.

or prefers it. Treatment is similar to that for advanced follicular lymphoma (see Chapter 41). One contrast in comparison to follicular lymphoma therapy is the response of Bruton's tyrosine kinase (BTK) inhibitors (e.g., ibrutinib). Ibrutinib is a valid option for patients with advanced-stage disease requiring therapy and intolerant to a more aggressive approach.

First-line treatment: Clinical trial; if not possible, consider either locoregional RT (palliative or disease control), single-agent or combination chemotherapy, or chemo-immunotherapy. If the patient is asymptomatic, then observation may be a reasonable approach. Follow up with esophagogastroduodenoscopy (EGD).

Relapsed/Refractory Disease (After Antibiotics)

After RT: In case biopsy is negative for lymphoma and *H. pylori*, then observe. If biopsy is positive for lymphoma, then consider further treatment as for follicular lymphoma (e.g., rituximab or chemo-immunotherapy). If *H. pylori* is positive, consider antibiotic treatment.

NONGASTRIC MALT LYMPHOMA

Management depends on the stage of disease at diagnosis and site of occurrence.

- Limited disease (stage I/II): Locoregional treatment with either RT or expectant management.
- Advanced disease (stage III/IV [1/3 of patients]): Immunotherapy or chemo-immunotherapy using similar management principles as in follicular lymphoma (see Chapter 41).

PRIMARY CUTANEOUS MZL

In this rare disorder, lymphoma presents only in the skin, and no extracutaneous site is present.

- Focal disease: Manage with RT over surgical excision or chemotherapy.
- Asymptomatic multifocal disease: Observation is reasonable.
- Symptomatic multifocal disease: Local control with intralesional steroids, RT, or surgical resection. Chemotherapy or chemoimmunotherapy can be considered as a last resort.

◾ POTENTIAL PRACTICE-CHANGING CLINICAL TRIALS

Given the success seen in the use of Lenalidomide in the treatment of indolent lymphoma, including MALT lymphoma, several studies are looking into the combination with novel targeted and immunotherapeutic agents. Lenalidomide and obinutuzumab have been shown to have an overall response rate of 80% to 100% in heavily treated indolent lymphoma. A single-agent trial of obinutuzumab is still recruiting (NCT03322865).

PI3K inhibitors have shown activity in indolent lymphoma, and many agents are currently approved for the treatment of follicular lymphoma. A combination study of copanlisib with rituximab (NCT03474744) is recruiting patients with MZL to evaluate whether the addition of CD20 inhibitor can improve outcomes. Other ongoing studies in MALT include umbralisib. Cellular therapy using chimeric antigen receptor (CAR-T) cells therapy is ongoing and enrolling patients with relapsed refractory MALT.

▨ REFERENCES FOR SUPPLEMENTAL READING

1. Sackmann M, Morgner A, Rudolph B, et al. Regression of gastric MALT lymphoma after eradication of *Helicobacter pylori* is predicted by endosonographic staging. MALT Lymphoma Study Group. *Gastroenterology.* 1997;113(4):1087–1090.

2. Zucca E, Arcaini L, Buske C, et al. Marginal zone lymphomas: ESMO Clinical Practice Guidelines for diagnosis, treatment and follow-up. *Ann Oncol.* 2020;31(1):17–29.

3. Kiesewetter B, Raderer M. Antibiotic therapy in nongastrointestinal MALT lymphoma: a review of the literature. *Blood.* 2013;122(8):1350–1357.

4. Zucca E, Bertoni F. The spectrum of MALT lymphoma at different sites: biological and therapeutic relevance. *Blood.* 2016;127(17):2082–2092.

5. National Comprehensive Cancer Network. *NCCN non-Hodgkin lymphoma guidelines 2015.* 2015. https://www.nccn.org/professionals/physician_gls/f_ guidelines.asp#nhl

46 Adult T-Cell Leukemia/ Lymphoma

Nikhil Mukhi and Lubomir Sokol

INTRODUCTION

Adult T-cell leukemia/lymphoma (ATLL) is a rare mature T-cell neoplasm caused by human T-cell lymphotropic virus type-1 (HTLV-1). The retrovirus is transmitted via breast feeding, sexual intercourse, or blood transfusions and is endemic to southern Japan, the Caribbean basin, Central/South America, tropical Africa, and northern Iran. In nonendemic areas, such as North America and Europe, it is seen in immigrant populations from affected areas.

HTLV-1 infection is asymptomatic in the majority of carriers, and malignant transformation is seen in 2% to 7% of infected individuals after a long latency. It is commonly seen in the sixth and seventh decades of life. HTLV-1 most frequently infects mature CD4+ T-cells, immunophenotypically most closely resembling Tregs. Transformed, malignant T-cells with clonally integrated HTLV-1 can be identified on peripheral blood smear by their characteristic flowerlike shaped nucleus (Figure 46.1). Compared to other peripheral T-cell lymphomas, ATLL has very poor 5-year overall survival (OS) rate of 14%. Clinically, it is classified into aggressive (acute and lymphomatous) and indolent (chronic, smoldering) subtypes.

DIAGNOSIS

- Presence of monoclonal T-cells expressing CD3, CD4, CD25, TCRαβ, and FOXP3+/– with loss of CD7, determined via flow cytometry (Figure 46.2) or lymph node histology and clonality studies with TCR gene rearrangement by using polymerase chain reaction (PCR).
- Presence of positive HTLV-1 serology.

Laboratory evaluation includes complete blood count (CBC) with differential, complete metabolic panel (CMP), and lactate dehydrogenase (LDH). Serologic evaluation of HTLV-1, hepatitis B/C, and human immunodeficiency virus–1/2 (HIV-1/2) should be done prior to treatment. Diagnostic workup includes contrast computed tomography (CT) scan of chest, abdomen, and pelvis or positron emission tomography/computed tomography (PET/CT) scan. In the absence of peripheral blood involvement, a lymph node biopsy should be performed. Bone marrow (BM) aspiration and biopsy and lumbar puncture are recommended for all patients prior to therapy initiation in order to determine the extent of disease involvement.

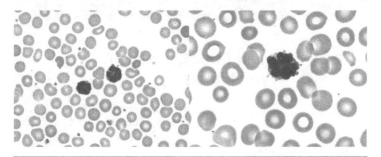

Figure 46.1 Characteristic "flowerlike" T-cells in ATLL: Several circulating atypical lymphoid cells were identified in a peripheral blood smear from a patient diagnosed with ATLL. The cells showed hyperchromasia, markedly irregular nuclear contour with lobated nuclei (flower-like cells), and an abundant amount of basophilic cytoplasm.

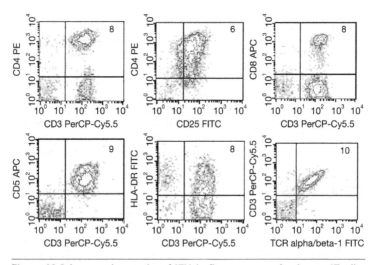

Figure 46.2 Immunophenotyping of ATLL by flow cytometry: An abnormal T-cell population is positive for CD3, CD4, CD5, CD25, HLA-DR (dim), and TCRαβ and negative for CD8 and CD7.

■ KEY DIAGNOSTIC DILEMMA

It is important to distinguish this entity from other peripheral T-cell lymphomas, such as angioimmunoblastic T-cell lymphoma (AITL), anaplastic large cell lymphoma (ALCL), mycosis fungoides/Sézary syndrome (MF/SS), and peripheral T-cell lymphoma not otherwise specified (PTCL NOS). Positive serology and ethnic background of the patient can help guide the diagnosis. AITL is very similar to ATLL except for the expression of CD10 cells in AITL. Similarly, ALCL is distinguished from ATLL by the presence of CD30 and Alk-1 expression in 70% of cases (see ALCL section). ATLL can mimic MF/SS with generalized erythrodermic skin involvement and circulating MF/Sézary cells in peripheral blood (see MF section). Lymphomatous subtype can also mimic PTCL NOS. Positive HTLV-1 serology and geographic origin of the patient are usually sufficient to distinguish these two entities, but, in some patients, HTLV-1 integration studies with Southern blotting or next-generation sequencing can be necessary for correct diagnosis.

▣ CLASSIFICATION

Shimoyama proposed diagnostic criteria to classify four clinical subtypes based on survival (Table 46.1; *Br J Haematol*. 1991;79(3):428–437).

▣ TREATMENT

Smoldering/chronic subtypes are considered indolent ATLL. Because of their relatively good prognosis, the most common strategy for these subtypes is "watchful waiting." A series of 17 patients from Japan used Zidovudine/Interferon-alfa (AZT/IFN) and had a 100% 5-year survival rate. A prospective trial is needed to further verify the findings.

Table 46.1 Clinical Subtypes in ATLL

Classification	Characteristics	Median Survival
Smoldering type	>5% abnormal lymphocytes, normal lymphocyte level (<4 × 10⁹/l), normal calcium level, LDH <1.5 × normal, no lymphadenopathy or involvement of liver, spleen, CNS. Skin or pulmonary lesions may be present.	>6.5 years
Chronic type	Absolute lymphocytosis (>4 × 10⁹/l) with T lymphocytes >3.5 × 10⁹/l, LDH >2 × normal limit. Lymphadenopathy, involvement of liver, spleen, skin and lung may be present.	24.3 months
Lymphomatous type	No lymphocytosis, 1% or less abnormal T-lymphocytes, and histologically proven lymphadenopathy with or without extranodal lesions.	10.2 months
Acute type	Remaining ATLL patients who have leukemic manifestation and tumor lesions but are not classified as any of the three other types.	6.2 months

ATLL, adult T-cell leukemia/lymphoma; CNS, central nervous system; LDH, lactate dehydrogenase.

Acute/lymphomatous subtypes are considered aggressive ATLL, and three treatment strategies have been suggested: (1) chemotherapy alone, (2) Interferon/Zidovudine, and (3) combination/sequential chemotherapy + Interferon/Zidovudine.

A variety of chemotherapy regimens, such as CHOP, DA-EPOCH, and Hyper-cyclophosphamide, vincristine, doxorubicin and dexamethasone alternating with cycles of methotrexate and cytarabine (CVAD), have been used. Despite aggressive treatments, the median survival for these ATLL subtypes is 6 to 13 months. The disease biology is widely considered to be different in Japanese and Caribbean populations. In the Japanese studies, the best results have been seen with LSG-15 regimen (vincristine, cyclophosphamide, doxorubicin, and prednisolone [VCAP]; doxorubicin, ranimustine, and prednisolone [AMP]; vindesine, etoposide, carboplatin, and prednisolone [VECP]), with an OS rate of 12.7 months and progression-free survival (PFS) rate of 7 months (Table 46.2).

In the United States, ATLL is primarily seen in immigrant populations from the Caribbean islands and Central and South America, and response data are largely available from retrospective studies (Table 46.3).

An alternative treatment option that has been explored in aggressive type is a combination of interferon-alfa with antiviral therapy. A meta-analysis reviewed the efficacy of AZT/IFN in aggressive ATLL. In lymphomatous subtype, first-line antiviral therapy only (*n* = 13) resulted in a significant survival disadvantage (median OS of 7 months). In acute subtype, first-line antiviral therapy only (*n* = 45) resulted in a significant survival advantage (median OS of 9 months).

Table 46.2 Clinical Trials and Outcomes in Aggressive ATLL

Trial	Regimen	Outcome
JCOG 8101	VEPA regimen	OS: 8 months
		4-year OS: 8.3%
JCOG 9801	LSG-15 (6 cycles)	OS: 12.7 months
		PFS: 7 months
		3-year OS: 24%
	CHOP (8 cycles)	OS: 10.9 months
		PFS: 5.4 months
		3-year OS: 13%
Hodson et al.	Chemotherapy + AZT/IFN	OS: 9 months

ATLL, adult T-cell leukemia/lymphoma; AZT/IFN, Zidovudine/Interferon-alfa; CHOP, cyclophosphamide, doxorubicin, vincristine, and prednisone; OS, overall survival; PFS, progression-free survival; VEPA, Vincristine, Cyclophosphamide, prednisone, and Doxorubicin.

Table 46.3 Retrospective Studies of Chemotherapy Regimens in ATLL		
Study	Regimen	Outcome
Phillips AA, et al., 2010[3]	CHOP-like regimen (68.5%)	ORR: 64.1 %
		OS: 24 weeks
Verma V, et al., 2015[4]	EPOCH	PFS: 4.6 months
		OS: 6.7 months

ATLL, adult T-cell leukemia/lymphoma; CHOP, cyclophosphamide, doxorubicin, vincristine, and prednisone; EPOCH, etoposide, cytoxan, doxorubicin, vincristine, and prednisone; ORR, overall response rate; OS, overall survival; PFS, progression-free survival.

Combination/sequential chemotherapy/IFN/AZT was studied prospectively and showed improvement in response rate from 49% to 81% as compared with chemotherapy alone. Median OS was 9 months: 7.5 months for acute and 10 months for lymphomatous subtype. Use of AZT/IFN-α at any time prolonged survival in acute ($p < .001$) and lymphomatous ATLL subtypes ($p < .001$) and was the sole factor associated with reduction in risk of death in aggressive ATLL.

Central nervous system (CNS) prophylaxis with intrathecal methotrexate is recommended for all patients because of the high risk of CNS involvement. The role of autologous and allogeneic hematopoietic stem cell transplantation is unclear in aggressive ATLL, as only small case series have not demonstrated a significant survival benefit. However, consolidation with allogeneic stem cell transplantation is considered in selected patients with chemotherapy-sensitive disease.

RELAPSED/REFRACTORY DISEASE

Chemokine receptor 4 (CCR4) is expressed in >90% of ATLL patients. Mogamulizumab is a humanized anti-CCR4 monoclonal antibody approved for relapsed and refractory ATLL in Japan. A phase 2 trial conducted in Japan showed ORR of 50%. However, this couldn't be replicated in a prospective trial in the United States, where ORR of only 11% was reported. Lenalidomide is another plausible treatment option that has been studied in phase 2 study in relapsed or refractory ATLL. It showed ORR of 42% in a Japanese trial, with a PFS of 3.8 months.

▨ POTENTIAL PRACTICE-CHANGING CLINICAL TRIALS

Brentuximab vedotin is a CD30+ antibody-drug conjugate (ADC) that is currently in clinical trial in relapsed refractory CD30+ lymphomas, including some ATL patients (NCT01703949). The JAK-1/2 inhibitor ruxolitinib is currently recruiting in a phase 2 trial in patients with smoldering or chronic ATLL types (NCT01712659). Cobomarsen, an miR-155 inhibitor, demonstrated improved overall survival in preliminary reports of a phase 1 study in patients with aggressive ATLL (NCT02580552).

▓ REFERENCES FOR SUPPLEMENTAL READING

1. Malpica L, Pimentel A, Reis IM, et al. Epidemiology, clinical features, and outcome of HTLV-1-related ATLL in an area of prevalence in the United States. *Blood Adv*. 2018;2(6):607–620.

2. Tsukasaki K, Utsunomiya A, Fukuda H, et al. VCAP-AMP-VECP compared with biweekly CHOP for adult T-cell leukemia-lymphoma: Japan Clinical Oncology Group Study JCOG9801. *J Clin Oncol*. 2007;25(34):5458–5464.

3. Phillips AA, Shapira I, Willim RD, et al. A critical analysis of prognostic factors in North American patients with human T-cell lymphotropic virus type-1-associated adult T-cell leukemia/lymphoma: a multicenter clinicopathologic experience and new prognostic score. *Cancer*. 2010;116(14):3438–3446.

4. Verma V, Mukhi N, Ahmed A, et al. Efficacy of dose adjusted infusional chemotherapy: etoposide, cytoxan, doxorubicin, vincristine and prednisone (EPOCH) in untreated adult T-cell leukemia lymphoma (ATL). *J Clin Oncol*. 2015;33(Suppl):e19527.

5. Hodson A, Crichton S, Montoto S, et al. Use of zidovudine and interferon alfa with chemotherapy improves survival in both acute and lymphoma subtypes of adult T-cell leukemia/lymphoma. *J Clin Oncol*. 2011;29(35):4696–4701.

47   Anaplastic Large Cell Lymphoma

Poorvi Desai, Ling Zhang, and Lubomir Sokol

▓ INTRODUCTION

Anaplastic large cell lymphomas (ALCLs) belong to the mature T-cell and natural killer–cell (NK-cell) neoplasms, according to the 2017 Revised World Health Organization (WHO) Classification of Tumors of the Hematopoietic and Lymphoid Tissues. WHO now recognizes four subtypes of ALCL: systemic ALK-positive (ALK+ ALCL), systemic ALK-negative (ALK– sALCL), primary cutaneous (PC-ALCL), and the provisional entity breast implant–associated (BIA-ALCL). ALK+ ALCL is characterized by a t(2;5)/*NPM1/ALK* translocation, accounting for approximately 80% of cases. It has a more favorable prognosis, with 5-year survival rate of 70% to 90% compared to ALK– sALCL, which has the same morphologic but distinct clinical and molecular features. A subset of ALK– sALCL with *DUSP*22/IRF4 chromosomal rearrangements (30%) has a survival rate similar to ALK+ ALCL; conversely, those with *TP*63 rearrangements (8%) have a more aggressive course. BIA-ALCL is recently recognized and has no known recurrent genetic aberrations, which is thought to develop as an immune reaction to textured silicone. PC-ALCLs are generally indolent and also ALK-negative. High CD30 expression, a hallmark of diagnosis of ALCL, has allowed use of the anti-CD30 antibody-drug conjugate brentuximab vedotin (BV) in both systemic and PC-ALCL forms.

▓ CLINICAL FEATURES/PRESENTATION

Patients with systemic ALCLs usually present with advanced stage III/IV disease with B symptoms and have a slight male predominance. ALK+ ALCL usually develops in the first three decades, while the mean age of diagnosis for ALK– sALCL is between 55 and 60 years. In ALK+ ALCL, extranodal sites are frequently involved, including skin, soft tissue, bone, liver, lung, bone marrow (BM), and central nervous system (CNS). Conversely, half of ALK– sALCL cases involve lymph nodes. PC-ALCL is generally indolent and rarely spreads extracutaneously. It typically presents as a solitary ulcerating tumor or several grouped nodules or papules. Median age at presentation is 60 years. BIA-ALCL is a rare but now widely recognized entity associated with textured silicone implants approximately 10 years after their placement. It includes two subgroups, one that presents as a seroma (effusion around the implant) and the other as a palpable indolent tumor that is generally confined to the breast but with occasional systemic involvement.

▣ DIAGNOSIS

According to the 2017 WHO classification, the distinction among different PTCLs requires the integration of the clinical picture, morphology, immunohistochemistry (IHC), flow cytometry, cytogenetics, and molecular biology. Morphologically, "hallmark" ALCL cells are large and atypical, with eccentric horseshoe- or kidney-shaped nuclei, intermediate nuclear:cytoplasmic ratio, and eosinophilic perinuclear clearing (Figure 47.1). Advanced molecular profiling has revealed constitutive *JAK/STAT* activation as one of the central pathogenic features of systemic ALCLs.

ALK protein expression using immunohistochemistry (IHC) (Figure 47.1) correlates almost exactly with the presence of a chromosomal rearrangement involving the *ALK* gene on chromosome 2p23 and the *NPM* gene on chromosome 5q35 (NPM/ALK, a novel chimeric protein) in 75% to 85% of patients. The remaining 15% to 25% of cases include variant rearrangements of the *ALK* gene with a multitude of partner genes. Given the high correlation, IHC has largely replaced fluorescence in situ hybridization (FISH) testing.

CD30 plays a central diagnostic role, as ALCL is almost always CD30-positive (Figure 47.1). ALCL cells are also frequently positive for expression of epithelial membrane antigen (EMA). There are five different morphologic patterns of ALK+ ALCL: common, lymphohistiocytic,

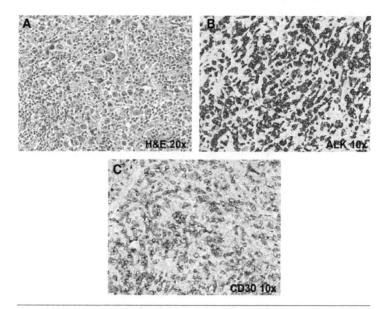

Figure 47.1 ALK+ ALCL: hematoxylin and eosin (H&E, 20×) shows hallmark cells with eccentric horseshoe- or kidney-shaped nuclei and intermediate nuclear: cytoplasmic ratio. Tumor cells are positive for ALK and CD30 (B–C, 1×).

small cell, Hodgkin-like, and composite. In contrast to ALK+ ALCL, no morphologic variants are recognized in ALK– sALCL. Pan-T-cell antigens, such as CD3, are more frequently expressed in ALK– sALCL than in ALK+ lymphoma. Two new gene rearrangements have been identified in ALK– sALCL (*DUSP22* and *TP63*), which aid in prognosis.

BIA-ALCL is a provisional entity per 2017 revised WHO classification of hematologic neoplasms separated into two different clinicopathologic subgroups, a seroma and a palpable tumor. In seromas, the capsule is commonly thickened, with a granular layer and adjacent fibrinoid material, but implants are usually intact. Palpable indolent tumors are generally confined to the breast but with fibrotic or chronic inflammatory background. In this second subtype, tumor cells are large, with abundant cytoplasm and vesicular multilobulated nuclei; typical hallmark cell morphology is rarely observed.

Diagnosis of PC-ALCL includes clinical and histologic criteria. Histologically, dense nodular dermal infiltrates resemble hallmark ALCL cells. Clusters of small reactive lymphocytes and eosinophils may be found within the surrounding tumor cells. PC-ALCL lacks EMA expression but is positive for cutaneous lymphocyte antigen HECA-452. In PC-ALCL, there must be absence of extracutaneous involvement or limited regional lymph node involvement.

▨ KEY DIAGNOSTIC DILEMMA

The failure to recognize specific morphologic variants of ALK+ ALCL can lead to misdiagnoses. Nodular sclerosis classical Hodgkin lymphoma (cHL) can be difficult to distinguish from Hodgkin-like variant ALK+ ALCL. ALCL shows a more diffuse, sheetlike staining pattern. Although cHL expresses CD30 and is B-cell-derived, it usually does not express typical B-cell markers, such as surface immunoglobulin, CD20, CD79a, or the common leukocyte antigen CD45. In contrast to ALCL, Hodgkin or Reed-Sternberg cells of cHL express weak PAX-5 and are typically EMA-negative. Thus, it is advisable to include EMA staining, with positivity prompting evaluation for ALK expression. Small-cell variant ALCL can morphologically mimic metastatic carcinoma. The lack of diffuse cytokeratin positivity (variable loss of T-cell markers), presence of ALK rearrangement, and characteristic strong and uniform CD30 expression (Figure 47.1) are key features in properly diagnosing ALCL.

Differentiating ALK– sALCL from Peripheral T-cell Lymphoma, Not Otherwise Specified (PTCL NOS) can be especially challenging. PTCL NOS has a more variable cytology, more heterogeneous and usually patchy and/or weaker expression of CD30, and more common CD2 and CD3 positivity than ALK– sALCL. It is typically ALK- and EMA-negative. The diagnosis of ALK– sALCL should be reserved for cases with morphologic and IHC features closely resembling the classic pattern of ALK+ ALCL.

Secondary involvement of ALK– sALCL in the skin can be difficult to distinguish from PC-ALCL. PC-ALCL is usually restricted to the skin but may also involve regional lymph nodes without indicating systemic disease. A systemic investigation with imaging studies is required in these cases. Positive IHC for ALK expression and presence of ALK rearrangement by FISH should prompt consideration of a cutaneous manifestation of systemic ALK+ ALCL.

▓ PROGNOSIS

The International Prognostic Index (IPI) is the most commonly used prognostic tool in PTCL, including ALCL. The IPI includes age, sex, Ann Arbor stage, number of extranodal sites, performance status, β2-microglobulin, and lactate dehydrogenase (LDH) elevation. The 5-year overall survival (OS) rates of ALK+ ALCL patients with low-risk IPI (0–1 risk factors), low-intermediate IPI (2 risk factors), high-intermediate IPI (3 risk factors), and high-risk IPI (4–5 risk factors) were 90%, 68%, 23%, and 33%, respectively. Importantly, survival of ALK+ ALCL dropped dramatically in patients with IPI scores of 3 or higher. It is critical to note that the majority of patients studied for IPI received an anthracycline-based combination chemotherapy without the use of anti-CD30 antibody-drug conjugate brentuximab vedotin, the new standard of care.

PC-ALCL is usually indolent and has an excellent prognosis (5-year survival rates of 76%–96%). Patients with BIA-ALCL generally show an excellent outcome, with 3-year OS of 100% and event-free survival (EFS) of 63%, but in a small proportion of patients (5%), relapsed/refractory disease is associated with poor prognosis.

More recently, novel chromosomal rearrangements other than with ALK+ have been identified as having prognostic significance. DUSP22 in normal T-cells acts as a negative regulator of the TCR signaling by inactivating the MAPK/ERK2 pathway. ALK– sALCLs with *DUSP22* rearrangements, present in 30% of cases, are associated with favorable prognoses similar to those of ALK+ sALCLs (5-year OS 90%). ALK– sALCLs with *TP63* rearrangements, presenting in 8% of cases, have a dismal outcome, with 5-year OS 17%. ALCLs without ALK, DUSP22, or TP63 rearrangements are now commonly referred to as "triple-negative" ALCLs and have an intermediate prognosis, with 5-year OS of 42%.

▓ TREATMENT

In the past, an anthracycline-based combination chemotherapy, such as cyclophosphamide, doxorubicin, vincristine, and prednisone (CHOP), was the standard therapy for aggressive lymphomas, including ALK+ ALCL. The addition of Etoposide (CHOEP) was thought to offer a potential benefit over CHOP, but this was mostly seen in more favorable (<60 years, ALK+) ALCL and was associated with greater toxicity in high-risk, elderly patients. The phase III 3 randomized study ECHELON-2 has set the new standard for CD30+ PTCL treatment by comparing Cyclophosphamide, Doxorubicin, and prednisone (CHP) plus anti-CD30 antibody-drug conjugate BV against the previous standard CHOP. Adding BV resulted in a 29% reduction in risk of progression-free survival (PFS) and 34% lower risk of death, with a

77% probability of survival at 36 months. Importantly, these improvements in survival came without an observed increase in toxicity.

An international, open-label, phase 3 trial ALCANZA compared BV to physicians' choice (oral methotrexate or bexarotene) and found that the proportion of patients achieving an objective global response lasting at least 4 months was 56.3% (36/64 patients) with BV, compared to 12.5% (8/64) with physicians' choice. This trial set the standard for BV as the preferred treatment for CD30-positive cutaneous T-cell lymphomas.

SYSTEMIC ALCL: PREFERRED TREATMENT
BV + CHP ± Radiation (ECHELON-2 Trial)

– Complete response (CR) or partial response (PR):
  - ALK+ ALCL or ALK– sALCL with *DUSP22* rearrangement
    - Complete planned course of treatment and observe.
  - ALK– sALCL without *DUSP22* rearrangement
    - Consider autologous stem cell transplant versus observation.
– Relapsed/refractory disease
    Second-line therapy-clinical trial or chemotherapies are listed below.
  - CR or PR: consider allogeneic hematopoetic stem cell transplant (HSCT).
  - Refractory or not a transplant candidate: Clinical trial or palliative treatment (chemotherapy, radiation therapy [RT], best supportive care)

SYSTEMIC ALCL: SECOND-LINE TREATMENTS
CHOP

CHOEP

Dose-adjusted EPOCH (Etoposide, Prednisone, Vincristine, Cyclophosphamide, and Doxorubicin)

BIA-ALCL
– Total capsulectomy and excision of associated mass with biopsy of suspicious nodes
– Consider removal of contralateral implants.
  - Localized disease to capsule/implant/breast
    - Complete excision: observation
    - Incomplete excision or regional lymph node (LN) involvement: Adjuvant treatment
  - Extended disease (stages II–IV): Adjuvant treatment
    - Adjuvant treatment options
      ○ BV ± CHP, CHOP, CHOEP, or DA-EPOCH

PC-ALCL

– Solitary or focally grouped lesions
  - Surgical excision ± radiation or radiation alone
– Multifocal lesions
  - BV (preferred, ALCANZA trial)
    - Methotrexate, pralatrexate, or systemic bexarotene/retinoids
– Regional node involvement (systemic ALCL ruled out)
  - BV ± radiation (preferred)
  - Radiation alone
  - Systemic treatment: BV + CHP, methotrexate or pralatrexate ± RT, CHOP or CHOEP ± RT
  - Romidepsin or belinostat
– CR: observation
– Relapsed/refractory disease: Repeat regimen or alternative regimen.

▓ POTENTIAL PRACTICE-CHANGING CLINICAL TRIALS

In the era of targeted therapy, gene-expression profiling may refine diagnostic classification, but it has not yet been validated for routine clinical use. A next-generation oral ALK/EGFR inhibitor, brigatinib, which has gained Food and Drug Administration (FDA) approval in ALK+ non-small-cell lung cancer, is being studied in relapsed or refractory ALK+ ALCL (NCT03719898). Two clinical trials involving anti-CD30 chimeric antigen receptor-T-cells are in process for relapsed/refractory CD30+ lymphoma (NCT03602157 and NCT02274584).

In pediatrics, a Children's Oncology Group study showed that relapsed/refractory ALK+ ALCL had a robust and sustained clinical response to the ALK inhibitor crizotinib. There is also a frontline randomized phase 2 pediatric trial comparing combination chemotherapy with either BV or crizotinib (NCT01979536).

▓ REFERENCES FOR SUPPLEMENTAL READING

1. NCCN Clinical Practice Guidelines in Oncology. *Non-Hodgkin's Lymphomas.* 2020. https://www.nccn.org/professionals/physician_gls/default.aspx
2. Hapgood G, Savage KJ. The biology and management of systemic anaplastic large cell lymphoma. *Blood.* 2015;126(1):17–25.
3. O'Connor OA, Bhagat G, Ganapathi K, et al. Changing the paradigms of treatment in peripheral T-cell lymphoma: from biology to clinical practice. *Clin Cancer Res.* 2014;20(20):5240–5254.
4. Montes-Mojarro IA, Steinhilber J, Bonzheim I, et al. The pathological spectrum of systemic anaplastic large cell lymphoma (ALCL). *Cancers.* 2018;10(4):107. doi: 10.3390/cancers10040107
5. Swerdlow SH, Campo E, Pileri SA, et al. The 2016 revision of the World Health Organization classification of lymphoid neoplasms. *Blood.* 2016;127(20):2375–2390. doi: 10.1182/blood-2016-01-643569

Extranodal Natural Killer/T-Cell Lymphoma

Joseph Clara and Lubomir Sokol

▆ INTRODUCTION

Extranodal natural killer/T-cell lymphoma (ENKTL) is an aggressive and distinct subtype of non-Hodgkin lymphoma (NHL) associated with Epstein–Barr virus (EBV) infection. It is uncommon in Western countries (<1% of all lymphomas), but more prevalent in Asia and Latin America (5%–15% of lymphomas), with a median age at diagnosis of 50 to 60 years and male-to-female ratio of approximately 2:1. ENKTL most frequently occurs as a localized disease involving the nasal cavity and paranasal sinuses, although it can involve extranasal sites, such as the skin, upper aerodigestive tract, and testis. Although it is predominantly extranodal, rare cases of disseminated disease may involve lymph nodes, bone marrow (BM), and peripheral blood, and these cases may overlap with aggressive natural killer–cell (NK-cell) leukemia (see Chapter 27). Despite a typically aggressive clinical course and overall poor prognosis, the incorporation of L-asparaginase into therapeutic regimens has resulted in substantial improvements in outcomes.

▆ DIAGNOSIS

2008 WORLD HEALTH ORGANIZATION (WHO) CLASSIFICATION HISTOPATHOLOGIC FEATURES OF ENKTL

- Histologic features: Polymorphic neoplastic lymphoid infiltrates, zonal necrosis, and angiocentric and angiodestructive growth pattern (Figure 48.1).
- Immunophenotype with surface CD3 (–), cytoplasmic CD3 (+), and CD56 (+). Positive EBV-encoded RNA (+) (EBER) by in situ hybridization (ISH) in almost all cases and cytotoxic molecules (granzyme B, perforin, T-cell intracellular antigen 1 [TIA-1]) (Figure 48.1).
- For CD56 (–) cases, cytotoxic molecules and EBER must be positive for the diagnosis.
- For definitive diagnosis in cases with atypical phenotypes, germline configuration of the T-cell receptor β and γ genes confirms NK-cell origin.

Diagnosis requires tissue biopsy, with specimens as large as possible due to frequent extensive necrosis. Contrast magnetic resonance imaging (MRI) or computed tomography (CT) scan of the affected area should be obtained as well as whole-body positron

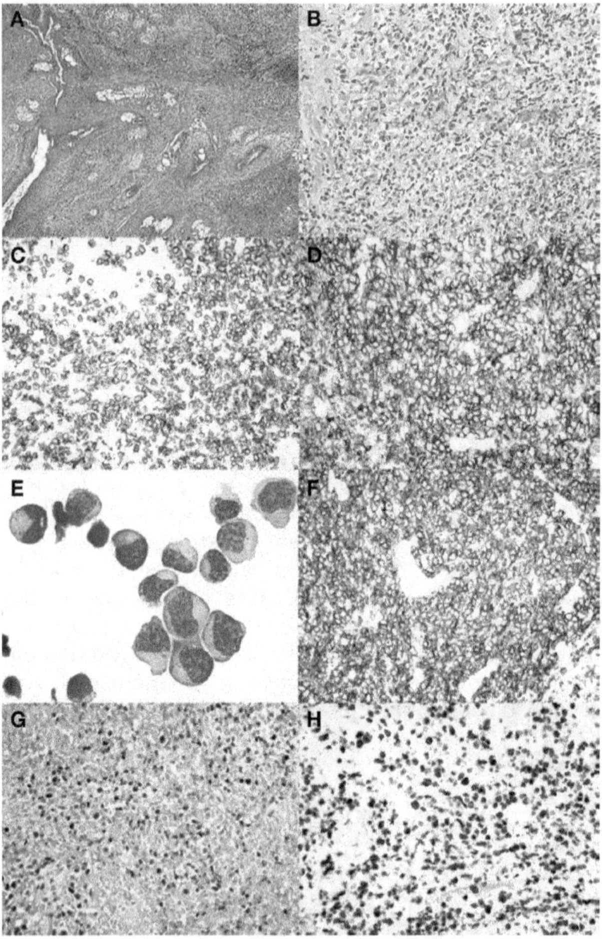

Figure 48.1 Histopathologic characteristics of ENKTL. Hematoxylin and eosin sections show a low-power view of intact squamous mucosa with submucosal atypical cell infiltrate (A, H&E, ×40). The atypical cells are medium to large, with dispersed to vesicular chromatin, irregular nuclear contours, and a certain amount of clear cytoplasm associated with hyaline fibrosis (B, H&E, ×100). Immunohistochemical stains (IHC) show these atypical cells to be positive for cytoplasmic CD3d and CD56 (C and D, respectively; immunoperoxidase ×200). Touch imprint demonstrates large atypical lymphoid cells with irregular nuclei, prominent nucleoli, and cytoplasmic reddish granules (E, WG ×1,000). IHC for CD2 is positive (F, immunoperoxidase ×200). EBER-ISH studies show the neoplastic NK cells are positive (G, ISH, ×200). The proliferation index by Ki-67 is high, up to 80% to 90% (H, immunoperoxidase ×200).

emission tomography (PET) scan. Nasal panendoscopy is recommended regardless of presenting site, and in cases with no apparent nasal disease, occult nasal involvement must be excluded by random nasopharyngeal biopsies and PET-CT scan. Workup also includes BM biopsies with EBER-ISH to assess for marrow involvement. Laboratory evaluation includes complete blood count (CBC) with differential, complete metabolic panel (CMP), and lactate dehydrogenase (LDH). Plasma-quantitative EBV DNA titer is a surrogate for tumor load and is quantified to assist with prognosis and serial analysis. Serologic testing for hepatitis B should also be done prior to the start of treatment.

▓ KEY DIAGNOSTIC DILEMMA

Although rare, ENKTL can present with isolated gastrointestinal (GI) tract involvement. Enteropathy-associated T-cell lymphoma (EATL) has a monomorphic variant, which expresses CD56 and can be EBV-positive. EATL expresses CD8 (>80%) and surface CD3. It also has adjacent enteropathy, where the intraepithelial lymphocytes share the same immunophenotype. ENKTL is CD8 and surface CD3-negative. This difference in immunophenotype can help distinguish these cases.

▓ PROGNOSIS

ENKTL is an aggressive malignancy. Although patients with limited-stage disease can have relatively good prognoses if treated with combined modality, disseminated ENKTL usually has a very poor prognosis (Tables 48.1–48.5). Prognostic assessment includes clinical staging and laboratory testing. Commonly utilized prognostic models include the International Prognostic Index (IPI) (Table 48.1), Korean Prognostic Index (KPI) (Table 48.2), and NK/T-Cell Lymphoma Prognostic Index (NKPI) (Table 48.3). More recent prognostic models are based on the contemporary use of non-anthracycline-based chemotherapy and may more accurately reflect prognosis in the modern era; PINK (prognostic index of natural killer lymphoma) (Table 48.4) and

Table 48.1 IPI for ENKTL

IPI	Risk	% 10-Year OS
0–1	Low	63.8 (IPI ≤1)
2	Low-intermediate	
3	High-intermediate	26.8 (IPI ≥2)
4–5	High	

ENKTL, extranodal natural killer/T-cell lymphoma; IPI, International Prognostic Index; LDH, lactate dehydrogenase; OS, overall survival.

1 point each for age >60 years, stage ≥ III, elevated LDH, Eastern Cooperative Oncology Group (ECOG) score ≥2, >1 extranodal site.

Table 48.2 KPI for ENKTL

Risk Group	Number of Factors	% 5-Year OS
1	0	80.9
2	1	64.2
3	2	34.4
4	3–4	6.6

ENKTL, extranodal natural killer/T-cell lymphoma; KPI, Korean Prognostic Index; LDH, lactate dehydrogenase; OS, overall survival.

Factors: B symptoms, stage ≥III, LDH ≥1 × upper normal limit, and regional lymph node (N1–N3, not M1) involvement according to tumor node metastasis (TNM) staging system.

Table 48.3 NKPI for ENKTL

Risk Group	Number of Factors	% 4-Year OS
1	0	55
2	1	33
3	2	15
4	3–4	6

ENKTL, extranodal natural killer/T-cell lymphoma; NKPI, NK/T-cell lymphoma prognostic index; OS, overall survival.

Factors: advanced stage ≥ III, ECOG ≥2, >1 location of extranodal involvement, non-nasal disease.

Table 48.4 PINK for ENKTL

Risk Group	Number of Factors	% 3-Year OS
Low	0	81
Intermediate	1	62
High	≥2	25

ENKTL, extranodal natural killer/T-cell lymphoma; PINK, Prognostic Index of Natural Killer Lymphoma; OS, overall survival.

Factors: age >60, advanced stage ≥III, non-nasal type, and distant lymph-node involvement.

PINK-E (Table 48.5) incorporate quantitative assessment of EBV-DNA. Other factors associated with a poor prognosis include high plasma levels of EBV DNA (>7.3 × 10^7 copies/mL), the presence of EBV-positive cells in BM, and local tumor invasion in stage IE and IIE disease. Serum concentrations of beta-2 microglobulin, soluble interleukin 2, and C-reactive protein are also being investigated as potential prognostic indicators.

Table 48.5 PINK-E for ENKTL

Risk Group	Number of Factors	% 3-Year OS
Low	0-2	81
Intermediate	2	55
High	≥3	28

ENKTL, extranodal natural killer/T-cell lymphoma; PINK-E, Prognostic Index of Natural Killer Lymphoma–Epstein–Barr virus; OS, overall survival.

Factors: age >60, advanced stage ≥III, non-nasal type, and distant lymph-node involvement, detectable Epstein–Barr virus DNA.

▓ TREATMENT

Treatment strategies for ENKTL are based on retrospective analyses and small phase 2 studies, and optimal therapy is yet to be established. Combined modality (radiation therapy [RT] and chemotherapy), either concurrent or sequential, is the mainstay approach for localized disease (stages I–II), as systemic chemotherapy is frontline treatment for disseminated disease (stages III–IV). In contrast to other types of NHL, RT should employ doses >50 Gray to a field extending beyond the visible macroscopic tumor volume. ENKTL exhibits resistance to anthracycline-based chemotherapy due to an expression of high P-glycoprotein concentration/multidrug resistance (MDR) phenotype. Chemotherapy selection, therefore, favors regimens of non-MDR-dependent agents, often incorporating L-asparaginase. Early or upfront RT plays an important role in improvement of overall survival (OS) and disease-free survival (DFS) rates in patients with limited-stage ENKTL.

No clinical trials have been conducted comparing different therapies head-to-head, but several preferable regimens are listed as follows. The utility of hematopoietic stem cell transplant (HSCT) remains undefined, although recent recommendations from the American Society for Blood and Marrow Transplantation provide some guidance. It supports the use of autologous HSCT in CR1 for disseminated disease and in relapsed chemosensitive ENKTL and allogeneic HSCT for advanced, relapsed, or refractory disease. All patients should be considered for clinical trial, particularly those with disseminated, relapsed, or refractory disease. In the absence of clinical trial, PD1 blockade has recently emerged as a promising treatment for patients who have failed L-asparaginase regimens. Monitoring after treatment includes plasma EBV DNA and PET-CT.

STAGES I–II NASAL NK/T-CELL LYMPHOMAS

- Dexamethasone, etoposide, ifosfamide, and carboplatin (2/3 DeVIC) with concurrent RT (complete response [CR] 77%, OS 78% at 2 years; *J Clin Oncol.* 2009;27(33):5594–5600).

- Cisplatin with concurrent RT followed by etoposide, ifosfamide, cisplatin, and dexamethasone (VIPD; CR 80%, OS 86% at 3 years; *J Clin Oncol.* 2009;27(35):6027–6032).
- L-asparaginase, vincristine, and prednisolone (LVP) with sandwiched RT (CR 81%, OS 89% at 2 years; *Cancer.* 2012;118(13):3294–3301).
- Dexamethasone, methotrexate, ifosfamide, *E. coli* L-asparaginase, and etoposide (SMILE) with sandwiched RT (CR 66%, OS 50% at 5 years, regimen-related mortality of 7%; *Blood.* 2012;120(15):2973–2980).
- Gemcitabine, *E. coli* L-asparaginase, and oxaliplatin (GELOX) with sandwiched RT in patients unable to tolerate intensive chemotherapy (CR 74%, OS 86% at 2 years; *Cancer.* 2013;119(2):348–355).
- Chemotherapy-unfit patients (serious medical comorbidities) with clearly localized nasal disease on PET-CT: RT alone (*Int J Radiat Oncol Biol Phys.* 2002;54(1):182–190; *J Clin Oncol.* 2006;24(1):181–189).
- Polyethylene glycol–asparaginase (PEG-asparaginase), gemcitabine, and oxaliplatin (P-GEMOX) followed by RT (CR 80%, OS 83% at 2 years; *Hematology.* 2017; 22:320–329).
- L-asparaginase, cisplatin, dexamethasone, and etoposide (LVDP) with sandwich RT and cisplatin (CR 83%, OS 70% at 3 years; *Oncotarget.* 2017;8:50155–50163).
- Concurrent L-asparaginase and cisplatin with RT, followed by methotrexate, etoposide, ifosfamide, dexamethasone, and L-asparaginase (MIDLE; CR 82% OS 82% at 3 years; *Oncotarget.* 2016;7:85584–85591).

LOCALIZED NONNASAL DISEASE AND DISSEMINATED DISEASE

- SMILE with or without involved-field radiotherapy (*Blood.* 2012;120(15):2973–2980; *Ann Oncol.* 2012;23(10):2703–2707; *J Clin Oncol.* 2011;29(33):4410–4416).
- Dexamethasone, cisplatin, gemcitabine, and PEG-asparaginase (DDGP; CR 71%, OS 90% at 1 year; *Clin Cancer Res.* 2016;22: 5223–5228).
- Consider allogenic or autologous HSCT if CR is achieved.

RELAPSED/REFRACTORY DISEASE

- Anti-PD1 therapy (Pembrolizumab: $N = 7$ patients; overall response rate (ORR) 100%, CR 71%, PR 29%; CR maintained at a median 6 months in all 5 patients achieving CR; *Blood.* 2017;129(17):2437–2442).
- SMILE (OS at 1 year 79% for relapsed and 25% for primary refractory; *J Clin Oncol.* 2011;29(33):4410–4416).
- L-asparaginase, methotrexate, and dexamethasone (AspaMetDex; *Blood.* 2011;117(6):1834–1839).

- PEG-asparaginase, gemcitabine, and oxaliplatin (P-GEMOX; CR 51%, OS 65% at 3 years; *Oncotarget*. 2016;7:29092–29101).
- Consider allogenic or autologous HSCT if CR is achieved.

▥ POTENTIAL PRACTICE-CHANGING CLINICAL TRIALS

The search for novel treatment strategies is ongoing due to the persistent overall poor prognosis, but it has been aided by the identification of several oncogenic pathways in ENKTL. An epigenetic approach using the proteasome inhibitor bortezomib and the histone deacetylase inhibitor (HDAC) panobinostat, in a phase 2 study in peripheral T-cell lymphoma, resulted in a partial response and stabilization of disease in two ENKTL patients with relapsed/refractory disease (*Lancet Haematol*. 2015;2(8):e326–e333). In addition, the anti-VEGF monoclonal antibody bevacizumab combined with gemcitabine, oxaliplatin, PEG-asparaginase, and dexamethasone is being evaluated as a first-line treatment (NCT01921790). Evaluation of the antibody-drug conjugate targeting CD30, brentuximab vedotin, is warranted, given that CD30 expression is detected in approximately 50% of ENKTL cases, and one trial including ENKTL patients has completed accrual (NCT01309789). T-cell immunotherapy using cytotoxic T-cell lymphocytes to target EBV antigens has demonstrated activity in ENKTL patients, and CD30-targeted CAR-T cells, not yet tested in ENKTL patients, may provide another immunotherapy option. CD38 expression has also been detected in ENKTL, and its strong expression associated with worse prognosis, also suggesting CD38 as a potential therapeutic target that is being investigated in a multicenter phase 2 trial (NCT02927925). PD1 blockade has recently shown tremendous promise in a series of patients having failed L-asparaginase regimens, and trials of anti-PD1 therapies in relapsed/refractory ENKTL are ongoing (NCT03107962 and NCT03021057). Some of the first randomized studies to compare different regimens are in the early stages, including a multicenter trial comparing gemcitabine, PEG-asparaginase, cisplatin, and dexamethasone (DDGP) with a modified SMILE regimen in stage III/IV disease (NCT01501149) and another comparing DDGP and VIPD both with RT and RT alone in stage I/II disease (NCT01501136).

▥ REFERENCES FOR SUPPLEMENTAL READING

1. Yamaguchi M. Advances in the treatment of extranodal NK/T-cell lymphoma, nasal type. *Blood*. 2018;131(23):2528–2540. doi: 10.1182/blood-2017-12-791418

2. Hu B, Oki Y. Novel immunotherapy options for extranodal NK/T-cell lymphoma. *Front Oncol*. 2018;8:139. doi: 10.3389/fonc.2018.00139

3. Harabuchi Y, Takahara M, Kishibi K, et al. Extranodal natural killer/T-cell lymphoma, nasal type: basic science and clinical progress. *Front Pediatr*. 2019;7:141. doi: 10.3389/fped.2019.00141

4. Haverkos B, Pan Z, Gru A, et al. Extranodal NK/T cell lymphoma, nasal type (ENKTL-NT): an update on epidemiology, clinical presentation, and natural history in North American and European cases. *Curr Hematol Malig Rep.* 2016;11(6):514–527. doi: 10.1007/s11899-016-0355-9

5. Kim S, Yoon D, Jaccard A, et al. A prognostic index for natural killer cell lymphoma after non-anthracycline-based treatment: a multicenter, retrospective analysis. *Lancet Oncol.* 2016;17(3):389–400. doi: 10.1016/S1470-2045(15)00533-1

Mycosis Fungoides

Vania Phuoc and Lubomir Sokol

▓ INTRODUCTION

Mycosis fungoides (MF) is the most common type of cutaneous T-cell lymphoma (CTCL), constituting approximately 50% of primary cutaneous lymphomas. The average age at presentation is 55 to 60 years, with a male predominance of 2:1, and highest incidence rates occur in African Americans (0.9/100,000). Elevated risk of MF has been associated with certain occupations, including painting, woodworking, farming, petrochemical, textile, and metal industries. Due to limited number of atypical malignant T-cells in skin, initial skin biopsies may be nondiagnostic. A waxing and waning "premycotic" period ranges from months to years, and repeat skin biopsies are usually necessary. Skin lesions can present as erythematous patches and plaques, papules, hypo- or hyperpigmented lesions, or generalized erythroderma, often accompanied by alopecia, palmar and/or plantar hyperkeratosis, ectropion, and dystrophic nail changes. Patch- and plaque-stage MF frequently occurs in a "bathing suit" distribution involving the trunk, but any body surface area may be affected. Sézary syndrome (SS) is a leukemic form of CTCL, traditionally with the triad of erythroderma, lymphadenopathy, and clonal T-cells with characteristic cerebriform nuclei (Sézary cells, Figure 49.1) in skin, lymph nodes, and blood. Pruritus is seen in a majority of MF patients and is especially severe in patients with SS. Lymphadenopathy is observed in about 11% of patients, but visceral organ metastasis is extremely rare at diagnosis.

Epidermotropism with intraepidermal aggregates of atypical malignant T-cells interacting with Langerhans cells (i.e., "Pautrier microabscesses") and infiltration of the basal layer by atypical "haloed" (perinuclear clearing) lymphocytes are characteristic pathologic features of MF/SS (Figure 49.1). Histologic variants of MF exist, including folliculotropic, pagetoid reticulosis, and granulomatous slack skin (GSS), each with different disease-specific survival rates. The disease-specific 5-year survival rate is often significantly worse for the folliculotropic variant compared to classical patch- or plaque-stage MF (*J Clin Oncol.* 2010;28(31):4730–4739), but a subgroup of folliculotropic MF can exhibit more indolent behavior similar to early-stage classic MF. Immunophenotyping is essential in the diagnostic process of these patients. MF cells commonly express CD2, CD3, CD4, and CD5, with the frequent loss of CD7 and CD26. SS cells have a similar CD4+ immunophenotype but demonstrate

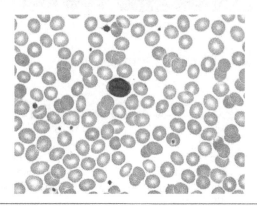

Figure 49.1 Sézary cell with typical cerebriform nucleus circulating in a patient with mycosis fungoides.

higher CCR4 (skin-homing receptor) and KIR3DL2 expressions. Flow cytometry diagnostic criteria for SS include an absolute Sezary cell count ≥1,000 cells/mcL or ≥1,000 cells/mcL with immunophenotypically abnormal CD4+/CD26– or CD4+/CD7– populations. Positive T-cell receptor (TCR) β and/or γ gene rearrangement clonality studies support a diagnosis of MF/SS. However, the presence of clonal TCR gene rearrangement in the absence of morphologically and phenotypically abnormal T-cell populations is not sufficient to diagnose MF. Modern molecular studies, including genome wide sequencing, have revealed numerous chromosomal abnormalities and gene mutations implicated in the pathogenesis of MF and SS (*Nat Genet.* 2015;47(12):1465–1470).

■ DIAGNOSIS

The European Organization for Research and Treatment of Cancer (EORTC) criteria for diagnosis uses a scoring system with at least 4 points required for the diagnosis of MF (*Blood.* 2007;110(6):1713–1722; Table 49.1).

Large-cell transformation is defined by the presence of ≥25% large lymphoid cells in the dermal infiltrate, and CD30 expression is present in approximately 40% to 50% of transformed MF.

■ KEY DIAGNOSTIC DILEMMA

The clinical presentation of MF, especially early stage, can mimic a diverse range of benign and malignant skin conditions. Patients with SS have an increased number of atypical lymphocytes with cerebriform nuclei in peripheral blood circulation, as shown in Figure 49.1; thus, the diagnosis can be established with flow cytometry. Other malignancies that may clinically mimic MF are primary cutaneous

Table 49.1 Clinicopathologic Diagnostic Criteria for MF

Criteria	Major Criteria (2 points)	Minor Criteria (1 point)
Persistent and/or progressive patches and plaques plus: • Non-sun-exposed location • Size/shape variation • Poikiloderma	Any 2	Any 1
Superficial lymphoid infiltrate plus: • Epidermotropism without spongiosis • Lymphoid atypia	Both	Either
Clonal TCR gene rearrangement	Not applicable	Present
Immunopathologic: • <50% CD2+, CD3+, and/or CD5+ T-cells • <10% CD7+ T-cells • Epidermal/dermal discordance of CD2, 3, 5, or 7	Not applicable	Any 1

MF, mycosis fungoides; TCR, T-cell receptor.

B-cell lymphoma, lymphomatoid papulosis, CD4+ small/medium pleomorphic T-cell lymphoproliferative disorder, cutaneous γ/δ T-cell lymphoma, adult T-cell leukemia/lymphoma, T-cell prolymphocytic leukemia, primary cutaneous anaplastic large-cell lymphoma, and subcutaneous panniculitis-like T-cell lymphoma (see Chapters 23 and 46). The history, physical exam, morphology, immunohistochemical (IHC), flow cytometry results, serology for HTLV-1 antibody, clonally rearranged TCR genes, and imaging studies may help distinguish MF from these conditions. Consultation in tertiary cancer centers with a cutaneous malignancy program may be necessary in cases with an inconclusive diagnosis.

■ STAGING

The Revised Tumor-Node-Metastasis-Blood (TNMB) staging system according to the International Society for Cutaneous Lymphomas (ISCL) and the Cutaneous Lymphoma Task Force of the EORTC is currently used for staging of MF/SS (Table 49.2). Patients are stratified into two clinical groups: early stage (stages IA–IIA) and advanced stage (stages IIB–IV). Approximately 70% of patients present with early-stage disease, and 30% present with advanced stages. Essential staging studies include complete blood count (CBC) with differential, complete metabolic panel (CMP) with lactate dehydrogenase (LDH), flow cytometry of peripheral blood with an appropriate T-cell antibody panel, TCR gene-rearrangement studies, and

Table 49.2 TNMB Staging System for MF

Stage		Description
I	A	<10% skin involvement (patches, plaques, papules) of total skin surface area (T1); no lymph-node involvement
	B	≥10% skin involvement (patches, plaques, papules) (T2); no lymph-node involvement
II	A	Skin involvement (T1 or T2) along with N1–N2 lymph-node involvement
	B	Skin involvement along with one or more tumors ≥1 cm in diameter (T3) with N0–N2 involvement
III		Skin involvement >80% (erythroderma) (T4) with low blood-tumor burden (<1,000/mcL Sézary cells), absent or early lymph-node involvement (N0–N2)
IV		High-circulating tumor burden (≥1,000/μL Sézary cells), advanced lymph-node involvement (N3), and/or visceral involvement (M1)
Lymph-node involvement pathologic criteria:		
N0		No abnormal lymph-node involvement
N1		Abnormal lymph nodes with no cerebriform cells, Dutch grade 1 or NCI LN 0–2
N2		Abnormal lymph nodes with scattered cerebriform cells, Dutch grade 2 or NCI LN 3
N3		Abnormal lymph nodes with several cerebriform cells/effacement of architecture, Dutch grade 3–4 or NCI LN 4
Blood involvement pathologic criteria:		
B0		Absence of blood involvement: ≤5% of peripheral blood lymphocytes by cytomorphology or <250/mcL by flow cytometry are malignant MF/Sézary cells or <15% CD4+/CD26– or CD4+/CD7– cells of total lymphocytes
B1		Low tumor burden: >5% of peripheral blood lymphocytes are atypical (Sézary) cells or >15% CD4+CD26– or CD4+CD7– of total lymphocytes but do not meet the criteria of B0 or B2
B2		High tumor burden: ≥1,000/mcL Sézary cells determined by cytomorphology or ≥1,000 CD4+CD26– or CD4+CD7– cells/mcL or other abnormal subset of T lymphocytes by flow cytometry with TCR gene rearrangement clone in blood identical to that in skin. Other criteria for high blood-tumor burden in CD4+ MF/SS include CD4+/CD7– cells ≥40% and CD4+CD26– cells ≥30%

MF, mycosis fungoides; NCI LN, National Cancer Institute Lymph Node; TCR, T-cell receptor; TNMB, Tumor-Node-Metastasis-Blood.

Source: Data from *Blood*. 2007;110(6):1713–1722; *J Clin Oncol*. 2011; 29:2598–2607; and NCCN Guidelines: Primary Cutaneous Lymphomas. Version 2.2020–April 10, 2020.

a contrast computed tomography (CT) scan of the chest, abdomen, and pelvis or a whole body positron emission tomography–computed tomography (PET-CT) scan. Bone marrow (BM) biopsy is not typically a part of staging for MF/SS but can be useful in patients with advanced stage and/or cytopenias.

▧ PROGNOSIS

MF is considered incurable with currently available skin-directed or systemic therapies. The overall survival (OS) rate by T stage at 5 years was 95% for T1, 87% for T2, 57% for T3, and 52% for T4 (*Clin Cancer Res*. 2012;18(18):5051–5060). Progression to a higher stage occurred in about 10% of patients, and death from disease was observed in 8.1% of all patients. OS and progression-free survival (PFS) are better for early-stage patients with patches (T1a/T2a) than with patches/plaques (T1b/T2b). Four factors (stage IV, age >60 years, large-cell transformation, and increased LDH) were independent prognostic markers for a worse survival rate in a novel prognostic index model for advanced stage MF (*J Clin Oncol*. 2015;33(32):3766–3773). Based on this model, three risk groups across stages revealed significantly different 5-year survival rates: low risk (0–1; 68%), intermediate risk (2; 44%), and high risk (3–4; 28%).

▧ TREATMENT

Disease involving <10% of the body surface area of skin (T1) with no nodal or visceral organ involvement (stage IA) is treated with skin-directed therapies, such as a topical corticosteroids, topical bexarotene, topical nitrogen mustard, phototherapy (narrow-band UV-B or psoralen-UV-A [PUVA]), and focal radiation therapy. Most of the skin-directed therapies have a very good response rate, but relapses are frequent (*J Am Acad Dermatol*. 2016;74(1):27–58). For patients with >10% skin involvement or nodal involvement (stage IB/IIA), skin-directed therapies remain the mainstay of treatment. However, in patients with stage IB/IIA refractory to these therapies, focal or total skin electron beam radiation therapy (EBRT) can be a very effective treatment modality, with a response rate of 80% to 100%. However, because most patients develop recurrent disease early after completion of radiation, a maintenance therapy is usually required. Patients with advanced-stage (IIB–IV) disease are usually treated with systemic therapies, such as oral bexarotene, interferon alfa, or histone deacetylase (HDAC) inhibitors, such as romidepsin and vorinostat. The anti-CD52 monoclonal antibody alemtuzumab is useful in patients with erythrodermic manifestation and blood involvement but not in patients with bulky nodal disease. Brentuximab vedotin (BV), an anti-CD30 monoclonal-antibody-drug conjugate, was evaluated in the phase 3 ALCANZA trial compared to physicians' choice of either oral methotrexate or bexarotene in patients with CD30+ MF or primary cutaneous anaplastic large-cell lymphoma, and overall response rates (ORR) lasting for at least 4 months and complete response (CR) rates were significantly higher for BV (56% [16% CR] vs. 13% [2% CR]; $p < .0001$). Peripheral neuropathy was the most common adverse event from BV in 67% of patients (*Lancet* 2017;390(10094):555–566). Mogamulizumab, a humanized anti-CCR4 monoclonal antibody, was compared to vorinostat in the phase 3 MAVORIC trial with relapsed/refractory (R/R) MF and SS, and mogamulizumab showed significantly higher ORR (28% vs. 5%) and PFS (8 months vs. 3 months) after median follow-up of 17 months. There was observed higher ORR in patients with SS than MF (37% vs. 21%) (*Lancet Oncol.* 2018;19(9):1192–1204). The anti-programmed cell death protein 1 (PD-1) immune checkpoint inhibitor pembrolizumab was evaluated in a phase 2 study of 24 patients with advanced R/R MF or SS, and ORR was 38%, with 2% CR and 29% partial response (PR). There was noted cutaneous flare reaction with transient worsening of erythroderma and pruritus in 53% of patients with SS, but the flare reaction did not result in treatment discontinuation and was not associated with clinical response (*J Clin Oncol.* 2020;38(1):20–28). Extracorporeal photopheresis (ECP) is a frontline modality for patients with SS and can be combined with systemic targeted or biological therapies, such as oral bexarotene, interferon alfa, and HDAC inhibitors. Monochemotherapy can be used sequentially in patients who do not respond or progress on biological therapy. Combined chemotherapy has been used for refractory advanced-stage disease, especially in patients with tumor stage or large-cell transformation. Prior systematic review and meta-analysis of allogeneic transplantation for MF and SS report OS 59%, PFS 36%, relapse rate 47%, and pooled non-relapse mortality rate 19% (*Biol Blood Marrow Transplant.* 2020;26(1):76–82). A summary of the treatment options is shown in Tables 49.3 and 49.4.

■ POTENTIAL PRACTICE-CHANGING CLINICAL TRIALS

The phase 2 REDIRECT trial in patients with R/R peripheral T-cell lymphoma or transformed MF is currently evaluating AFM13, a first-in-class tetravalent, bi-specific innate cell engager that binds CD30 on tumor cells to CD16A on natural killer (NK) cells and macrophages (NCT04101331). An ongoing phase 1/2 trial in patients with R/R peripheral T-cell lymphoma including CTCL uses immune checkpoint inhibitor durvalumab as monotherapy or in combination with lenalidomide (NCT03011814). Talimogene laherparepvec, a genetically modified herpes simplex virus 1 (HSV) oncolytic virus, is being studied in combination with anti-PD-1 agent nivolumab in a phase 2 study in refractory MF, SS, and other cutaneous malignancies (NCT02978625). There is an ongoing phase 1 study of administration of T lymphocytes coexpressing the CD30 chimeric antigen receptor (CAR) and CCR4

Table 49.3 Treatment Modalities for MF by Stage

Stage	Treatment	OR (%)	CR (%)
Early stage			
IA–IIA	Topical corticosteroids	94	63
	Topical carmustine	98	86
	Topical nitrogen mustard	70–80	10–25
	Topical retinoids	40–65	20
	Electron beam therapy	100	40–98
	UV B	90	83
	PUVA	90–100	90
IB/IIA	Topical corticosteroids/ carmustine	77	31
	Topical nitrogen mustard	50–70	12
	Electron beam therapy	80–90	40–98
	UV B/PUVA	71	22
Advanced stage			
	Electron beam therapy	44–74	39
	Bexarotene	45–55	10–20
	Interferon	53–74	21–35
	HDAC inhibitors (romidepsin/vorinostat)	30–35	6
	PUVA	95	30–70
	Alemtuzumab	55	32
	Brentuximab vedotin	56	16
	Mogamulizumab	28	3
	Pembrolizumab	38	2
	ECP	41	21

CR, complete response; ECP, extracorporeal photopheresis; HDAC, histone deacetylase; MF, mycosis fungoides; OR, overall response; PUVA, psoralen ultraviolet A.

for R/R CD30+ CTCL (NCT03602157). Two phase 1 studies with CD4 CAR T-cell therapy in R/R CD4+ T-cell malignancies are ongoing in the United States and China (NCT04162340, NCT03829540). The phase 2 TELLOMAK trial is evaluating IPH4102/lacutamab, an anti-KIR3DL2 monoclonal antibody, as monotherapy or in combination with chemotherapy in patients with advanced T-cell lymphomas, including MF and SS (NCT03902184).

Table 49.4 Chemotherapy Regimens for the Treatment of MF

Chemotherapy	OR (%)	CR (%)
Pegylated liposomal doxorubicin*	56–84	20–42
Pentostatin[†]	40–55	14
Pralatrexate[‡]	45	4
Gemcitabine[§]	40–70	8–23
Methotrexate[ˡ]	58	41
CHOP[¶]	95	29
COMP[#ˡ**]	100	57
Interferon-alfa + oral isotretinoin followed by electron-beam therapy[††]	85	60

CHOP, cyclophosphamide, vincristine, prednisone, and doxorubicin; COMP, cyclophosphamide, vincristine, methotrexate, and prednisone; CR, complete response; MF, mycosis fungoides; OR, overall response.
*J Clin Oncol. 2012;30(33):4091–4097. [†]J Clin Oncol. 1992;10(12):1907.
[‡]Blood. 2012;119(18):4115. [§]Ann Oncol. 2010;21(4):860. [ˡ]J Am Acad Dermatol. 1996;34(4):626. [¶]Cancer Treat Rep. 1979;63(4):647. [#]Am J Clin Oncol. 1984;7(5):453.
[††]J Am Acad Dermatol. 1991;24:247.

■ REFERENCES FOR SUPPLEMENTAL READING

1. Willemze R, Cerroni L, Kempf W, et al. The 2018 update of the WHO-EORTC classification for primary cutaneous lymphomas. *Blood.* 2019;133(16):1703–1714.

2. Hristov AC, Tejasvi T, Wilcox RA. Mycosis fungoides and Sezary syndrome: 2019 update on diagnosis, risk-stratification, and management. *Am J Hematol.* 2019;94(9):1027–1041.

3. Prince HM, Kim YH, Horwitz SM, et al. Brentuximab vedotin or physician's choice in CD30-positive cutaneous T-cell lymphoma (ALCANZA): an international, open-label, randomised, phase 3, multicentre trial. *Lancet.* 2017;390(10094):555–566. doi: 10.1016/S0140-6736(17)31266-7

4. Kim YH, Bagot M, Pinter-Brown L, et al. Mogamulizumab versus vorinostat in previously treated cutaneous T-cell lymphoma (MAVORIC): an international, open-label, randomised controlled phase 3 trial. *Lancet Oncol.* 2018;19(9):1192–1204. doi: 10.1016/S1470-2045(18)30379-6

5. Khodadoust MS, Rook AH, Procu P, et al. Pembrolizumab in relapsed and refractory mycosis fungoides and Sezary syndrome: a multicenter phase II study. *J Clin Oncol.* 2020;38(1):20–28. doi: 10.1200/JCO.19.01056

50 Hepatosplenic T-Cell Lymphoma

Walter Hanel and Narendranath Epperla

▪ INTRODUCTION

Hepatosplenic T-cell lymphoma (HSTCL) is an aggressive, mature T-cell lymphoma that is very rare and accounts for about 1.4% of all cases of T-cell lymphomas. It was initially reported as a distinct entity in 1990 after a detailed description of two cases. Since then, there has been increased recognition of the disease and clinicopathologic features. In a study of the National Cancer Database, between 1998 and 2011, there were 185 patients with newly diagnosed HSTCL. A malignant proliferation of cytotoxic T-cells predominantly of the gamma-delta ($\gamma\delta$) T-cell receptor type is seen, with only a small subset of cases being of the alpha-beta ($\alpha\beta$) type. Intrasinusoidal infiltration of spleen, liver, and bone marrow (BM) is another characteristic feature of HSTCL. The disease mainly affects adolescents and young adults, with a median age of 35 years and male predominance. Although the majority of cases arise de novo, there is an association of HSTCL with prolonged antigenic stimulation or long-term immunosuppression due to solid organ transplantation therapy (approximately 20% of cases). The largest at-risk specific patient population that has been described is young patients with inflammatory bowel disease (IBD) on immunosuppression. In men with IBD younger than 35 years, the absolute risk is estimated to be 1:7,404 on thiopurine monotherapy and 1:3,534 on combination thiopurine + anti-tumor necrosis factor (TNF) therapy, with 80% of cases occurring after 2 years on therapy. This led to the recommendation to limit combination immunosuppressive therapy to <2 years in this population to avoid this deadly complication.

The most common presentation of HSTCL includes fever, fatigue, weight loss, and abdominal discomfort as a result of hepatosplenomegaly. Liver involvement may lead to jaundice in some patients and bleeding diathesis in others, with coagulopathy from factor deficiencies likely contributing. Severe anemia and thrombocytopenia are common due to splenic sequestration. Hepatosplenomegaly (typically with an absence of generalized lymphadenopathy) is the most notable physical examination finding. HSTCL has an aggressive clinical course, with a median overall survival (OS) of only 16 months.

■ DIAGNOSIS

The most common laboratory findings typically include pancytopenia, abnormal liver function tests (i.e., elevated aspartate transaminase [AST], alanine transaminase [ALT], and alkaline phosphatase [ALP]), and lactate dehydrogenase (LDH). In particular, thrombocytopenia seems to directly correlate with disease burden. Recurrent thrombocytopenia in patients who achieved complete remission (CR) may be suggestive of disease relapse (Table 50.1). With disease progression, the neoplastic lymphocytes in circulation may increase in

Table 50.1 Diagnosis of HSTCL	
Initial diagnostic evaluations	Hematologic parameters: • CBC may show anemia (84% of cases), leukocytopenia (45% of cases), and thrombocytopenia (85% of cases)
	• Other notable parameters include: • Elevated LDH (62% of cases) • Abnormal liver-function test (43% of cases) • Hepatitis B/C, HIV-1/2, and EBV are infrequently associated with HSTCL.
Histopathology	• Small to medium-sized cells lack distinct nucleoli and have scant pale, nongranular cytoplasm. Atypia in the form of a large cell or blastic cytology can signal the progression of the disease. • Splenic (98%) and hepatic involvement (80%) are characteristic. BM involvement is present in 66% (sinusoidal infiltration, often subtle) of cases, while lymph node involvement is rare. • Spleen: diffuse invasion of red pulp, no visible macroscopic lesions, with normal to reduced bulk of white pulp • HSTCL actively secretes cytokines, including TNF-α, which can subsequently lead to erythrophagocytosis via histiocyte activation.
Immunophenotype	• Flow cytometry has a central role for diagnosis. • CD2+, CD3+, CD4−, CD5−, CD7+, CD8±, CD56± • TCRγδ is the most common receptor noted. • Cytoplasmic granules expressed: TIA1, granzyme M, but lack perforin and granzyme B • One or more NK cell markers (CD16, CD56, CD57) are usually seen.
Cytogenetics	• Combination of isochromosome 7q with trisomy 8 is commonly seen in HSTCL.

BM, bone marrow; CBC, complete blood count; EBV, Epstein–Barr virus; HIV, human immunodeficiency virus; HSTCL, hepatosplenic T-cell lymphoma; LDH, lactate dehydrogenase; NK, natural killer.

number and size and can lead to a leukemic phase (i.e., in terminal stages, HSTCL may resemble acute leukemia).

■ KEY DIAGNOSTIC DILEMMA

Once T-cell or natural killer–cell (NK-cell) lineage has been established, a diagnosis of mature T-cell or NK-cell neoplasm is further determined by the constellation of flow cytometric, immunohistochemical, and genetic findings. Within the spectrum of mature T-/NK-cell lymphomas, the major diagnostic challenge lies in differentiating HSTCL from other γδ T-cell neoplasms, such as primary cutaneous γδ T-cell lymphoma and γδ subtype of T-cell large granular lymphocyte (LGL) leukemia (see Chapter 26). Clinical presentation with skin lesions is not characteristic for HSTCL, and an indolent course with a lack of massive hepatosplenomegaly is seen in the γδ subtype of T-cell LGL leukemia. The LGL leukemic clone typically expresses CD57, granzyme B, and perforin. The BM of HSTCL, if involved, will have a sinusoidal expansion, with T-cells negative for cytotoxic granules. Aggressive NK-cell leukemia should also be considered in the differential diagnosis (see Chapter 27). This disease lacks surface CD3 but is positive for cytoplasmic CD3ε and CD56. As demonstrated in other T-cell lymphomas, a clonal T-cell receptor gene γ or β rearrangement can usually be demonstrated in HSTCL. The presence of isochromosome 7q in a majority of cases further supports the diagnosis of HSTCL.

■ PROGNOSIS

HSTCL portends an aggressive course with resistance to anthracycline-based chemotherapy. CR is uncommon. Median 5-year failure-free survival (FFS) and OS rates were found to be 0% and 7%, respectively, in an international cohort of HSTCL patients. Negative prognostic factors deduced from small retrospective series include male sex, absence of TCR gene rearrangement, and lack of obtaining CR to induction therapy. Thrombocytopenia and the occurrence of hemophagocytic syndrome are associated with a more aggressive clinical course (see Chapter 52). HSTCL arising in the post-transplant setting is associated with even poorer outcomes. Patients with Crohn's disease–associated HSTCL have only an 8-month median survival. It is unclear whether this is due to the biology of HSTCL in this subset of patients versus other comorbidities.

■ TREATMENT

Due to the low prevalence of HSTCL, there is a paucity of prospective clinical trials and no standard treatment guidelines. Much of the therapeutic data are presently anecdotal, as no randomized controlled studies of HSTCL exist. The patients with relapsed disease are usually chemorefractory, and salvage may not be feasible due to compromised organ function, cytopenias, or declining performance

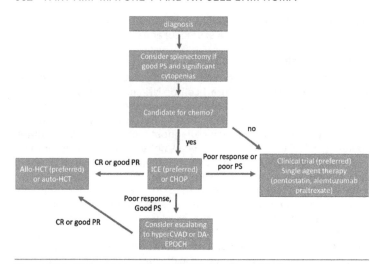

Figure 50.1 Treatment algorithm for HSTCL (frontline setting).

Allo, allogeneic; Auto, autologous; CHOP, cyclophosphamide, doxorubicin, vincristine, and prednisone; CR, complete response; HSTCL, hepatosplenic T-cell lymphoma; PR, partial response; PS, performance status.

status. Unlike certain cases of B-cell post-transplant lymphoprolif-erative disorder (PTLD), there have been no published case reports of spontaneous regression of HSTCL following the withdrawal of immunosuppression as sole therapy. This is consistent with its over-all infrequent association with Epstein–Barr virus (EBV), and thus cytotoxic therapy is considered the mainstay of treatment in this population, just as in de novo cases. The choice of chemotherapy reg-imens as well as the decision for BM transplant in the upfront setting is weighed against the patient's age, performance status, previous transplant status, and degree and duration of immunosuppression. In addition to supportive therapy, splenectomy can be considered in cases of severe thrombocytopenia. By correcting thrombocytopenia, early splenectomy may allow more effective delivery of systemic che-motherapy (*Ann Surg Oncol.* 2009;16(7):2014).

A treatment algorithm is presented to summarize the treatment approach in newly diagnosed HSTCL (Figure 50.1), and a discussion of the data for these recommendations follows.

Treatment with cyclophosphamide, doxorubicin, vincristine, and prednisone (CHOP) in the first-line setting has shown limited benefit overall, with OS of just 16 months (*Blood.* 2003;102(13):4261–4269). Thus, as is the case for peripheral T-cell lymphoma (PTCL), it is clear that CHOP has limitations in the treatment for HSTCL and that other treatment approaches are needed. A single institutional retrospective study provided interesting data suggesting that the use of the non-CHOP regimens, such as ifosfamide, carboplatin, and etoposide (ICE) or ifosfamide, etoposide, and cytarabine (IVAC), resulted in a higher chance of CR compared to CHOP (50% vs. 25%), despite having a similar overall response rate (ORR) of 75% (*Clin Lymphoma Myeloma Leuk.* 2103;13(1):8–14). Of note, 2 of the 3 patients who did not achieve CR with CHOP went on to receive ICE and subsequently achieved CR. This ultimately resulted in less time to transplant in chemosensitive cases, potentially resulting in a better chance of long-term remission with the use of a regimen other than CHOP.

There is less experience with more intense induction regimens, such as Hyper-Cyclophosphamide, vincristine, doxorubicin, and dexamethasone (CVAD) or Etoposide, prednisone, oncovin, cyclophosphamide, and doxorubicin (EPOCH). One case report described a long-term remission with Hyper-CVAD along with a reduction in immunosuppression in a patient with a history of a prior solid organ transplant (*Am J Hematol.* 2008;83(4):330–333). In the MD Anderson Cancer Center (MDACC) experience, a similar regimen, Hyper-CVID-Doxil (fractionated Cytoxan, liposomal doxorubicin, vincristine, dexamethasone alternating with methotrexate and cytarabine) showed ORR of 100% with CR of 75% among 4 patients (*Ann Oncol.* 2009;20:1080–1085), 3 of whom went on to transplant.

Treatment with the purine analog (pentostatin) has shown striking results in case reports, with some leading to CR with long-term remission following transplant (*Haematologica.* 2005;90:ECR14; *Br J Haematol.* 2002;117:995–996). However, other series have shown more limited activity (*Ann Oncol.* 2009;20:1080–1085). Pentostatin may be a reasonable alternative for patients who cannot tolerate combination chemotherapy.

CONSOLIDATION TREATMENT AFTER FRONTLINE THERAPY

After frontline therapy for HSTCL, consolidation therapy with BM transplant should be considered for all transplant-eligible patients, with a preference for allogeneic hematopoietic cell transplantation (allo-HCT).

Auto-HCT versus Allo-HCT

The Center for International Blood and Marrow Transplant Research (CIBMTR) compared OS between auto-HCT and allo-HCT in patients with HSTCL. The preliminary data revealed the probability of OS at 1 year after auto-HCT to be 88%, compared with 68% after allo-HCT, although not statistically significant (*Clin Lymphoma Myeloma Leuk.* 2013;13(4):360–369). However, the risk of relapse was noted to be significantly lower with allo-HCT, albeit with higher treatment-related mortality. Patients who underwent auto-HCT appeared to have greater chemotherapy sensitivity and less advanced disease, making outcome comparisons between these two HCT groups difficult (*J Clin Oncol.* 2013;31(25):3100–3109). A recent study published by the European Bone Marrow Transplant (EBMT) group showed that patients with HSTCL (*n* = 25) who underwent allo-HCT (n = 18) had long-term disease control compared to those who underwent auto-HCT (n = 7). With a median follow-up of 36 months, 50% of patients (n = 9) were alive after allo-HCT. Of the patients who died, only one patient died due to relapse. In contrast, 71% of patients (n = 5) who underwent auto-HCT died (*Leukemia*. 2015;29:686–688).

RELAPSED/REFRACTORY HSTCL—WHAT ARE THE OPTIONS?

There is no standard therapeutic option for patients with relapsed or progressive disease, although systemic chemotherapy using an alternative first-line regimen can be done. Allo-HCT is suitable for individual clinical use, provided the patient did not undergo allo-HCT after frontline therapy. However, the relapsed state is usually chemotherapy refractory, and preference is for a clinical trial, if possible. In recent years, several new therapeutic agents have become available for the treatment of PTCL in patients with advanced, relapsed, or refractory disease, some of which have efficacy data specifically in HSTCL.

1. **Alemtuzumab:** Among PTCL subtypes, HSTCL is associated with high levels of CD52 expression, the target of alemtuzumab. Positive treatment outcomes have been reported in a few single-case studies in HSCTL with alemtuzumab in combination with cladribine, fludarabine, or as salvage therapy in a treatment-refractory case of HSTCL (*Leuk Lymphoma*. 2004;45:1673–1675; *Eur J Haematol*. 2006;76:531–534; *Ann Oncol*. 2008;19:1025–1026).

2. **Pralatrexate:** Pralatrexate is an antifolate agent approved by the Food and Drug Administration (FDA) for patients with refractory PTCL. Pralatrexate has shown efficacy (n = 1) in refractory HSTCL with a durable CR such that the patient could undergo allo-HCT (*Ann Surg Oncol*. 2009;16:2014–2017).

3. **Histone deacetylase (HDAC) inhibitors:** HDAC inhibitors induce histone acetylation and have shown activity in various hematologic malignancies. Interestingly, ARID1B, a component of the SWI/SNF chromatin remodeling complex, is a commonly mutated protein in HSCTL, suggesting that epigenetic dysregulation may play an important role in HSCTL pathogenesis. Romidepsin, a potent class I HDAC inhibitor, showed ORR of 38% in a phase 2 study with relapsed/refractory (R/R) PTCL patients (there was only 1 patient with HSTCL in that study). Similarly, belinostat, a potent pan-HDAC inhibitor, has also shown ORR of 26% in R/R PTCL patients, although 0 of 2 patients with HSTCL responded (*Blood*. 2011;117:5827–5834; *J Clin Oncol*. 2015;33:2492–2499).

4. **Brentuximab vedotin:** This is an anti-CD30 antibody conjugated to a potent antimicrotubule agent, monomethyl auristatin E (MMAE). In CD30+ PTCL, ORR was 41%. Although CD30 positivity is uncommon in HSTCL, this could be a potential option in cases with CD30 positivity (*Blood*. 2014;123:3095–3100).

NEW TREATMENTS ON THE HORIZON

Several novel agents and combinations are showing promise in other mature T-cell lymphomas but have yet to be tested in HSTCL.

1. **Hypomethylating agents:** A remarkable degree of synergism has been shown with the DNA hypomethylating agent 5-azacytidine along with romidepsin in T-cell lymphoma cell lines, leading to a phase 2 study (NCT01998035) of this combination in a mixed population of newly diagnosed or R/R T-cell lymphomas (none of which was HSTCL) Preliminary results presented in abstract form at the 2019 International Conference on Malignant Lymphoma showed ORR of 68% and CR of 42%.

2. **Antibody therapies:** CD47 is a cell-surface glycoprotein that functions as an inhibitory signal for macrophage phagocytosis. Thus, antibody binding to CD47 can inactivate this signal, leading to phagocytic lymphoma cell death. Like other cancers, CD47 is heterogeneously expressed across many primary T-cell lymphomas, providing a new therapeutic target in these diseases (*Blood*. 2019;134(17):1430–1440). Magrolimab is a CD47 antibody studied in B-cell non-Hodgkin lymphoma (NHL) in combination with Rituximab, which showed ORR of 50% and CR of 36% (*N Engl J Med*. 2018;379(18):1711–1721). Given the macrophage-rich environment of the spleen and liver, this therapy may have activity in HSTCL.

   CD37 expression is found in >80% of B- and T-cell lymphomas as well as in certain cases of HSTCL. AGS67E is a fully human anti-CD37 conjugated to monomethyl auristatin A and studied as a single agent in a clinical trial of 50 patients with B- and T-cell lymphomas (NCT02175433), with ORR of 22% and CR of 14%.

3. **Cellular therapies:** Despite the inherent limitations in the use of chimeric antigen receptor T (CAR-T) therapy for T-cell lymphomas, there are cellular therapy approaches that may circumvent these limitations. CD30+–directed CAR-T cells are offering new hope for R/R CD30+ lymphomas. Two clinical trials investigating CD30-directed CAR-T cells demonstrated safety and responses in HL and ALCL (*J Clin Invest*. 2017;127(9):3462–3471; *Clin Cancer Res*. 2017;23(5):1156–1166). As discussed previously, CD30 expression on HSCTL is uncommon but if present could be a potentially curative option in refractory disease. NK-cell redirection therapy with BiKEs (bispecific killer-cell engagers) with CD30 as a target is currently in a phase 2 clinical trial (NCT02321592). Perhaps BiKEs may have a future in HSTCL, with the gamma or delta T-cell receptor serving as a target for NK bridging.

▧ REFERENCES FOR SUPPLEMENTAL READING

1. Foppoli M, Andres J, Ferreri M. Gamma-delta T-cell lymphoma. *Eur J Haematol*. 2015;94(3):206–218.

2. Ferreri AJ, Govi S, Pileri SA. Hepatosplenic gamma-delta T-cell lymphoma. *Crit Rev Oncol Hematol.* 2012;83(2):283–292.

3. Visnyei K, Grossbard M, Shapira I. Hepatosplenic γδ T-cell lymphoma: An overview. *Clin Lymphoma Myeloma Leuk.* 2013;13(4):360–369.

4. Wilson WH, Beaven AW, Savage KJ, et al. Hepatosplenic T-cell lymphoma: clinicopathological features and treatment outcomes: report from the North American peripheral T-cell lymphoma consortium. *Blood.* 2013;122(21):3032.

5. Vose J, Armitage J, Weisenburger D. International T-cell lymphoma project. International peripheral T-cell and natural killer/T-cell lymphoma study: pathology findings and clinical outcomes. *J Clin Oncol.* 2008;26(25):4124–4130.

51 Langerhans Cell Histiocytosis, Erdheim-Chester Disease, Rosai-Dorfman Disease, and Histiocytic Sarcoma

Sameem Abedin and Ehab Atallah

■ INTRODUCTION

The histiocytic/dendritic cell neoplasms are a group of diseases characterized by an abnormal accumulation of cells derived from macrophages or dendritic cells within various tissues of the body. These disorders occur in both children and adults, and more than 100 different subtypes have been described. Langerhans cell histiocytosis (LCH) and Erdheim-Chester disease (ECD) are the most common disorders and are characterized by clonal mutations involving the mitogen-activated protein kinase (MAPK) pathway. LCH occurs in various organs but most commonly affects the bones (80%), skin (25%), and lymphatic system or lungs (15% each). In adults, lung involvement is more common than in children due to increased history of smoking. The annual incidence ranges from 5 to 9 in 1 million in children under the age of 15, to 1 in 1 million in children and adults over 15 years of age. ECD, on the other hand, is more commonly seen in middle-aged adults (mean age: 55–60 years). ECD involves the bone in >95% of cases and commonly also involves the heart (50%) and central nervous system (CNS; 25%). Clinically, both disorders may lead to the development of diabetes insipidus (DI), in up to 30% of cases. Rarer histiocyte disorders include Rosai-Dorfman disease (RDD) and histiocytic sarcoma (HS), a non-Langerhans histiocyte disorder of unclear etiology. Unlike LCH, HS less commonly is associated with the BRAF V600E mutation. Further, HS has been described in association with hematologic neoplasms, including follicular lymphoma (FL), acute lymphoblastic leukemia (ALL), and acute myeloid leukemia (AML).

On recognition of these disorders, evaluation of disease location and burden and molecular characterization are of critical importance to guide both prognostication and treatment.

■ DIAGNOSIS

Due to the rarity and heterogeneity in presentation of histiocytic/dendritic cell neoplasms, diagnosis is often a challenge. Diagnosis requires both biopsy of involved tissue and assessment of clinical and radiographic features. Clinical context is required to separate possible pathologic lesions from reactive tissue due to other causes, including infection, and other malignancies.

MORPHOLOGY

LCH is characterized by histiocytes with coffee bean– or kidney-shaped nuclei. While LCH can be recognized based on morphologic appearance, its identity must be confirmed either by positive immunohistochemistry staining for CD1a and CD207 or by the presence of Birbeck granules under electron microscopy. ECD is characterized by infiltration of tissues by foamy mononucleated histiocytes with small nuclei. Touton cells or multinucleated histiocytes may be observed, and fibrosis is present in most cases (see Figure 51.1). In ECD, features of both LCH and ECD may be present. Another histiocyte disorder, RDD, should be distinguished from LCH. Morphologically, RDD is characterized by multinucleated S100+ histiocytes, with evidence of emperipolesis, or engulfment of erythrocytes, plasma cells, or lymphocytes by histiocytes (see Figure 51.2). Finally, histiocytic sarcoma morphologically presents as a diffusely infiltrative process, with large, irregular cells expressing histiocytic markers, but without B-cell or T-cell–related markers, LCH markers, follicular dendritic cell markers, epithelial markers, or myeloid-cell markers.

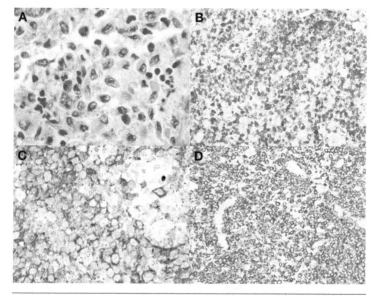

Figure 51.1 LCH: A. Microscopic examination reveals a big collection of Langerhans cells admixed with background mature eosinophils. Eosinophilic micro-abscesses can often be identified but not shown here. The present Langerhans cells are characterized with large cell size, irregular nuclei, nuclear cloves, inconspicuous nucleoli, and pale amphophilic cytoplasm (H&E, 600×). B. Immunostain with anti-S100 (B), CD1a (C), and Langerin/CD207 (D) antibodies highlight these LCH cells (immunoperoxidase, 200×, 600×, and 200×, respectively), supporting the diagnosis of LCH.

H&E, hematoxylin and eosin; LCH, Langerhans cell histiocytosis.

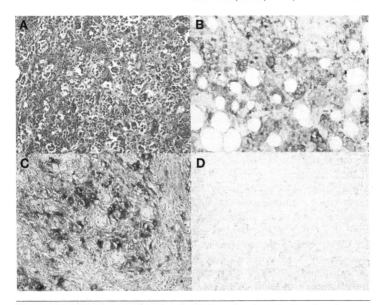

Figure 51.2 RDD: hematoxylin and eosin (H&E) section through a lymph node shows complete effacement of normal nodal architecture and replacement by sheets of epithelial histiocytes with an eosinophilic or clear cytoplasm engulfing numerous small mature lymphocytes, neutrophils, and occasional eosinophils, namely emperipolesis. Mature plasma cells are noted in the background (H&E, 200×). B. Immunostain with CD163 highlights large histiocytes that contain CD163-negative cells, including small lymphocytes and neutrophils (immunoperoxidase, 200×). C and D. The large histiocytes are also positive for S100 (C) but negative for CD1a (D), distinguishing it from LCH (immunoperoxidase, 200×).

H&E, hematoxylin and eosin; LCH, Langerhans cell histiocytosis; RDD, Rosai-Dorfman disease.

IMMUNOPHENOTYPE
Typical immunophenotype by indeterminate cell histiocytosis (ICH):
- LCH: CD1a (+), CD207(+)
- ECD: CD68 (+), CD163 (+), +/− S100 (+), CD1a (−)
- RDD: S100 (+), CD1a (−), CD207(−)
- HS: (+) for one or more (CD163, CD68, or lysozyme), absent of CD1a, CD21, CD23, CD35, pan-cytokeratin, EMA, HMB-45, Melan A, tyrosinase, MiTF, CD13, CD33, MPO

SOMATIC MUTATIONS
In both LCH and ECD, recurrent *BRAF*V600E mutations are observed in 50% of cases. Other mutations involving the MAPK pathway have been observed, including mutations involving *N/KRAS*, *MAP2K1*, and *ARAF*. Overall, more than 80% of LCH patients and up to 100% of

ECD cases have been reported to have mutations involving the MAPK pathway, and these are useful studies to confirm difficult LCH or ECD diagnoses. *NRAS*, *KRAS*, *MAP2K1*, and *ARAF* mutations have been identified in some forms of RDD. While less common, *BRAF* V600E and *MAP2K1* mutations have been reported in HS.

ADDITIONAL WORKUP

Once the diagnosis of LCH or ECD has been determined, baseline laboratory and radiographic studies are required to help determine an appropriate therapeutic approach. Required laboratory studies include a complete blood count (CBC) with differential; complete metabolic panel (CMP); coagulation studies, including prothrombin time (PT)/partial thromboplastin time (PTT)/international normalized ratio (INR); and an erythrocyte sedimentation rate (ESR). Assessment is important, as LCH patients with anemia and thrombocytopenia in addition to those with hypoalbuminemia can have a worse outcome. Endocrinopathies should be assessed if suspected. Finally, if polydipsia or polyuria is reported, early morning urine-specific gravity and osmolality should be obtained, and a water-deprivation test should be performed, if possible. DI is the most frequent endocrinopathy in LCH. Due to improved sensitivity and ability to monitor treatment response, positron emission tomography/computed tomography (PET/CT) scan has supplanted the chest radiograph and skeletal radiograph survey in the initial evaluation for both LCH and ECD. In the case of suspected lung involvement, high-resolution computed tomography (CT) scan of the lung should be considered to assess for typical cysts and nodular findings of LCH. In ECD, if cardiac involvement is suspected, a cardiac magnetic resonance imaging (MRI) scan should be obtained. If CNS involvement or craniofacial bone lesions are suspected, an MRI of the head should be pursued. If vertebral lesions are suspected, an MRI of the spine should also be obtained to assess for soft-tissue lesions and to exclude cord compression.

▨ KEY DIAGNOSTIC DILEMMA

LCH shares presentation and pathologic features with other histiocyte disorders, including ICH, RDD, and ECD. Immunohistochemistry can help differentiate between these disorders. Furthermore, LCH has been associated with various blood cancers, including RDD, ECD, Hodgkin disease, and acute leukemia.

▨ PROGNOSIS

The prognosis of both LCH and ECD depends on the site and extent of disease. In LCH, patients with unifocal disease generally have an excellent prognosis. Previously, in multifocal LCH, 60% of patients have had a chronic course, 30% of patients achieved complete remission (CR), and 10% of patients died from the disease (*J Pediatr*. 1975;87(2):184–189). Through improved understanding of these disorders, recent reported 5-year survival rates are estimated at more than 80%. One of the most important prognostic indicators for multifocal LCH is disease location.

Patients who risk organ involvement, which includes CNS involvement or pulmonary involvement, have worse long-term outcomes. In ECD, older age and involvement of the CNS or lungs are associated with the worst outcomes. There is also an increased incidence of overlapping myeloid neoplasm in patients with ECD (10%).

▧ TREATMENT

A. Langerhans Cell Histiocytosis: Treatment recommendations are based on site and extension of disease. Unlike pediatric LCH, there is no standard first-line therapy in adults. Clinical trials should be considered, if available.

SUGGESTED FIRST-LINE APPROACH

1. Single-System LCH (SS-LCH):
   - Local therapy (resection or irradiation), prednisone, or vinblastine + prednisone
2. Primary Pulmonary LCH:
   - Smoking cessation and steroids in symptomatic patients
   - Chemotherapy (Cladribine) for progressive disease
3. SS-LCH with multifocal lesions, SS-LCH with "special-site" lesions, multisystem LCH (MS-LCH):
   - Cladribine: 5 mg/m^2 for days 1 to 5, q28 days (*Blood.* 2019; 134(Suppl1):4189)
   - Cytarabine: 100 mg/m^2 for days 1 to 5, q28 days (*PLoS One.* 2012;7(8):e43257)
   - Vinblastine + prednisone: Pediatric standard, not commonly used in adult management

RECURRENT DISEASE

1. Chemotherapy:
   - Limited skin/bone/lymph node: Hydroxyurea (*Blood.* 2016;128(20): 2462–2465)
   - Multisystem and CNS risk: Cladribine/Cytarabine (*Blood.* 2015;126(12):1415–1423) or Clofarabine (*Pediatr Blood Cancer.* 2014;61(3):479–487)
2. Targeted agents:
   - BRAF inhibitor: Vemurafenib (*JAMA Oncol.* 2018;4(3):384)

B. Erdheim Chester Disease: ECD represents as an indolent disorder, and watchful waiting is appropriate for most patients. Treatment is reserved for impending end-organ dysfunction, CNS involvement, or symptomatic disease. Patients should be evaluated every 3 to 6 months or more frequently, as organ dysfunction and symptoms require.

POTENTIAL THERAPIES

1. Targeted agents:
   - BRAF inhibitor: Vemurafenib (*JAMA Oncol.* 2018;4(3):384)
   - MEK inhibitor: Trametinib or cobimetinib (*Cancer Discov.* 2016;6(2):154–165; *BJH.* 2018;180:147–166)
2. Chemotherapy:
   - Cladribine (*JAMA Oncol.* 2017;3(9):1253–1256)
   - Interferon alfa (*Blood.* 2011;117(10):2778)

C. Rosai-Dorfman Disease: RDD management is largely driven by patient presentation and circumstance. Uncomplicated cases or unifocal disease that has been resected can be observed. The following are commonly considered options for symptomatic disease (*Blood.* 2018;131(26):2877–2890):

- Corticosteroids: 1 mg/kg followed by taper
- Radiotherapy: 30 to 50 Gy
- Cladribine 5 mg/m^2 D1 to D5, q28d

D. Histiocytic Sarcoma:

1. Unifocal disease: Surgical resection or radiotherapy: 30 to 50 Gy
   - Multisystem disease: Ifosfamide, carboplatin, etoposide (ICE); cyclophosphamide, doxorubicin, vincristine, and prednisone (CHOP)

▓ POTENTIAL PRACTICE-CHANGING CLINICAL TRIALS

The molecular characterization of LCH and ECD has led to clinical trials underway studying the effect of novel targeted agents. Current trials include the addition of Vemurafenib (BRAF inhibitor) to chemotherapy (NCT03585686). Further study of cobimetinib for both refractory LCH and ECD (NCT04079179) and the combination of dabrafenib with trametinib for ECD (NCT03794297) are underway. In the future, targeted agents may overtake traditional chemotherapy as initial therapy for Langerhans disorders. Non-targeted trials with novel agents continue and are important, particularly in the case of HS. Lenalidomide is another novel agent currently under investigation for LCH, ECD, and HS (NCT02523040). Finally, in HS, immunotherapy with pembrolizumab is under current investigation (NCT03316573).

▓ REFERENCES FOR SUPPLEMENTAL READING

1. Girschikofsky M, Arico M, Castillo D, et al. Management of adult patients with Langerhans cell histiocytosis: recommendations from an expert panel on behalf of Euro-Histio-Net. *Orphanet J Rare Dis.* 2013;8:72.
2. Diamond EL, Durham BH, Haroche J, et al. Diverse and targetable kinase alterations drive histiocytic neoplasms. *Cancer Discov.* 2016;6(2):154–165.

3. Emile J-F, Abla O, Fraitag S, et al. Revised classification of histiocytoses and neoplasms of the macrophage-dendritic cell lineages. *Blood*. 2016;127:2672–2681.

4. Goyal G, Young JR, Koster MJ, et al. The Mayo Clinic histiocytosis working group consensus statement for the diagnosis and evaluation of adult patients with histiocytic neoplasms: Erdheim-Chester disease, Langerhans cell histiocytosis, and Rosai-Dorfman disease. *Mayo Clin Proc*. 2019;94:2054–2071.

52 Hemophagocytic Lymphohistiocytosis

Hilda Ding and Lubomir Sokol

▓ INTRODUCTION

Hemophagocytic lymphohistiocytosis (HLH) is a life-threatening hyperinflammatory syndrome characterized by systemic immune activation and subsequent pathologic inflammation. It is an entity first defined in pediatrics that has been increasingly recognized in adults. About 40% of HLH cases are estimated to occur in adults, with an incidence as high as 1 in 2,000 adult admissions at tertiary medical centers. Median age of diagnosis is the fifth to sixth decades of life.

HLH can be familial or acquired, both culminating in a common pathologic inflammatory pathway. Familial HLH mostly occurs in the pediatric population, though it can be seen in young adults. These patients often have a family history and/or a genetic defect leading to cytotoxic T-cell and natural killer–cell (NK-cell) dysfunction. Familial HLH associated with gene defects (e.g., *PRF1, UNC13D, STX11*, and *STXBP2*) is often triggered by infections. Associated syndromes in familial HLH include type 2 Griscelli syndrome, Chédiak-Higashi syndrome, and X-linked lymphoproliferative syndromes. Adults often have acquired HLH, where malignancy, autoimmunity, and infection are common triggers. Lymphoma is the most commonly associated malignancy, including such entities as anaplastic large cell lymphoma, subcutaneous panniculitis-like T-cell lymphoma, and NK-cell lymphoma. Epstein–Barr virus (EBV), human immunodeficiency virus (HIV), and cytomegalovirus (CMV) are common viral triggers of acquired HLH. Moreover, *Mycobacterium tuberculosis* and *Rickettsia* spp. are reported as the most common bacterial etiologies of HLH. *Leishmaniasis* and *Histoplasmosis* are frequently implicated parasitic and fungal infections associated with HLH. It is important to note that HLH can also occur after hematopoietic stem cell transplant (HSCT), as these patients are in a state of immune reconstitution, whereby risks of infection and graft-versus-host disease (GVHD) can culminate in excessive immune activation. Common presentations of HSCT-associated HLH include fever, cytopenias, and hepatosplenomegaly. In adults, pulmonary involvement is also common. Elevated triglyceride levels, low fibrinogen, elevated ferritin, phagocytosis by activated macrophages, and elevated soluble interleukin receptor alpha (sIL-2R) are common laboratory features (see below). Outcomes are variable and based on the precipitating condition. However, untreated HLH is uniformly fatal.

■ DIAGNOSIS

Diagnostic criteria have been established by consensus at the Histiocyte Society, which was used initially for patient enrollment into clinical trials (see the following section). Diagnostic investigation assesses molecular markers of inflammation, functional lymphocyte cytotoxicity, and genetic testing when warranted. Laboratory evaluation includes complete blood count (CBC) with differential, lipid panel, fibrinogen levels, liver-function testing, serum albumin, lactate dehydrogenase (LDH), ferritin levels, bone marrow (BM) biopsy and aspirate, tissue biopsy, and molecular testing. It is important to note that hemophagocytosis alone is not pathognomonic or sufficient for the diagnosis of HLH. Other common manifestations, though not part of the diagnostic criteria, include edema, rash, transaminitis, hypoalbuminemia, hyperbilirubinemia, elevated LDH, hyponatremia, and other lipid abnormalities. Central nervous system (CNS) involvement can be present; thus, a magnetic resonance imaging (MRI) brain scan and lumbar puncture should be considered in patients with neurological symptoms. Recent studies have devised a score predictive of HLH risks in adults that uses clinical, biologic, and cytologic variables (HScore, Table 52.1). It was developed from a retrospective cohort of adult HLH patients, where a score of ≤90 correlates with low probability (<1%), and ≥250 correlates with a high probability (>99%) of HLH.

Table 52.1 HScore (also available at http://saintantoine.aphp.fr/score/)

Parameter	Number of Points (Criteria for Scoring)
Known underlying immunosuppression	0 (no) or 18 (yes)
Temperature (°C)	0 (<38.4), 33 (38.4–39.4), or 49 (>39.4)
Organomegaly	0 (no), 23 (hepatomegaly or splenomegaly), or 38 (hepatomegaly and splenomegaly)
Number of cytopenias	0 (1 lineage), 24 (2 lineages), or 34 (3 lineages)
Ferritin (ng/dL)	0 (<2,000), 25 (2,000–6,000), or 50 (>6,000)
Triglycerides (mmol/L)	0 (<1.5), 44 (1.5–4), or 64 (>4)
Fibrinogen (g/dL)	0 (>2.5) or 30 (≤2.5)
Serum glutamic oxaloacetic transaminase (IU/L)	0 (<30) or 19 (≥30)
Hemophagocytosis on aspirate	0 (no) or 35 (yes)

DIAGNOSTIC CRITERIA USED IN THE HLH-2004 TRIAL (*PEDIATR BLOOD CANCER.* 2007;48:124–131)

A. A molecular diagnosis consistent with HLH

OR

B. Five of the eight following findings:

1. Fever

2. Splenomegaly

3. Cytopenias affecting at least two of three hematopoietic lineages:

   a. Hemoglobin <9 g/dL

   b. Platelets <100 k/mcL

   c. Neutrophils <1 × 10^3/mL

4. Hypertriglyceridemia (fasting, >265 mg/dL) and/or hypofibrino-genemia (<150 mg/dL)

5. Hemophagocytosis in BM, spleen, liver, or lymph nodes

6. Low or absent NK-cell activity

7. Ferritin >500 ng/mL

8. Elevated soluble CD25 (soluble IL-2 receptor alpha)

▓ KEY DIAGNOSTIC DILEMMA

Diagnosing HLH depends on clinical, laboratory, and histopatholog-ical findings. Although hemophagocytosis is a prominent feature of HLH, it can also be seen in other disorders. Therefore, it is not pathog-nomonic for HLH and can actually be absent in BM biopsy evaluation of HLH patients. Though the negative predictive value of a normal ferritin level remains reliable, an elevated ferritin level (>50,000 mcg/L) is not found to be as specific or sensitive for adults (*Blood.* 2015;125(10):1548–1552). This is due to other pathologic processes that also contribute to an elevated ferritin level, such as liver failure, renal failure, hematologic malignancy, infections, or rheumatologic conditions (Figures 52.1 and 52.2). In some cases, lymphoma can be difficult to diagnose and detect in the setting of HLH; therefore, repet-itive tissue sampling, imaging, and consultations with pathologists experienced in lymphoma may be needed.

▓ PROGNOSIS

Outcomes are variable and based on underlying conditions but are worse in adults, especially those with malignancy, with a reported mortality rate as high as 66% (*Mayo Clin Proc.* 2014;89(4):484–492). Other reported poor prognostic factors are increasing age, male sex, thrombocytopenia (<40 k/mcL), presentation with spleno-megaly, active EBV infection, disseminated intravascular coag-ulopathy (DIC), fever not subsiding within 3 days of diagnosis, ferritin >50,000 ng/mL, hypoalbuminemia, organ failure, and

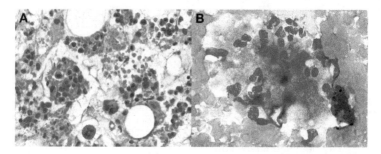

Figure 52.1 Bone marrow (BM) core biopsy demonstrates numerous enlarged histiocytes with hemophagocytosis (engulfment of nRBCs, lymphocytes, myeloid precursors, and platelets into the cytoplasm), which results in reduced normal hematopoiesis (A, hematoxylin and eosin [H&E], ×600). BM aspirate with a giant histiocyte with hematopoietic elements (B, Wright-Giemsa, ×1,000).

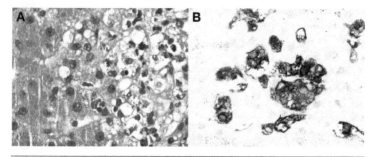

Figure 52.2 Liver biopsy from the same patient demonstrates an aggregate of histiocytes with the same phenomenon (A, hematoxylin and eosin [H&E], ×600 total magnification), highlighted by the histiocytic marker CD68 (B, immunoperoxidase, ×600).

lack of etoposide during management. Survival is <10% without immunochemotherapy.

▧ TREATMENT

HSCT is recommended for patients with familial HLH as the only definitive treatment where remission prior to transplant is associated with better outcomes. Goals of treatment for familial and acquired HLH are aimed at controlling hyperinflammation and treating underlying triggers. Treatment protocols for acquired HLH and control of familial HLH prior to transplant include HLH-94 and HLH-2004 (Figures 52.3 and 52.4). Treatment recommendations are derived from pediatric data and based on expert opinions to target hyperinflammation and the underlying condition, which includes immunochemotherapy and/ or HSCT. These therapeutic strategies target cytotoxic T-lymphocytes, NK-cells, and macrophages, resulting in the suppression of cytokines.

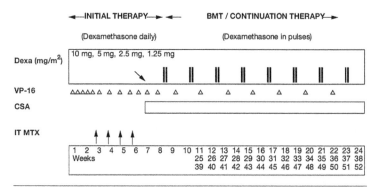

Figure 52.3 Treatment schema per HLH-1994. Dexa: daily dexamethasone (10 g/m²
for 2 weeks followed by 5 mg/m² for 2 weeks, 2.5 mg/m² for 2 weeks, 1.25 mg/m²
for 1 week, and 1 week of taper; pulses given as 10 mg/m² daily for 3 days). VP-16:
Etoposide 150-mg/m² IV.

BMT, bone marrow transplant; CNS, central nervous system; CSA, Cyclosporin A aiming for trough levels in the blood of 200 mcg/L; Dexa, dexamethasone; HLH, hemophagocytic lymphohistiocytosis; IT, intrathecal; IT therapy,
intrathecal methotrexate for patients with CNS disease.

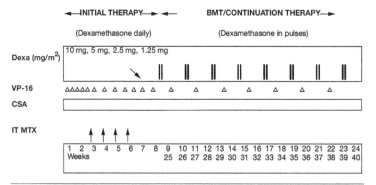

Figure 52.4 Treatment schema per HLH-2004. Regimen is the same as HLH-1994,
except CSA from initiation of therapy and hydrocortisone are given in addition
to methotrexate IT with CNS disease.

BMT, bone marrow transplant; CNS, central nervous system; CSA, cyclosporin A; Dexa, dexamethasone; IT, intrathecal; VP-16, etoposide.

Agents used include corticosteroids, such as dexamethasone/methyl-
prednisolone, etoposide, intrathecal methotrexate, cyclosporine, and
intravenous immunoglobulins (IVIG). The main difference between
the two protocols is that cyclosporine is initiated at Week 9 in HLH-
94, as compared to the onset of treatment in HLH-2004. As a result,
due to nephrotoxicity, cyclosporine is not recommended in the initial weeks of presentation. Therefore, HLH-94 is often better tolerated
in adults and should be used as initial therapy. However, in adults,

there is no standard of care, and a single agent is often chosen from the preceding as treatment based on the patient's clinical course. In adults, only expert opinions and retrospective observational studies are available. Etoposide has been shown to target activated T-cells and macrophages and suppress inflammatory cytokines. Intrathecal methotrexate is recommended for CNS involvement but rarely used in adults. Such agents as corticosteroids and cyclosporine have immunosuppressive activity, whereas IVIG is used to address immune deficiency and as an anti-inflammatory agent. Other immunotherapeutic agents, such as rituximab, anakinra (interleukin-1 [IL-1] receptor inhibitor), and tocilizumab (interleukin-6 receptor [IL-6] inhibitor), have also been used. The German Adult HLH Registry is a valuable resource for consultation (www.hlh-registry.org). Overall treatment requires extensive supportive care and individualized treatment strategies due to variable manifestations and underlying triggers, especially as most data stem from pediatric trials, and few studies exist for adult patients with HLH.

▦ RELAPSE/REFRACTORY DISEASE

While HSCT is the definitive treatment for patients with familial HLH, this is also the treatment of choice for patients with relapse or refractory acquired HLH. However, HSCT may not always be feasible for every patient. Emapalumab is a monoclonal immunoglobulin G1 antibody directed against interferon gamma that was approved by the Food and Drug Administration (FDA) in 2018 for adult and pediatric patients with primary HLH with refractory, recurrent, or progressive disease or intolerance with conventional HLH therapy based on a multicenter, open-label, single-arm trial. It has been shown to reverse previously refractory HLH and did not seem to impair the control of infections in these patients.

▦ POTENTIAL PRACTICE-CHANGING CLINICAL TRIALS

Current clinical trials targeting inflammation while minimizing treatment's effect on cytopenias are ongoing by assessing the addition of tocilizumab (IL-6 inhibitor) and alemtuzumab (anti-CD52 monoclonal antibody) to the standard induction regimen with etoposide/dexamethasone (NCT02385110). Ruxolitinib, an oral JAK1 and JAK2 inhibitor, has been shown to be active and well tolerated in a series of patients with HLH in an ongoing phase 2 clinical trial (NCT02400463). Programmed cell death-1 (PD-1) blockade utilizing Nivolumab has also shown promise in the treatment of HLH, specifically those associated with EBV. In a series of patients with EBV-HLH, a number of patients achieved complete response. Additionally, there is currently a phase 3 clinical trial investigating the use of PD-1 antibody and lenalidomide for EBV-HLH (NCT04084626).

▧ REFERENCES FOR SUPPLEMENTAL READING

1. Fardet L, Galicier L, Lambotte O, et al. Development and validation of the HScore, a score for the diagnosis of reactive hemophagocytic syndrome. *Arthritis Rheumatol.* 2014;66(9):2613–2620.

2. La Rosee P, Horne A, Hines M, et al. Recommendations for the management of hemophagocytic lymphohistiocytosis in adults. *Blood.* 2019; 133(23):2465–2477.

3. Nikiforow S, Berliner N. The unique aspects of presentation and diagnosis of hemophagocytic lymphohistiocytosis in adults. *ASH Hematology.* 2015; (1):183–189.

4. Schram AM, Berliner N. How I treat hemophagocytic lymphohistiocytosis in the adult patient. *Blood.* 2015;125(19):2908–2914.

5. Vallurupalli M, Berliner N. Emapalumab for the treatment of relapsed/refractory hemophagocytic lymphohistiocytosis. *Blood.* 2019;134(21):1783–1786.

53 Autologous Hematopoietic Cell Transplantation

Hemant S. Murthy and Mohamed A. Kharfan-Dabaja

▓ INTRODUCTION

Autologous hematopoietic cell transplantation (auto-HCT) entails using progenitor hematopoietic cells (also known as a hematopoietic cell graft) from the patient, after administering high-dose chemotherapy or chemoradiotherapy, to restore hematopoietic cell recovery from the resulting myelotoxicity. The procedure is comprises the conditioning regimen, prescribed for its high tumoricidal effect; the infusion of collected stem cells from the patient to restore hematopoiesis after myelosuppression exerted by the conditioning regimen; and supportive measures, such as transfusion support and infection prophylaxis, to prevent potential complications. Given the advances in supportive measures, nowadays the anticipated treatment-related mortality (TRM) from an autologous transplant is relatively low, ranging from 2% to 5%. Many transplant centers even perform auto-HCT on an outpatient basis, which begins with identification of patients suitable for transplantation by disease indication (Table 53.1) and by assessment for the patients' associated comorbidities. This is followed by stem cell mobilization and collection, after which comes the administration of conditioning regimen preceding autologous stem cell infusion. Following infusion of collected progenitor hematopoietic cells, supportive measures are instituted to manage resulting cytopenias, prevent occurrence of infections, and manage complications and toxicities until engraftment ensues. Following engraftment, patients are generally discharged home once they are able to meet their caloric demand and recover their performance status to at least be able to perform activities of daily living.

▓ PRE-TRANSPLANT WORKUP

High-dose therapy (HDT) and auto-HCT can be associated with short- and long-term toxicities. With improvement in supportive care, these toxicities are better tolerated and relatively well managed, allowing even older patients, some older than 70 years of age, to be considered for the procedure. Patients who are candidates for auto-HCT must demonstrate not only evidence of chemosensitive disease pre-transplantation but adequate organ function and performance status prior to the procedure.

Table 53.1 Indication for Auto-HCT and Disease State Based on 2020 Guidelines from American Society for Transplantation and Cellular Therapy (ASTCT)

Plasma Cell Disorders	
Multiple myeloma	Initial response (CR, VGPR, or PR), relapsed/refractory disease, relapse following prior autologous stem cell transplant
Tandem transplantation	Not recommended outside clinical trial setting;
	Prospective randomized phase 3 study BMT CTN 0702 (Stadmauer et al. *J Clin Oncol.* 2019;37(7):589–597) showed no improvement in PFS or OS with tandem auto-HCT compared to single auto-HCT. Retrospective analysis by EBMT showed benefit of tandem auto-HCT compared to single auto-HCT only in MM with high-risk cytogenetics and extramedullary disease (Gagelmann et al. *Biol Blood Marrow Transplant.* 2019;25(11):2134–2142). Auto-allo HCT failed to show benefit in two separate meta-analyses (Kharfan-Dabaja MA, et al. *J Hematol Oncol.* 2013;6:2; Armeson et al. *Bone Marrow Transplant.* 2013;48(4):562–567) with higher TRM.
Plasma cell leukemia	Initial response (CR, VGPR, or PR), relapsed/refractory disease
Primary amyloidosis	Initial response (CR, VGPR, or PR), relapsed/refractory disease. See Chapter 31.
Lymphoma	
Hodgkin lymphoma	Chemosensitive relapsed/refractory disease
Diffuse large B-cell lymphoma	Chemosensitive relapsed disease
Mantle-cell lymphoma	First objective response (complete, partial)
Peripheral T-cell lymphoma	First remission, chemosensitive relapse/refractory disease
Burkitts lymphoma	First remission
Other	
Acute promyelocytic leukemia	CR2 in molecular remission (refer to Chapter 19)
Germ-cell tumor	Relapse/refractory disease

(*continued*)

Table 53.1 Indication for Auto-HCT and Disease State Based on 2020 Guidelines from American Society for Transplantation and Cellular Therapy (ASTCT) (continued)

Plasma Cell Disorders	
Severe systemic scleroderma	Adults (18–69 years of age) with scleroderma for 5 years or fewer with pulmonary or renal involvement. Randomized phase 3 data (KM Sullivan et al. *N Engl J Med.* 2018;378: 35–47) and systematic review (Host L, et al. *Clin Exper Rheum.* 2017;35(106):198–207) showed auto-HCT recipients had significantly higher likelihood of improving skin sclerosis and disease activity and preserving lung function. ASTCT recommends auto-HCT as standard of care for patients with severe systemic sclerosis (Sullivan KM, et al. *Biol Blood Marrow Transplant.* 2018;24(10):1961–1964).

auto-HCT: autologous hematopoietic cell transplantation; ASBMT, American Society for Blood and Marrow Transplantation; CR, complete response; EBMT, European Society for Blood and Marrow Transplantation; EFS, event free survival; MM, multiple myeloma; OS, overall survival; PFS, progression-free survival; PR, partial response; RR, response ratio; TRM, treatment-related mortality; VGPR, very good partial remission.

ASSESSMENT OF COMORBIDITIES

Outcomes of auto-HCT might be predicted based on the overall health of a patient prior to undergoing the procedure. As HDT can affect various organ functions throughout the entire process, it is important to assess the pre-transplantation health status of the patient when considering them for the procedure. Various pre-transplant comorbidity scoring models exist for assessing pre-transplant risk and potential impact on outcomes, with examples including the Charlson Comorbidity Index and the Cumulative Illness Rating Scale. The Hematopoietic Cell Transplantation Comorbidity Index (HCT-CI) developed by Sorror et al. in 2005 remains a widely accepted pre-transplant comorbidity prognostication tool. It comprises 17 specific comorbidity assessments (Sorror et al. *Blood.* 2005;106(8):2912–2919). Studies conducted by the Center for International Blood and Marrow Transplant Research (CIBMTR) have validated HCT-CI in auto-HCT (Saad et al. *Biol Blood Marrow Transplant.* 2014;20(3):402–408; Sorror et al. *Biol Blood Marrow Transplant.* 2015;21(8):1479–1487), although it is not a perfect model, and future research is focused on better defining disease-specific risk of transplantation.

VITAL ORGAN TESTING

Below are the more standard tests that are required for patients prior to undergoing auto-HCT:

1. Assessment of performance status: Eastern Cooperative Oncology Group (ECOG), Karnofsky score

2. Cardiac: Electrocardiogram (EKG), echocardiogram, or multigated acquisition (MUGA) scan

3. Pulmonary: Chest X-ray, arterial blood gases, and pulmonary function testing

4. Renal: serum creatinine, creatinine clearance

5. Hepatic: serum liver-function tests (bilirubin, aspartate transaminase, alanine aminotransferase)

6. Infection: hepatitis B/C, human immunodeficiency virus (HIV) I and II Ab,* Human T-lymphotropic virus (HTLV) 1-2, cytomegalovirus (CMV), Epstein–Barr virus (EBV), herpes simplex virus I/II, Varicella zoster virus. *HIV-positive patients should receive CD4 count and viral load (VL) via reverse transcription polymerase chain reaction (RT-PCR); CD4 <100 per mm^3, VL <10,000 copies per mL tolerate auto-HCT well (*Bone Marrow Transplant.* 2010;45(8):1259–1268).

7. Psychosocial evaluation

8. Caregiver support (typically for first 4–6 weeks post-auto-HCT)

Post-transplant outcomes could also be influenced by intensity of the conditioning regimen and peri-transplant anti-infectious prophylaxis. Each case must be evaluated on an individual basis and in conjunction with all pre-transplantation information.

RESTAGING EXAMS (DISEASE SPECIFIC)

Typically, restaging exams are necessary prior to proceeding to transplantation to document that there has been evidence of an objective response to ensure the auto-HCT will have a beneficial effect. Imaging, such as computed tomography (CT) or positron emission tomography (PET) scans, is performed prior to proceeding to transplantation for lymphomas. A bone marrow (BM) biopsy prior to proceeding to transplant is typically warranted, usually within 30 days of admission for auto-HCT. Lumbar punctures are not typical components of restaging exams except in cases of prior meningeal involvement or in clinical conditions that predispose to high risk of central nervous system (CNS) relapse. Additional tests for multiple myeloma (MM) are used, including serum/urine protein electrophoresis and serum-free κ/λ ratio.

■ STEM CELL PROCESSING

Hematopoietic progenitor cells (HPC) are immature cells that are capable of multilineage blood-cell formation and differentiation when transplanted back into the host, as is the case with auto-HCT. These cells, when infused intravenously, migrate to the marrow and, through interactions with extracellular matrix, stem cell niche, and extracellular signals, adhere, expand, and differentiate, providing hematologic and immune reconstitution. CD34+ is frequently used as a marker of HPC, allowing for the identification and quantification of HPC via flow cytometry.

MOBILIZATION AND COLLECTION

HPC collected from peripheral blood via apheresis (HPC-A) is preferred for stem cell collection and mobilization. For single autologous transplant, a minimum of 2×10^6 CD34+/kg body weight is generally required for safe autologous engrafting. Granulocyte colony-stimulating factor (G-CSF) mobilization is the standard regimen, able to mobilize sufficient CD34+ cells with relatively well-tolerated toxicities. While there are varieties between institutions pertaining to mobilization regimens, one commonly accepted regimen is G-CSF doses of 5 to 10 mcg/kg subcutaneously, administered daily for minimum of 4 days and collection providing that target CD34+ is met, followed by collection via apheresis. Our target is 2 to 5 million CD34+ cells/kg for patients in complete response (CR) or very good partial remission (VGPR) and 4 to 10 million CD34+ cells/kg for partial response (PR) or less. Failure to achieve a target CD34+ has been reported, ranging from 10% to 20% in myeloma and lymphoma patients. Risk factors identified for poor mobilization include older age (age ≥65); heavily pretreated patients; prior pelvic radiation; certain regimens, such as Hyper-CVAD or prolonged lenalidomide exposure (≥4 cycles of lenalidomide-containing regimen); and/or a wash-out period of <3 weeks from the most recent dose of lenalidomine or hypocellular marrow. For poor mobilizers, or those at high risk for poor mobilization, plerixafor, a bicyclam inhibitor that blocks CXCR4 and facilitates release of HPC from marrow to bloodstream, has been shown to be effective. Its widespread use is limited by its cost, and thus it is mostly used within a risk-adapted model for cost-effectiveness. Another option is chemomobilization, which utilizes the white blood cell (WBC) nadir and subsequent count recovery, augmented with G-CSF administration, to maximize HPC mobilization. In myeloma, single-agent cyclophosphamide (2–5 g/m^2) or etoposide (375 mg/m^2) has been used, yielding successful outcomes in poor mobilizers. In lymphoma, chemomobilization is generally planned following the second or third cycle of a salvage regimen, with G-CSF administered during count recovery, allowing for successful stem cell collection with minimal delays and easy coordination with salvage therapy. The drawbacks of chemomobilization include expected toxicities associated with chemotherapies as well as lack of predictability when planning apheresis for collection.

▓ CONDITIONING REGIMENS (TABLE 53.2)

Table 53.2 Common Autologous Transplant Conditioning Regimens

Regimen	Disease	Dosage and Timing
Melphalan	Multiple myeloma	200 mg/m² administered either day −2, or day −1
		140 mg/m² can be used for patients with renal insufficiency or numerous comorbidities.
Busulfan-Melphalan	Myeloma	Busulfan PK targeted AUC 5,000 mmol-min daily day −7 to −4; Melphalan 70 mg/m² day −2 to −1
BEAC	Lymphoma	BCNU 300 mg/m² day −6
		Etoposide 800 mg/m² daily day −6 to −3
		Cytarabine 800 mg/m² daily day −6 to −3
		Cyclophosphamide 35 mg/kg daily day −6 to −3
BEAM	Lymphoma	BCNU 300 mg/m² day −7
		Etoposide 200 mg/m² daily day −5 to −2
		Cytarabine 400 mg/m² daily day −5 to −2
		Melphalan 140 mg/m² day −1
Cy-VP-16-TBI	Lymphoma	TBI 1,200 cGy (divided into 10–12 fractions) day −8 to −5
		Etoposide 60 mg/kg day −4
		Cyclophosphamide 100 mg/kg day −2
CBV	Lymphoma	BCNU 15 mg/kg day −6
		Etoposide 60 mg/kg day −4
		Cyclophosphamide 100 mg/kg day −2
TBC	Primary CNS lymphoma	Thiotepa 250 mg/m² daily day −9 to −7
		Busulfan 0.6–0.8 mg/kg every 6 hours on days −6 to −4
		Cyclophosphamide 60 mg/kg daily days −3 and −2
BCNU-Thiotepa	CNS lymphoma	carmustine 400 mg/m² on day −6
		thiotepa 5 mg/kg every 12 hours on days −5 and −4
Carboplatin/etoposide	Germ-cell tumor	Carboplatin AUC 7–8 day −4 to −2

(continued)

Table 53.2 Common Autologous Transplant Conditioning Regimens (continued)

Regimen	Disease	Dosage and Timing
		Etoposide 400 mg/m² day −4 to −2 (planned tandem transplant 3 following two cycles of Taxol-ifosphamide)
Cy-ATG-TBI	Systemic scleroderma	TBI 400 cGy daily on day −5 and −4 (lungs and kidneys shielded from transmission of >200 cGy)
		Cyclophosphamide 60 mg/kg day −3 and −2
		Equine anti-thymocyte globulin 15 mg/kg day −5, −3, −1, +1, +3 and +5

AUC, area under the curve; BCNU, carmustine; cGy, centi-gray; CNS, central nervous system; PK, pharmacokinetic; TBI, total body irradiation.

ENGRAFTMENT

Engraftment is defined as sustained absolute neutrophil count (ANC) >500/mcL and platelet count >20,000/mcL without transfusion support. Typically for auto-HCT with peripheral blood stem cells (PBSC), time to engraftment on average ranges from 10 to 14 days from the day of infusion of cells.

TRANSPLANT COMPLICATIONS

Patients undergoing auto-HCT remain at high risk of infectious complications. Factors that increase risk include a prolonged period of myelosuppression secondary to conditioning, development of mucositis, and indwelling catheters. Incidence of *Clostridium difficile*–associated diarrhea (CDAD) among recipients of hematopoietic stem cell transplantation (HSCT) is reported to be 5 to 9 times higher compared to the general hospitalized population (Guddati et al. *Int J Hematol*. 2014;99;758–765). Neutropenic fevers in the setting of ASCT must be managed aggressively, with prompt evaluation and initiation of empiric broad spectrum antibiotic coverage targeting gram-negative coverage (e.g., cefepime, piperacillin/tazobactam, or carbapenems). Prophylaxis strategies for infections include prevention of bacterial and viral pathogens, while fungal prophylaxis in auto-HCT is reserved for those with anticipated prolonged neutropenia, with mucosal damage from intense conditioning regimens, or who have received purine analogs (Table 53.3).[5] Cytomegalovirus (CMV)-directed therapy or surveillance is not typically instituted to auto-HCT recipients, unless otherwise indicated by history or prior chemotherapy exposure. *Clostridium difficile*–prevention trials are ongoing and currently not recommended outside clinical trial.

Table 53.3 Anti-Infection Prophylaxis and Duration of Therapy

Microbe Type	Prophylaxis	Duration
Bacterial (gram-negative)	Ciprofloxacin, levofloxacin	From day +0 until recovery from neutropenia
Viral (HSV)	Acyclovir, valacyclovir	From start of conditioning until day +365 to prevent late HSV reactivation
Fungal (*Candida*)	Fluconazole, micafungin, voriconazole	From start of conditioning until engraftment (~30 days after auto-HCT) or until 7 days after ANC >1,000 cells/mm³

ANC, absolute neutrophil count; auto-HCT, autologous hematopoietic cell transplantation; HSV, herpes simplex virus.

Table 53.4 CTCAE Mucositis Grade Severity

Grade	Symptoms
1	Asymptomatic or mild symptoms
2	Moderate pain; no interference with solid food intake
3	Severe pain; interferance with oral intake
4	Life-threatening consequence; urgent intervention indicated (i.e., intubation)

CTCAE, Common Terminology Criteria for Adverse Events.

Source: Adapted from Cancer Therapy Evaluation Program, Common Terminology Criteria for Adverse Events, Version 3.0, DCTD, NCI, NIH, DHHS.

Mucositis occurs when chemotherapy affects the rapidly divided epithelial cells lining the entire gastrointestinal tract. Typically, the onset of symptoms may occur within 7 to 10 days following initiation of conditioning regimen and can persist until engraftment. Mucositis may vary in severity (Table 53.4). Mucositis treatment is geared toward palliation of symptoms, including topical agents (viscous lidocaine, magic mouthwash, morphine rinses) and intravenous pain medications for severe intractable pain. Parenteral nutrition and even intubation may be warranted in severe cases.

ENGRAFTMENT SYNDROME

Engraftment syndrome (ES) is generally characterized by high fevers (>39 °C), diffuse erythematous rash, and pulmonary injury (infiltrates, pulmonary edema) in the absence of other causes (e.g., infections or drug reactions). It has been reported in large series, occurring in 7% to 10% of all auto-HCT for MM and lymphoma (*Biol Blood Marrow Transplant.* 2015;21(12):2061–2068). ES is usually self-limiting, and steroids are generally prescribed to achieve resolution of symptoms more rapidly.

■ POST-TRANSPLANT CARE

VACCINATION (TABLE 53.5)

PREVENTION STRATEGIES: MAINTENANCE AND SURVEILLANCE

Maintenance and post-transplantation consolidation therapy are aimed at reducing the risk of relapse following ASCT. The most prominent example of the success of post-transplant maintenance therapy is in MM, with lenalidomide following auto-HCT (*N Engl J Med.* 2012;366(19):1770–1781; *N Engl J Med.* 2014;371(10):895–905; see Chapter 26). Ixazomib, an oral proteasome inhibitor, also showed reduction of progression and improved PFS in TOURMALINE-MM3 prospective randomized placebo controlled phase 3 study (Dimopoulos et al. *Lancet.* 2019;393(10168):253–264). Further studies are ongoing with other myeloma-specific therapies in the maintenance setting, including combination lenalidomide with subcutaneous daratumumab, which is currently being studied in a large randomized phase 3 trial.

Until recently, there has been limited success with post-transplant therapy in lymphomas. The ATHERA trial, an international, multicenter, randomized study, demonstrated a significant reduction in progression-free survival in patients with Hodgkin lymphoma at high risk for relapse who received brentuximab vedotin, an antibody-drug

Table 53.5 Typical Post-HCT Vaccination Schedule			
Vaccine	Form	Dose	Time After HCT
Haemophilus influenza type B	Conjugate polysaccharide	3	6–12 months
Streptococcus pneumonia	Conjugate polysaccharide	3	3–6 months
DPT	Toxoid	3	6–12 months
Influenza	Inactivated	1 (annually)	4–6 months
Hepatitis B	Inactivated	3	6–12 months
MMR	Live attenuated	1	24 months
Polio	Inactivated	3	6–12 months

DPT, diphtheria, pertussis, tetanus; HCT, hematopoietic cell transplantation; MMR, measles, mumps, rubella.

conjugate directed to the protein CD30, given every 3 weeks for up to 16 cycles following auto-HCT (*Lancet.* 2015;385(9980):1853–1862). Rituximab, an anti-CD20 monoclonal antibody, has had mixed results in the maintenance setting, with improvement in progression-free survival but not overall survival in mantle cell and follicular lymphomas (*Blood.* 2014;124(21):146; *J Clin Oncol.* 2013;31(13):1624–1630). Rituximab maintenance, however, demonstrated no benefit post-auto-HCT for diffuse large B-cell lymphoma based on results of the CORAL study (*J Clin Oncol.* 2012;30(36):4462–4469). As newer agents are becoming available, including checkpoint inhibitors and therapies targeting B-cell–signaling pathways, there are numerous ongoing clinical trials seeking to improve survival outcomes for diffuse large B-cell lymphoma in the maintenance setting.

▨ REFERENCES FOR SUPPLEMENTAL READING

1. Appelbaum FR, Forman SJ, Negrin RS, et al. *Thomas' Hematopoietic Cell Transplantation: Stem Cell Transplantation* (5th ed.). John Wiley & Sons; 2015.

2. Wingard JR, Gastineau DA, Leather HL, et al. *Hematopoietic Stem Cell Transplantation: A Handbook for Clinicians* (2nd ed.). American Association of Blood Banks (AABB); 2015.

3. Kanate AS, Majhail NS, Savani BN, et al. Indications for hematopoietic cell transplantation and immune effector cell therapy: guidelines from the American society for transplantation and cellular therapy. *Biol Blood Marrow Transplant.* 2020;26(7):1247–1256.

4. Hamadani M, Craig M, Awan FT, et al. How we approach patient evaluation for hematopoietic stem cell transplantation. *Bone Marrow Transplant.* 2010;45(8):1259–1268.

5. Tomblyn M, Chiller T, Einsele H, et al. Guidelines for preventing infectious complications among hematopoietic cell transplantation recipients: a global perspective. *Biol Blood Marrow Transplant.* 2009;15:1143–1238.

54 Allogeneic Hematopoietic Cell Transplantation

Hemant S. Murthy, Taiga Nishihori,
and Mohamed A. Kharfan-Dabaja

▓ INTRODUCTION

Allogeneic hematopoietic cell transplantation (allo-HCT) entails using progenitor hematopoietic cells from a related or an unrelated donor. While similar to autologous transplantation in the aspect of utilization of conditioning chemotherapy or chemoradiotherapy, it differs in that the histocompatibility differences between donor and recipient provide the ability to correct defective hematopoiesis, provide immunotherapy, and promote graft-versus-malignancy effect. This is often counterbalanced by the increased risk of transplant-associated morbidity, which includes but is not limited to graft rejection and graft-versus-host disease (GVHD) as well as a higher risk of treatment-related mortality.

Consideration of allo-HCT based on disease state is shown in Table 54.1.

▓ PRE-TRANSPLANT WORKUP

The pre-transplant workup for the recipient of an allograft is relatively similar to the workup for autologous hematopoietic cell transplantation (see Chapter 53). The HCT-comorbidity index (HCT-CI) was initially developed by Sorror et al. in 2005 and later adjusted for age contributing as a poor prognostic factor in 2014 (*J Clin Oncol.* 2014;32(29):3249–3256). It remains a widely used pre-transplant comorbidity prognostication tool. It comprises 17 specific comorbid assessments, including cardiac (coronary artery disease, arrhythmias), pulmonary, renal, rheumatologic, endocrine (diabetes, obesity), gastrointestinal (GI; peptic ulcer disease, inflammatory bowel disease, and hepatic), neurologic (prior cerebrovascular accident [CVA]), prior solid tumor, ongoing infection, and mental health. It has been validated in all transplantations for malignancies in both auto- and allo-HCT, with higher scores (HCT-CT ≥3) predictive of decreased overall survival (OS) rates and increased treatment-related mortality rates (*Biol Blood Marrow Transplant.* 2015;21(8):1479–1487). Vital organ testing (see Chapter 53) is also necessary prior to proceeding with allo-HCT. Adequate renal, pulmonary, hepatic, and cardiac organ function is required to proceed with allo-HCT as well as appropriate psychosocial evaluation.

Table 54.1 Indication for Allo-HCT and Disease State Based on 2020 Guidelines from American Society for Transplantation and Cellular Therapy (ASTCT)

Leukemia/MDS	
Acute myeloid leukemia	Good risk t(8;21), t(16;16)/inv(16)—CR2
	Intermediate risk, high risk, and secondary AML–CR1
Chronic myeloid leukemia	Chronic phase—TKI resistant or intolerant
	Accelerated phase/blast phase
Myelodysplastic syndrome	Intermediate—2/high risk by IPSS (can consider in low/intermediate risk refractory to therapy)
Lymphoid Malignancies	
Acute lymphoblastic leukemia	Adults—CR1 (standard, high risk)
DLBCL, mantle cell lymphoma, T-cell lymphomas	Relapse following auto-HCT; primary refractory, CR2 or greater
Chronic lymphocytic leukemia	Lack of response or evidence of disease progression after BCR and/or Bcl-2 inhibitor therapy
	Refractory to 2 or more lines of therapy disease and responsive to BCR or Bcl-2 inhibitor therapy
	Richter transformation after achieving an objective response to anthracycline-based chemotherapy
	Recommendations based on expert panel of CLL experts convened as part of ASTCT Clinical Practice Guidelines Committee (Kharfan-Dabaja et al. *Biol Blood Marrow Transplant*. 2016;22(12):2117–2125. doi: 10.1016/j.bbmt.2016.09.013)
Follicular lymphoma	Primary refractory, CR2 or beyond, relapse following auto-HCT, transformation to high-grade lymphoma
Myeloproliferative Neoplasms	
Myelofibrosis and MDS-MPN overlap syndromes	Primary—(intermediate, high risk); secondary
BM Failure Syndrome	
Severe aplastic anemia	Newly diagnosed (matched sibling available), relapse/refractory
SCD	Recommended for eligible patients age 18 or younger

(*continued*)

Table 54.1 Indication for Allo-HCT and Disease State Based on 2020 Guidelines from American Society for Transplantation and Cellular Therapy (ASTCT) (continued)

Leukemia/MDS	
Thalassemia	Not currently recommended for adults outside clinical trial
	Currently allo-HSCT for SCD is covered by Medicare only for beneficiaries with severe, symptomatic SCD who participate in an approved prospective clinical study. Clinical trials through CIBMTR and a phase 3 randomized study comparing allo-HCT to standard of care (BMT CTN 1503-STRIDE) are ongoing.

allo-, allogeneic; ASBMT, American Society for Blood and Marrow Transplantation; ASTCT, American Society for Transplantation and Cellular Therapies; auto-, autologous; Bcl, B-cell lymphoma; BCR, B-cell receptor; BM, bone marrow; CIBMTR, Center for International Blood and Marrow Transplant Research; CLL, chronic lymphocytic leukemia; CR, complete response; DLBCL, diffuse large B-cell lymphoma; HCT, hematopoietic cell transplantation; inv, inversion; IPSS, International Prognostic Scoring System; MDS, myelodysplastic syndrome; MPN, myeloproliferative neoplasm; SCD, sickle cell disease; t, translocation; TKI, tyrosine kinase inhibitor.

▨ DONOR SELECTION

Donor selection is a vital component of allo-HCT. Primarily, donor selection hinges on compatibility based on the human leukocyte antigen (HLA) system, with siblings being the more ideal, fully matched HLA donor. In the absence of matched-related donors (MRD), other donor sources are considered, including unrelated donors through established registries and alternative sources, such as haploidentical donors and umbilical cord blood. Other factors play a role in donor selection as well, including donor age, sex (i.e., multiparous female), ABO compatibility, health status, cytomegalovirus (CMV) serology, and urgency of transplantation.

HLA-MATCHING

The HLA complexes are located on the short arm of chromosome 6 and sorted into major histocompatibility class (MHC) I antigens (HLA-A, HLA-B, HLA-C) and MHC II antigens (HLA-DP, HLA-DQ, HLA-DR). These loci are inherited as complete haplotypes from each parent, so full siblings carry an approximately one-in-four chance of being a full HLA match.

MRD VERSUS UNRELATED DONORS

Full HLA-matched siblings have historically been considered the preferable donor source. Earlier studies would test for matching in HLA-A, B, and DRB1. Today, ideal sibling donors are 8/8 MRD. The more

Table 54.2 HLA Locus and Implication If Mismatch Occurs Between Donor and Recipient[2]

HLA Locus	Impact of Mismatch
A	Decreased OS, increased TRM, increased acute GVHD
B	Increased acute GVHD
C	Decreased OS, increased TRM, increased acute GVHD
DRB1	Decreased survival, increased acute GVHD
DQ/DQB1	Unclear impact, no apparent significance for OS or TRM; possible increased acute GVHD
DPB1	Decreased OS, increased TRM in nonpermissive mismatch* compared to match or permissive mismatch

*Based on T-cell-epitope groups (*Blood*. 2014;124(16):2596–2606).

GVHD, graft-versus-host disease; HLA, human leukocyte antigen; OS, overall survival; TRM, treatment-related mortality.

HLA mismatches in HLA-A, B, C, and DR between donor and recipient exist, the worse the outcomes in terms of survival, treatment-related mortality, and acute GVHD (Table 54.2). Historically, use of matched unrelated donors (MUD) has resulted in inferior outcomes (*N Engl J Med*. 1989;320(4):197–204). However, marked improvements in treatment-related mortality and fewer differences in outcomes between MRD and MUD have been reported recently, credited in large part to improved HLA matching between donors and recipients with higher-resolution technology.

ALTERNATIVE DONOR SOURCES

At times, allo-HCT candidates may not have fully HLA-matched siblings, or fully matched unrelated donors may not be secured from the donor registries. This is particularly notable in African American or Hispanic patients and other minorities who are disproportionately underrepresented in donor registries compared to Caucasians and/or patients of European descent.

When a sibling or matched unrelated donor is not identified, alternative donor sources are sought, two examples of this being haploidentical donors and umbilical cord blood. Haploidentical transplantation (Haplo = half) refers to mismatched-related transplant in which a donor shares a haplotype with the recipient. Haploidentical donors possess the same set of HLA genes on one of the two number 6 chromosomes (4/8 HLA match). Parents are always a half-match for their biological children and vice versa, while full siblings have a 50% chance of being a half-match. With the availability of a haploidentical pool of donors coupled with the advent of post-transplant cyclophosphamide for GVHD prophylaxis, haploidentical transplantations are the most rapidly increasing transplant modality in the world today.

Retrospective registry data have shown comparable outcomes between haploidentical and unrelated donor transplantation for AML (*Blood*. 2015;126(8):1033–1040), while lymphoma survival and mortality outcomes were similar for haploidentical, matched related, and matched unrelated allogeneic transplants, though with less incidence of GVHD in haploidentical transplants. (Dreger et al. *Blood Adv*. 2019;3(3):360–369). Haploidentical transplantation may potentially be a feasible option in relapsed high-risk multiple myeloma. A study by the European Society of Blood and Marrow Transplant (EBMT) and Center for International Blood and Marrow Transplant Research (CIBMTR) reported 2-year OS of 48% and non-relapse mortality (NRM) of 21%, supporting further investigation of haploidentical transplantation in myeloma (Sahebi et al. *Biol Blood Marrow Transplant*. 2019;25(2):335–342). Further studies are ongoing, including a multicenter prospective study of haploidentical transplantation for severe aplastic anemia being conducted by the Bone Marrow Transplant Clinical Trial Network (BMT CTN).

Umbilical cord blood refers to the blood-forming stem cells obtained from the umbilical cord and placenta following delivery. The cord blood units are frozen, stored, and accessible, allowing for expedited transplantation when no suitable sibling or unrelated donors are identified. The immune cells are more naïve, allowing for less adverse interactions between donor and recipient and permitting more HLA mismatch (typically 4/6 HLA match). Cord units contain small amounts of stem cells, so two cord units are commonly used for adult transplantation (although only one unit will engraft). Delayed immune reconstitution and late engraftment remain prominent complications.

GRAFT SOURCE (BONE MARROW VS. PERIPHERAL BLOOD STEM CELLS)

Since the advent of allo-HCT, hematopoietic progenitor cells (HPC) have been traditionally harvested from the bone marrow (BM) of HLA-compatible donors. Utilization of filgrastim-stimulated peripheral blood stem cells (PBSC) was born from studies showing that increased BM cell dose was associated with faster and more robust engraftment and the ability to collect higher doses of HPC using PB. The BMT CTN 0201, a landmark phase 3 multicenter randomized trial, compared PBSC to BM as the graft source in recipients of unrelated donors.[5] While PBSC was associated with reduced risk of graft failure and increased risk of chronic GVHD, no significant survival differences were described. Due to the ease of collection of PBSC from donors, PBSC has become the preferred graft source for hematopoietic cell transplantation. One notable exception worth mentioning is aplastic anemia, for which, due to increased GVHD with PBSC, BM remains the preferred cell source.

■ CONDITIONING REGIMENS

Conditioning regimens, which combine chemotherapy and/or chemo-radiotherapy, aim not only at reducing or eliminating tumor burden but also at facilitating engraftment of donor hematopoietic cells. The focus of these regimens is to be immunosuppressive to prevent graft rejection and to limit non-hematologic toxicities. Conditioning regimens are classified according to the intensity of the regimen on the recipient as myeloablative, nonmyeloablative, or reduced intensity.[3] Higher-intensity regimens are typically associated with lower rates of relapse, but often at the expense of increased rates of toxicities and, consequently, higher NRM. Common myeloablative regimens include combinations of busulfan (16 mg/kg) with cyclophosphamide (100–200 mg/kg) and cyclophosphamide with total body irradiation (TBI) (5–12 Gy). Fludarabine with pharmacokinetic-targeted busulfan (dosed to area under the curve [AUC] of 5,300 mcm/min [*Bone Marrow Transplant.* 2011;46(11):1418–1425]), is one of the most commonly used myeloablative conditioning regimens. Commonly, reduced intensity/nonmyeloablative regimens are combined with fludarabine, with examples including fludarabine-TBI (2 Gy), the Seattle Flu-2 Gy TBI regimen (*Blood.* 2003;101:1620–1629), fludarabine-cyclophosphamide, fludarabine-busulfan, or fludarabine-melphalan.

■ GRAFT-VERSUS-HOST DISEASE

GVHD represents one of the most common and significant complications that arise from allo-HCT, and it is one of the leading causes of treatment-related morbidity and mortality. It derives from the effects of HLA incompatibility between donor and recipient in the setting of inflammation, resulting in tissue damage of various manifestations. Based on timing and symptom profile, GVHD is further classified as acute, chronic, or overlap, which has features of both acute and chronic GVHD.

Acute GVHD historically refers to any GVHD symptoms that would arise prior to 100 days post HCT or donor lymphocyte infusion (DLI). Acute GVHD typically affects the skin, GI tract, and liver, and it is thought to develop as a result of tissue damage from conditioning chemotherapy, leading to donor T-cell activation and followed by an effector phase, characterized by cytotoxic T-cell responses against host tissues. Strategies for prevention of acute GVHD include better donor and graft selection, choice of conditioning intensity, graft manipulation, and pharmacologic prophylaxis. The earliest GVHD prophylaxis was methotrexate (MTX) followed by single-agent cyclosporine (CSA). The combination of MTX-CSA was then studied and found to have improved survival in MRD (*N Engl J Med.* 1986;314(12):729–735). Tacrolimus (TAC) was evaluated in combination with MTX and showed a decrease in acute GVHD when compared to CSA-MTX in a randomized multicenter phase 3 trial (*Blood.* 1998;92(7):2303–2314). Currently, TAC-MTX and MTX-CSA are two of the most commonly used GVHD prevention regimens, although multiple novel therapeutic strategies are underway (Table 54.3).

Post-transplantation cyclophosphamide (PTCy) is emerging as a commonly used GVHD prevention strategy these days. Typically in combination with calcineurin inhibitors (TAC or CSA) and

Table 54.3 GVHD Prophylaxis Strategies

	Mechanism of Action	Complications
T-cell depletion	*In vivo:* peritransplantation antithymocyte globulin or alemtuzumab purge both donor and recipient T-cells	Delayed immune reconstitution
	Ex vivo: physical separation of T-cells from graft; positive selection of CD34+; negative selection of T-cells via monoclonal T-cell antibodies	Graft failure
		EBV-mediated PTLD
		High rate of CMV reactivation
Cyclosporine	Inhibition of calcineurin (responsible for IL-2 mediated T-cell expansion)	Nephrotoxicity, TMA, PRES, hypomagnesaemia
TAC	Inhibition of calcineurin	Similar to cyclosporine
MTX	Dihydrofolate reductase inhibition	Prolonged time to engraftment, mucositis, increased toxicity with fluid retention, myelosuppression
Sirolimus	mTOR inhibitor	Hyperlipidemia, hepatotoxicity, VOD, TMA (when used with TAC or cyclosporine), mild myelosuppression
Post-transplant cyclophosphamide (PTCy)	Alkylating agent (administered typically on day +3, +4)	Hemorrhagic cystitis, SIADH
Mycophenolate mofetil	Inhibition of IMP dehydrogenase	GI toxicity (nausea vomiting, diarrhea), mild myelosuppression

CMV, cytomegalovirus; EBV, Epstein–Barr virus; GVHD, graft-versus-host disease; IL, interleukin; IMP, inosine monophosphate; mTOR, mammalian target of rapamycin; MTX, methotrexate; PTCy, post-transplant cyclophosphamide; PLTD, posttransplant lymphoproliferative disorders; PRES, posterior reversible encephalopathy syndrome; SIADH, syndrome of inappropriate antidiuretic hormone secretion; TAC, tacrolimus; TMA; thrombotic microangiopathy; VOD, veno-occlusive disease.

mycophenolate mofetil (MMF), its use has expanded outside hap-loidentical transplantation and has been or currently studied in other donor transplants, including matched-related, matched-unrelated, and mismatch-unrelated allogeneic transplantation. Recently, a phase 2 randomized GVHD prevention study confirmed the superior benefit of PTCy in GvHD-free relapse-free survival rates (Bola-nos-Meade et al. *Lancet Haematol.* 2019;6(3):e132–e143). Recently, the HOVON-96 prospective randomized, multicenter, phase 3 trial comparing PTCy to CSA-based GVHD prevention in MRD and MUD allo-HCT reported significant reduction in severe acute and chronic GVHD without affecting relapse (De Jong CE, et al. *Blood.* 2019;134(Suppl1):1. doi: 10.1182/blood-2019-124659). Another phase 3 study comparing GVHD prevention with PTCy to TAC/MTX (BMT CTN 1703 study) is ongoing.

Once acute GVHD is confirmed, treatment must be instituted promptly. Aside from grade 1 GVHD, which can be treated with topical agents alone, the standard first-line therapy is corticosteroids (meth-ylprednisolone, dose up to 2 mg/kg/day). Treatment is continued until complete response (CR) is achieved, but it is tapered as clinically permissible. For steroid refractory acute GVHD, other immunosuppression agents have been used as treatment, including MTX, sirolimus, TAC, pentostatin, MMF, and budesonide/beclomethasone (for GI GVHD). Extracorporeal photopheresis (ECP) was shown in a meta-analysis to have high response rates in skin and GI acute GVHD, with little ECP-related mortality (*Biol Blood Marrow Transplant.* 2014;20(11):1677–1686). Recently, ruxolitinib was approved and currently is the only Food and Drug Administration–approved (FDA-approved) agent for steroid refractory acute GVHD. This was based on the REACH1 clinical trial, which demonstrated overall response rate (ORR) of 57% and CR of 31% in those with severe steroid refractory acute GVHD (*Biol Blood Marrow Transplant.* 2019;25(3):S52. doi: 10.1016/j.bbmt.2018.12.130).

Chronic GVHD can affect multiple organs and often involves multiple locations simultaneously. Sites involved include skin, nails, scalp, mouth, eyes, genitalia, GI, liver, lung, muscles, and joints, with hematopoietic and other manifestations, such as pericardial and/or pleural effusions, and neuropathy. Risk factors of developing chronic GVHD are essentially the same as acute GVHD; however, the presence of acute GVHD substantially increases the risk of developing chronic GVHD. The National Institutes of Health (NIH) consensus criteria describe severity and staging, both organ-specific and global staging. Treatment of chronic GVHD is similar to acute GVHD, with standard first-line therapy being corticosteroids. Ibruti-nib currently is the only FDA-approved agent for chronic GVHD. This was based on results from a phase 2 clinical trial and is indicated as second-line therapy for steroid-refractory or steroid-resistant cGVHD (Miklos D, et al. *Blood.* 2017;130(21):2243–2250. doi: 10.1182/blood-2017-07-793786).

▓ INFECTION

Prophylaxis strategies for prevention of infections, such as bacterial (particularly gram-negative organisms), viral (herpes simplex virus [HSV] reactivation, Table 54.4), and fungal (*Candida, Aspergillus*, and *Pneumocystis jirovecii*), are commonly undertaken. Typically, initiation of anti-bacterial prophylaxis starts at the time of neutropenia and is continued until engraftment is achieved. For HSV prophylaxis, it

Table 54.4 Viral Infections in Allo-HCT

Virus	Clinical Manifestation	Treatment
CMV	High risk of reactivation in seropositive host and in seronegative host with seropositive donor	Induction IV ganciclovir or IV foscarnet therapy followed by prolonged maintenance period once CMV is undetectable
	Can cause pneumonia, retinitis, hepatitis, and GI involvement	Prophylaxis: Letermovir 480 mg daily until day +100; dose reduced to 240 mg when used with CSA
EBV	Increased risk in T-cell depleted allografts	Anti-CD20 therapy (rituximab); EBV-derived CTL
	Localized or disseminated tumors often aggressive, rapidly progressive, fevers, lymphadenopathy, CNS involvement	
HHV-6	Reactivation occurs in 30%–70% of allo-HCT. Increased risk in cord blood, mismatch unrelated. Males > females	Only treat if HHV-6 encephalitis
	Can present as encephalitis, seizures, with or without hyponatremia. Detected via PCR in blood and/or CSF	Foscarnet, ganciclovir first line; cidofovir second line; seizure prophylaxis with levetiracetam
BK virus	Reactivation occurs in almost half of allo-HCT; increased risk with HLA mismatch, cord blood, alemtuzumab conditioning	Cidofovir (intravesical). Reduce immunosuppressive therapy
	Hemorrhagic cystitis-mild hematuria to urinary clots and severe hematuria. Nephropathy requiring hemodialysis (rare)	

(continued)

Table 54.4 Viral Infections in Allo-HCT (continued)

Virus	Clinical Manifestation	Treatment
Adenovirus	Increased risk in cord blood and T-cell depletion (Table 54.3). Presents as pneumonitis, hepatitis, or colitis. Also, hemorrhagic cystitis or adenoviral keratoconjunctivitis	Cidofovir, ribavirin
		If refractory, adenovirus specific (CTL)
HSV 1, 2, VZV	High risk of reactivation in first year following HCT. High risk with T-cell depletion	IV acyclovir, PO valacyclovir; second line/acyclovir resistance-foscarnet
	Presents as disseminated skin lesions or more severe with organ involvement, including ocular, hepatic	Prophylaxis: acyclovir (800-mg PO BID) or Valacyclovir (1,000 mg PO daily) x 1 year post-HCT

allo-HCT, allogeneic hematopoietic cell transplantation; BID, twice a day; CMV, cytomegalovirus; CNS, central nervous system; CSA, cyclosporine; CSF, cerebrospinal fluid; CTL, cytotoxic T-lymphocyte therapy; EBV, Epstein–Barr virus; GI, gastrointestinal; HCT, hematopoietic cell transplantation; HHV, human herpes virus; HLA, human leukocyte antigen; HSV, herpes simplex virus; PCR, polymerase chain reaction; PO, by mouth; VZV, varicella zoster virus.

is generally continued for at least 12 months, given the risk of late HSV reactivation. For prophylaxis against CMV reactivation, letermovir is an antiviral drug that inhibits the CMV-terminase complex and was recently FDA-approved based on a placebo control phase 3 study in which letermovir patients had less clinically significant CMV infection than those receiving placebo (Marty et al. *N Engl J Med.* 2017;377(25):2433–2444).

■ OTHER TOXICITIES/COMPLICATIONS

Veno-Occlusive Disease/Sinusoidal Obstruction Syndrome

Hepatic veno-occlusive disease/sinusoidal obstruction syndrome (VOD/SOS) is described as damage to sinusoidal endothelial cells and hepatocytes, which can lead to portal fibrosis, cirrhosis, and fulminant hepatic failure (Table 54.5). VOD affects up to 15% of allo-HCT patients but occurs rarely with auto-HCT. Risk for VOD development includes older age, myeloablative conditioning, prior hepatic injury, prior gemtuzumab-ozogamicin exposure, tumor involvement, or iron overload. The Baltimore diagnostic criteria for VOD require serum bilirubin >2 mg/dL within 21 days of transplant and at least two of the following: hepatomegaly, >5% weight gain from baseline, or presences

Table 54.5 Other Late Post-Transplant Complications and Screening/Preventive Measures

Complication	Screening Tool
Secondary malignancy	Age-appropriate screening, including mammogram, colonoscopy, Pap smear, routine skin examinations; avoid prolonged sun exposure
Sexual dysfunction/infertility	Regular assessments, FSH/LH testing, counseling
Endocrine (hypothyroidism, hypogonadism)	Thyroid-function testing, FSH/LH
Cardiovascular (CHF, CAD, hyperlipidemia)	Assessment of cumulative anthracycline dose and chest radiation
	EKG, 2-D echo, fasting lipid profile, early management of cardiac risk factors, such as diabetes, hypertension
Skeletal-osteoporosis, avascular necrosis	DEXA scans, MRI earlier screening with prolonged steroid use, vitamin D levels and supplementation; bisphosphonate therapy
Psychologic (depression, anxiety, fatigue)	Routine psychologic evaluation of patient assessments of family and caregivers; refer to support networks

CAD, coronary artery disease; CHF, congestive heart failure; DEXA, dual X-ray absorptiometry; EKG, electrocardiogram; FSH/LH, follicular-stimulating hormone/luteinizing hormone; MRI, magnetic resonance imaging.

of ascites. Abdominal ultrasound demonstrating reversal of portal flow can also aid in diagnosis. Currently, the standard preventive approach to VOD/SOS is ursodiol prophylaxis, based on a placebo-controlled study (*Ann Intern Med*. 1998;128:975–981). Treatment of VOD is limited, with defibrotide being the most promising agent available. In March 2016, the FDA approved defibrotide for VOD/SOS with renal or pulmonary dysfunction based on improvement in CR rates and day +100 survival compared to historical control (*Blood*. 2016;127(13):1656–1665).

PULMONARY TOXICITIES

Patients undergoing allo-HCT are at risk for various pulmonary complications, including fluid overload and opportunistic respiratory viruses (e.g., respiratory syncytial virus [RSV]). Serious and often fatal complications are diffuse alveolar hemorrhage (DAH) and bronchiolitis obliterans (BO). DAH is a rare, life-threatening disorder that is characterized by the acute onset of alveolar infiltrates on radiologic evaluation and hypoxemia. Typically seen within the first 100 days of allo-HCT, risks of incidence include older age, myeloablative conditioning, and use of TBI-containing regimens. Treatment of DAH involves the use of high-dose steroids (methylprednisolone >1,000 mg/day), but approximately 25% of those with DAH survive past day +100 (*Biol Blood Marrow Transplant*. 2006;12(10):1038–1046). BO represents a late complication of allo-HCT, occurring in only about 15% of all allogeneic transplants, characterized by small airway injury and inflammation that are progressive and often irreversible. BO is considered a pulmonary manifestation of chronic GVHD. Treatment for BO is limited, with localized FAM therapy (inhaled fluticasone propionate, azithromycin, and montelukast) showing the best results for reducing the likelihood of treatment failure (*Bone Marrow Transplant*. 2011;46(10):1369–1373; *Biol Blood Marrow Transplant*. 2016;22(4):710–716). Active treatment for chronic GVHD should be continued in patients with BO.

RELAPSE
The success of allo-HCT can be demonstrated by assessment and confirmation of disease response, which is disease-specific, and by assessing percentage of donor chimerism. The latter is performed in the BM or in peripheral blood (CD 3 [T-cell] and CD33 [myeloid]). Based on detection and comparison of DNA short tandem repeat (STR) regions in the recipient and donor after transplantation, one can differentiate and quantify donor and recipient components in the post-transplant sample obtained from the patient (host). Strategies for targeting impending relapse (or high risk of relapse) are typically disease-specific. For example, hypomethylating agents are being investigated for MDS/AML. One therapy that can be useful in such a scenario is DLI. First described for CML in 1997 (*J Clin Oncol*. 1997;15(2):433–444), its role is to directly confer a graft-versus-malignancy effect by the infusion of allo-reactive donor lymphocytes. It has shown benefit in treatment of relapse, prevention of relapse, and instances of mixed-donor chimerism to help restore full-donor chimerism. One notable downside to this therapy is the increased risk and incidence of GVHD, and it is not typically administered to patients with ongoing active GVHD.

GRAFT FAILURE
Graft failure represents a rare but serious complication of HCT. Primary graft failure is defined by failure to achieve a neutrophil count >500/mcL by day +28 despite utilization of growth factors (day +42 for cord blood transplant). Secondary graft failure refers to a neutrophil count that falls below 500/mcL after engraftment has already been achieved. This can occur due to viral infections, medications, GVHD, or autologous reconstitution. Typically, this is treated with growth factors or a boost of donor stem cells; however, if refractory, DLI or even a second allo-HCT may be necessary.

▓ REFERENCES FOR SUPPLEMENTAL READING

1. Appelbaum FR, Forman SJ, Negrin RS, et al. *Thomas' Hematopoietic Cell Transplantation: Stem Cell Transplantation* (5th ed.). John Wiley & Sons; 2015.

2. Lee SJ, Klein J, Haagenson M, et al. High-resolution donor-recipient HLA matching contributes to the success of unrelated donor marrow transplantation. *Blood*. 2007;110(13):4576-4583.

3. Bacigalupo A, Ballen K, Rizzo D, et al. Defining the intensity of conditioning regimens: working definitions. *Biol Blood Marrow Transplant*. 2009;15(12):1628–1633.

4. Sorror ML, Maris MB, Storb R, et al. Hematopoietic cell transplantation (HCT)-specific comorbidity index: a new tool for risk assessment before allogeneic HCT. *Blood*. 2005;106(8):2912–2919.

5. Anasetti C, Logan BR, Lee SJ, et al. Peripheral-blood stem cells versus bone marrow from unrelated donors. *N Engl J Med*. 2012; 367(16):1487–1496.

55 CAR-T Overview and Novel Cellular Therapeutic Options, Including TCR Gene Transfers

Cristian I. Rodríguez Arocho, Marco L. Davila,

and David A. Sallman

▓ INTRODUCTION

In order to understand current advances in cellular therapy, we need to understand how the immune system fights cancer. This chapter focuses on the role of the adaptive immune system against tumors and how we can manipulate the body's immune system to eradicate tumors through immunotherapy. We are going to briefly discuss chimeric antigen receptor therapy (CAR-T), T-cell receptor therapy (TCR-T), tumor mechanism of resistance, and future directions.

Adaptive immunity can be divided into cellular and humoral immune-mediated response. Lymphocytes are responsible for the induction of these immune responses. T-cell lymphocytes are mainly responsible for activation of cellular immunity, and B-cell lymphocytes for the activation of humoral immunity. T-cell lymphocytes are composed of CD4 helper and CD8 cytotoxic lymphocytes. T-cell lymphocytes each carry a T-cell receptor (TCR) that recognizes proteins presented by major histocompatibility complex (MHC). CD4 T lymphocytes recognize antigen peptides on MHC class II, and CD8 T lymphocytes recognize antigen peptides on MHC class I; hence, the activation of T lymphocytes is MHC-restricted. T helper 1 cells (TH1) drive the clonal expansion of CD8 T-cells by secretion of interferon gamma (IFN-γ) and interleukin-2 (IL2); when activated, they become cytotoxic T lymphocytes (CTL). CTL has become a crucial target for cancer immunotherapy due to its antigen-specific cytotoxicity, activation of apoptosis cascade, and secretion of antitumor cytokines, such as IFN-γ (Maher & Davies, 2004). CTL activation against a tumor antigen requires interaction between TCR and antigen-presenting cells through MHC class I interaction. A second costimulatory signal is required for activation of CTL. Known costimulatory domains include CD28, 4-1BB, ICOS, CD27, OX40, MYD88-CD40, and KIR2DS2.[4] From these, CD28 and 4-1BB are the most clinically relevant, because there are two Food and Drug Administration–approved (FDA-approved) types of CAR-T cell therapy with one of these costimulatory domains.

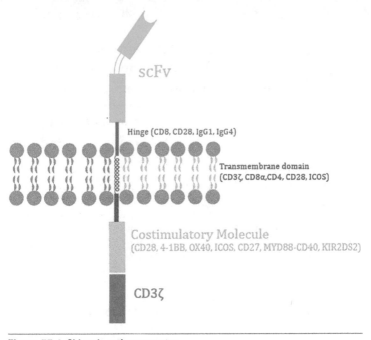

Figure 55.1 Chimeric antigen receptor.

scFv, single chain Fragment variant.

▨ CHIMERIC ANTIGEN RECEPTOR (CAR)

"Chimera" refers to having two different genetic components on the same organism. Through genetic engineering, synthetic receptors can be integrated on cells of interest. For example, T-cells can be engineered to express a receptor that targets a specific antigen in order to enhance antitumoral activity.

CAR STRUCTURE

In general, CAR is composed of an extracellular domain, transmembrane domain, and intracellular activation domain (see Figure 55.1). The extracellular domain is composed of a binding domain and a hinge. The most common binding domain used consists of single chain Fragment variant (scFv) immunoglobulin-derived (murine or human) that targets extracellular specific antigens independent of MHC. Other binding domains exist but are beyond the discussion of this chapter. The hinge provides stability and can be composed of amino-acid sequences from CD8, CD28, IgG1, or IgG4. The transmembrane domain provides stability and functionality to CAR and is usually derived from CD3ζ, CD28, CD4, or CD8α. The intracellular domain is composed of costimulatory domain (can be more than one) and activation domain. The intracellular domain plays an importance role in CAR expansion, proliferation, and persistence. First-generation CARs had short life spans and *in vivo* activity due to lack of costimulatory domains. Second-generation CARs have costimulatory domains and have demonstrated in vivo expansion, persistence, and cytotoxicity. The most commonly used costimulatory domains are CD28 and 4-1BB.[5]

Currently, there are two second-generation FDA-approved CAR-T cells targeting CD19, Yescarta® (axicabtagene ciloleucel or axi-cel) and Kymriah® (tisagenlecleucel or tis-cel), which are discussed in detail in Chapter 56. Both therapies are approved as third-line therapy for relapse/refractory diffuse large B-cell lymphoma (DLBCL), transformed follicular lymphoma (DLBCL arising from follicular lymphoma), and high-grade B-cell lymphoma. Axi-cel is also approved for primary mediastinal B-cell lymphoma. Tis-cel is the only approved CAR-T cell for patients up to 25 years old with relapse/refractory B-cell acute lymphoblastic lymphoma (B-ALL) after 2 or more lines of systemic therapy. Both have murine-derived scFv that targets CD19 antigen. Axi-cel transmembrane and costimulatory domain are composed of a CD28 molecule. On the other hand, tis-cel transmembrane domain is composed of a CD8α molecule, and the costimulatory domain is a 4-1BB molecule. In general, around 40% long-term complete response (CR) has been observed in patients with relapse/refractory DLBCL (compared with 7% CR to the next line of therapy; Crump et al., 2017; Schuster, 2019),[2] while 80% CR has been observed in patients with B-ALL. However, most patients required bridging with allogeneic bone marrow (BM) transplant, because median event-free survival is around 6 months, with the most durable responses occurring in patients with low BM blast burden, that is, <5%.[3]

Ongoing clinical trials are evaluating CAR-T cells targeting B-cell maturation antigen (BCMA) (for myeloma), CD22 (for B-ALL), WT1 (for acute myeloid leukemia [AML]), CD33/CD123 (for AML), NKG2D (for AML), and mesothelin (solid tumors), among others. Ongoing trials are also evaluating the efficacy and safety of natural killer (NK) cells genetically modified to express anti-CD19 CAR, and results are promising (Liu et al., 2020).

Currently there is ongoing investigation evaluating the safety and efficacy of the humanized anti-CD19 CAR-T cell called Hu19-CD828Z (Brudno et al., 2020). Hu19-CD828Z has a humanized scFv with a CD8 hinge and transmembrane domain, CD28 costimulatory domain, and CD3ζ activation domain. Third-generation CAR is under clinical investigation; the main difference from a second-generation CAR is the addition of a second costimulatory domain. Fourth-generation CAR is also under investigation; the main difference from a second-generation CAR is the addition of the intracellular molecule IL-12, and it is known as T-cell redirected for universal cytokine-mediated killing (TRUCKs).

PRODUCTION OF AUTOLOGOUS CARS AND GENETIC TRANSFER

The first step in manufacturing a CAR-T cell requires collecting T-cells by leukapheresis. After collection, T-cells are sent to a specialized laboratory for purification, culture, activation, and genetic engineering. Vectors are used to deliver and incorporate the desired CAR into the T-cell, a process called "transduction." Most common vectors are viral due to high transfer ability and efficacy, although non-viral vectors are also used (e.g., Sleeping Beauty transposon system and mRNA transfection). Retroviruses (including lentivirus) and adenoviruses are commonly used vectors. Axi-cel CAR-T cell was manufactured by using a retrovirus, and tis-cel was manufactured by using a lentivirus. Both products are manufactured by using autologous T-cells and on average take from 17 to 30 days from leukapheresis to delivery and infusion. This is very important, because patients requiring a CAR-T cell are refractory or have relapsed disease after more than two lines of therapy. Bridging therapy (including steroids, chemotherapy, and/ or targeted therapy) can be considered after leukapheresis but should be avoided 7 days prior to collection and 5 days prior to infusion of CAR-T cells. For more discussion, see Chapter 56. Novel transduction process (e.g., Sleeping Beauty) can lead to CAR generation in as few as 2 days, which may have benefit for patients who require urgent therapy.

CONDITIONING THERAPY PRIOR TO CAR-T CELLS

Lymphodepletive chemotherapy is likely required for in vivo expansion and has been incorporated into all CAR-T platforms where significant efficacy has occurred, although some clinical trials are evaluating CAR-T therapy with or without lymphodepletion. Fludarabine (range 25–30 mg/m^2) and cyclophosphamide (range 250–500 mg/m^2) daily for 3 days is the most common chemotherapy regimen used for CAR-T cell expansion. It is usually administered 5 days prior to infusion of the CAR-T product.

ALLOGENEIC CARS

Allogeneic CARs are of special interest, because these might have potential advantages over autologous CARs. One potential advantage of allogeneic CAR-T cells is the immediate availability of product (off shelf), thereby eliminating the time for manufacturing. Importantly, relapsed/refractory patients who have been exposed to chemotherapy, particularly lymphotoxic chemotherapy, have intrinsic dysfunction in the lymphocytes as well as other impairment directly related to the underlying disease. Thus, allogenic products from normal donors could have improved efficacy. Other potential benefits are redosing and combination of different CAR-T cells. Potential side effects related to allogeneic CAR-T cells include graft-versus-host disease (GVHD) and rapid elimination due to graft or CAR-T cell rejection by alloimmunization. Several approaches are under investigation in order to avoid GVHD, including $\alpha\beta$ TCR receptor "knockdown" to avoid allo-reactive T-cells, use of virus-specific memory T-cells, and use of non$\alpha\beta$ T- cells. Strategies to prevent immune destruction of allogeneic CAR-T cells include avoiding donor-specific antibodies (DSAs) and T-cell depletion by using anti-CD52 antibodies.[1] Ongoing clinical trials are evaluating the use of allogeneic CAR-T cells targeting CD19, CD22, BCMA, CD123, NKG2D, mesothelin, and CD3, among others.

GENE EDITING

Nucleases are defined as enzymes that degrade nucleic acids; they can be DNA-specific, RNA-specific, or both). Nucleases can be used to knockout genes. The main nucleases for precise gene editing include Zinc-finger nucleases, transcriptor activator–like effector nucleases (TALENs), megaTALs, and the clustered regularly interspaced short palindromic repeats (CRISPR) system. One example is the use of TALEN to knock out the T-cell receptor constant α chain (TRAC) to disrupt the $\alpha\beta$ TCR receptor. This can be used to manufacture a TCR-deficient allogeneic CAR-T cell and potentially avoid GVHD. TALEN can also be used to knock out CD52 antigen and make the CAR-T cell resistant to anti-CD52 antibodies (long half-life) that can be used for deeper lymphodepletion prior to infusion of CAR-T cell (to avoid host vs. graft rejection of CAR-T cells). CAR-T cells deficient in TCR and CD52 failed to induce GVHD in a mouse model and were resistant to Alemtuzumab (anti-52 monoclonal antibody).[1] Suicide genes can also be incorporated into CARs to eliminate the CAR-T cells when severe side effects of treatment occur.[1]

MECHANISM OF RESISTANCE AND CHALLENGES

The first challenge starts with collection of cells and manufacturing. Adequate manufacturing of autologous CAR-T cells ranges from 89% to 99%. T-cells' quality might be affected by disease; for example, patients with chronic lymphocytic leukemia (CLL) on average are older than patients with B-ALL, making their T-cells chronologically older and less responsive than younger T-cells. The experience in the use of anti-CD19 CAR-T cells with CLL is limited, but in general the efficacy is lower than in B-ALL and DLBCL patients. CR is reported on average from 20% to 30%. Data need to be evaluated carefully, because patients who required CAR-T for CLL are older and less fit, have received many lines of therapy (including ibrutinib, venetoclax, and allogeneic BM transplant), and also have Richter's transformation (Lemal & Tournilhac, 2019). Ongoing trials for CLL are evaluating CAR-T cell antitumor efficacy in combination with ibrutinib. Early results suggest that ibrutinib increases the overall response rate and progression-free survival rate when given concurrently with anti-CD19 CAR-T cell and may decrease cytokine release syndrome (CRS) (Gauthier et al., 2020).

Side effects related to CAR-T cells can be related to chemotherapy and collateral damage from activation of CAR-T cells. Once CAR-T cells are circulating, they identify the target cell, activate, secrete cytokines, and start the apoptosis cascade. This leads to antigen release that can be presented to endogenous T-cells by antigen-presenting cells and augments the anti-tumoral response. Cytokine release can be associated with systemic side effects, such as fever, tachycardia, hypotension, hypoxia, organ damage, and disseminated intravascular coagulation (DIC), among others. The constellation of symptoms is also known as CRS and occurs on average 3 days after infusion. Other potential side effects include neurological toxicity (confusion, aphasia, seizures, brain edema), which can present concurrently with CRS but on average happens 4 to 6 days post CAR-T cell infusion and can last from 14 to 17 days.

▓ TCR THERAPY

CAR-T cells target extracellular antigens in a non-MHC-restrictive way, but most proteins are expressed inside cells, making them unavailable for CAR-T cells. Studies have shown unsatisfactory results with CAR-T cells against solid organ tumors. TCR-T cell therapy requires genetic manipulation of native TCR in order to increase the binding affinity against a specific antigen (see Figure 55.2). TCR-T then relies on interaction with the MHC protein complex. This allows targeting intracellular and extracellular tumor antigens in an MHC-restrictive way. In general, human tumor antigens can be divided into shared tumor antigens and unique tumor antigens. Cancer testis antigen (CT antigen) is classified under shared tumor antigens and is the most common research target for TCR-T, becausee many tumors overexpress the CT antigen, while normal tissue rarely expresses it. Targeting shared tumor antigens with TCR-T can potentially target normal tissue, causing detrimental effects, a phenomenon called "on target/off tumor" effect. Most common antigens targeted on clinical trials are NY-ESO-1, MART-1, WT1, MAGE-A4, and gp100, among others. All of these mentioned antigens are categorized as shared-tumor antigens. Most common tumors evaluated in clinical trials are melanoma, GI cancer, leukemia, lung cancer, and sarcoma. Challenges with TCR-T include on target/off tumor damage, tumor immunosuppressive microenvironment, trafficking, limited persistence, high cost of targeting unique tumor antigens, and tumor heterogeneity, among others. Most current clinical trials are in phase 1, with more results expected in 2021.[6]

▓ FUTURE DIRECTIONS

Multiple myeloma is of special interest, and we are expecting FDA approval for a CAR-T cell against B-cell maturation antigen (BCMA). Early results suggest durable and high percentage of response in

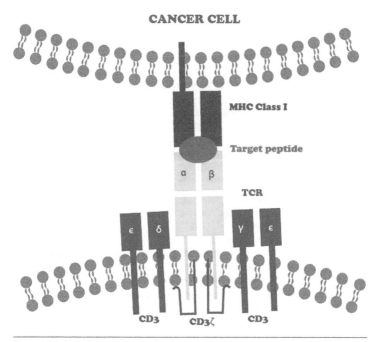

Figure 55.2 T-cell receptor.

MHC, major histocompatibility complex; TCR, T-cell receptor.

heavily pretreated patients, including high-risk cytogenetics (Raje et al., 2019). Results from ZUMA-2 suggest that patients with relapse refractory mantle cell lymphoma might benefit from CD19 CAR-T cell therapy, and FDA approval is expected during 2020 or early 2021. Early results of anti-CD19 CAR-T cells for relapse refractory follicular lymphoma suggest high rates of CR, although longer follow-up is needed. PD-1 disruptive CAR-T cells for solid tumors are under investigation. As mentioned earlier, the use of ibrutinib with anti-CD19 CAR-T cells is under investigation for CLL and DLBCL. T-cell malignancy is a huge challenge due to potential outcomes of using CAR-T cells against similar T-cell antigens. Potential outcomes include T-cell aplasia (from targeting a T-cell antigen on normal T-cells), product contamination (production of a CAR-T cell by using a tumor cell) with potential antigen masking, and fratricide (CAR-T cells targeting other CAR-T cells sharing the same targeted antigen) (Fleischer, Spencer, & Raikar, 2019). CAR-T cell therapy targeting CD33, CD123, and NKG2D is under clinical trial for relapse/refractory AML patients. Ongoing clinical trials are evaluating the use of bi-specific CAR-T cells, with the goal of targeting more than one tumor-associated antigen, increasing efficacy, and decreasing the potential for on target/off tumor effect as well as ideally decreasing the risk of relapse. The use of dual targeting to CD19 and CD22 to reduce antigen escape is of special interest for patients with B-ALL. CAR-T cells targeting CD13 and TIM3 are under investigation for treatment of AML. Dual-targeting CAR-T cells can decrease the on target/off tumor effect by sparing cells that do not express both antigens. For example, CD13 is a myeloid antigen highly expressed in AML but also on normal hematopoietic stem cells (HSCs). TIM3 has been shown to highly express in AML but in very low concentrations in normal HSCs. A dual CAR-T cell will be activated only when it encounters antigens, decreasing on target/off tumor effects and sparing cells that only express one of the antigens.

▩ REFERENCES FOR SUPPLEMENTAL READING

1. Depil S, Duchateau P, Grupp SA, et al. "Off-the-shelf" allogeneic CART cells: development and challenges. *Nat Rev Drug Discov*. 2020;19(3):185–199. doi: 10.1038/s41573-019-0051-2

2. Locke FL, Ghobadi A, Jacobson CA, et al. Long-term safety and activity of axicabtagene ciloleucel in refractory large B-cell lymphoma (ZUMA-1): a single-arm, multicenter, phase 1–2 trial. *Lancet Oncol*. 2019;20(1):31–42. doi: 10.1016/s1470-2045(18)30864-7

3. Park JH, Riviere I, Gonen M, et al. Long-term follow-up of CD19 CAR therapy in acute lymphoblastic leukemia. *N Engl J Med*. 2018;378(5):449–459. doi: 10.1056/NEJMoa1709919

4. Rafiq S, Hackett CS, Brentjens RJ. Engineering strategies to overcome the current roadblocks in CAR T cell therapy. *Nat Rev Clin Oncol*. 2020; 17(3):147–167. doi: 10.1038/s41571-019-0297-y

5. Zhang C, Liu J, Zhong JF, et al. Engineering CAR-T cells. *Biomark Res*. 2017;5:22. doi: 10.1186/s40364-017-0102-y

6. Zhang J, Wang L. The emerging world of TCR-T cell trials against cancer: a systematic review. *Technol Cancer Res Treat*. 2019;18:1533033819831068. doi: 10.1177/1533033819831068

56   CD19 CAR T-Cell Therapy

Michael D. Jain, Brigett D. Brandjes,

and Frederick L. Locke

▓ INTRODUCTION

The outcomes of patients with aggressive B-cell malignancies that are relapsed or refractory (R/R) to chemotherapy are historically poor. Recently, chimeric antigen receptor (CAR) T-cell therapies have been approved for the treatment of R/R large B-cell lymphomas (LBCL) and B-acute lymphoblastic leukemia (B-ALL). The impact of CAR T-cell therapy has been substantial, considering that it can support durable complete remissions (CR) in heavily pretreated patients. A CAR is an engineered protein that includes an extracellular receptor against a tumor surface marker, transmembrane and hinge regions, and intracellular domains to support signal transduction. For approved CAR products, CD19 is targeted by using an antibody fragment (scFv), and intracellular signaling is activated using a part of the T-cell receptor (CD3ξ) and a costimulatory domain, such as CD28 or 4-1BB.[1,2] Thus, when the gene encoding the CAR is introduced into a T-cell via a viral vector, the CAR protein is expressed. What is now a CAR T-cell has the capacity to recognize CD19 and, upon binding event, initiate signaling that leads to T-cell activation, proliferation, and cytotoxic activity. Only B-cells express CD19, and almost all B-cell malignancies invariably express CD19, thereby minimizing potential for off-tumor, on-target toxicities.

Production of approved CAR T-cell products starts with a patient's autologous T-cells, which are collected by having the patient undergo apheresis and collection of peripheral blood mononuclear cells (PBMCs), which are then shipped to a certified manufacturing facility. T-cells are then grown in vitro, undergoing activation, CAR gene transfer using a viral vector, expansion, and quality and sterility testing, prior to returning to the treating facility as a frozen product.[1] It is required that patients receive chemotherapy (typically with fludarabine and cyclophosphamide) to deplete existing lymphocytes and to optimize the homeostatic cytokine environment prior to CAR T-cell infusion. Without lymphodepleting chemotherapy prior to adoptive transfer, CAR T-cell proliferation in the patient is typically poor. We discuss pivotal trial toxicity and efficacy results with the two currently U.S. Food and Drug Administration–approved (FDA-approved) CD19 CAR T-cell products and another product being evaluated for approval at the time of this writing. Toxicities related to this therapy include cytokine release syndrome (CRS) and neurotoxicity, which are reviewed in more detail in Chapter 57.

▓ TISAGENLECLEUCEL

Tisagenlecleucel (tisa-cel) manufacturing uses a CD3 selection step that enriches for T-cells. The CAR transgene is inserted into the T-cell by using a lentivirus vector and includes the anti-CD19 single-chain variable fragment (scFv), CD3ξ, and 4-1BB costimulation domain.

The first CAR T-cell approved by the FDA was tisa-cel, in August 2017, for pediatric and young adult patients up to 25 years of age with B-ALL that is primary refractory or in second or later relapse. ELIANA is the phase 2 multicenter global trial that reported 92 enrolled and 75 infused pediatric and young adult patients.[2] Patients were heavily pretreated, with 61% of the infused patients having received a prior allogenic stem cell transplant. The median total dose of viable CAR T-cells was 1.0×10^8 (range, 0.03×10^8 to 2.6×10^8 cells). Most patients (71 of 75) received lymphodepletion chemotherapy with fludarabine and cyclophosphamide. Overall response rate (ORR) was 81%, with 60% attaining CR and 50% remaining in remission at 12 months. Relapse-free survival was 80% at 6 months and 59% at 12 months in those who responded to treatment. A total of 2 deaths occurred within 30 days after infusion; one was due to cerebral hemorrhage secondary to coagulopathy, and the other was from progressive disease. CRS occurred at a median onset of 3 days and was reported in 77% of patients, with 46% ≥ Grade 3. Neurotoxicity occurred in 40% of patients, with Grade 3 reported in 13%; there were no Grade 4 neurologic events noted.

Tisa-cel was approved in May 2018 for a second indication of R/R LBCL after two or more lines of systemic chemotherapy based on the JULIET trial. Among LBCL variants, the JULIET trial did not include patients with primary mediastinal B-cell lymphoma (PMBCL). In this open-label, multicenter, international phase 2 trial, 168 patients underwent apheresis, 111 patients received CAR T-cell infusion, and data were reported on 93 infused patients at data cutoff (median dose, 3.0×10^8 CAR-positive viable T-cells; range, 0.1×10^8 to 6.0×10^8).[3] Prior to receiving cells, patients received a 3-day lymphodepletion regimen consisting of fludarabine 25 mg/m^2 and cyclophosphamide 250 mg/m^2 or benadmustine 90 mg/m^2 for 2 days. ORR was 52%, and 40% of patients achieved CR at a median follow-up of 14 months. No deaths were attributed to tisa-cel therapy, though 3 patients died due to disease progression within the first 30 days. CRS occurred at a median onset of day 3 and occurred in 58% of patients, with Grade ≥3 in 22%. Neurotoxicity was reported in 21% of patients, with Grade ≥3 in 11%. Follow-up analysis has identified that 43% remain alive at 18 months after treatment.

◼ AXICABTAGENE CILOLEUCEL

Axicabtagene ciloleucel (axi-cel) is a CD19-targeted product that includes a CD3ζ intracellular domain paired with a CD28 co-stimulatory domain. During axi-cel production, in contrast with tisa-cel, T-cells are not selected. After T-cell activation, the unfractionated apheresis product is transduced with the CAR by using a gammaretroviral vector.

Axi-cel was approved by the U.S. FDA in October 2017 based on the ZUMA-1 trial. This was a single-arm, multicenter, phase 1/2 clinical trial for adults (≥18 years old) with relapsed/refractory diffuse large B-cell lymphoma (DLBCL) not otherwise specified, high-grade lymphoma, PMBCL, high-grade B-cell lymphoma, and LBCL transformed from follicular lymphoma after two or more lines of therapy. The approval for PMBCL is unique to axi-cel. Patients in ZUMA-1 received three days of lymphodepletion consisting of cyclophosphamide 500 mg/m^2 and fludarabine 30 mg/m^2 prior to CAR T-cell infusion (2 × 10^6 CAR T-cells per kg of body weight). The median axi-cel time to infusion was 17 days, and bridging chemotherapy was excluded. A total of 119 patients was enrolled, and 108 (7 in phase 1, 101 in phase 2) received the product. At median follow-up of 27.1 months, ORR was 83%, with 58% of patients attaining CR. At last follow-up, 39% of patients remained in remission, with 50% still alive. This highlights that axi-cel leads to durable CR in a proportion of treated patients, although it is not known yet whether this represents cure. ZUMA-1 also reported that 93% of patients experienced CRS at a median onset of day 2, with 11% being Grade ≥3. Neurological events were reported in 65% of patients, with 32% being Grade ≥3. Non-relapse mortality was reported at 3% in the first 30 days; deaths were due to hemophagocytic lymphohistiocytosis (HLH), cardiac arrest, and one instance of Grade 4 CRS/encephalopathy along with intracranial bleeding not attributed to axi-cel.

◼ LISOCABTAGENE MARALEUCEL

Though not currently approved by the FDA, lisocabtagene maraleucel (liso-cel) has demonstrated promising results with significant treatment responses and low toxicity rates. As a CAR T-cell product, it is similar to tisa-cel ,with the CAR including a 4-1BB costimulatory domain and gene transfer occurring with a lentivirus. However, it is unique among all CAR T-cell products in that it is infused as a fixed 1:1 CD4:CD8 T-cell ratio, with each delivered in a separate vial. The median time from apheresis to infusion was 24 days.

The pivotal registrational trial for liso-cel is TRANSCEND-001.[4] This multicenter trial was conducted in three phases: dose finding (60 patients), dose expansion (83 patients), and dose confirmation (126 patients). There were three different dose levels tested—DL1 0.5 × 10^8, DL2 1 × 10^8, and DL3 1.5 × 10^8—and DL2 was selected for the confirmation phase. Patients underwent lymphodepletion with cyclophosphamide 300 mg/m^2 and fludarabine 30 mg/m^2 for 3 days. At the three different dose levels, a total of 344 patients was leukapheresed, and 294 were infused. Among patients receiving liso-cel, 25 received product that did not conform to manufacturing standards. Reported analysis was conducted on 256 evaluable patients (out of a total of 269) receiving the conforming product. In the reported subset, ORR was 73%, and CR was attained in 53%, with 12-month progression-free survival (PFS) and overall survival (OS) rates of 44% and 58%, respectively. Severe CRS Grade 3/4 was reported in only 2% of patients, with no patients having Grade 5. Neurotoxicity was reported at ≥Grade 3 in 10% of patients. Four patients noted Grade 5 treatment-emergent adverse events due to liso-cel and lymphodepletion (diffuse alveolar hemorrhage, pulmonary hemorrhage, multiorgan failure, and cardiomyopathy). It should be noted that toxicity management has evolved over time, and the lower reported rates of severe toxicity with liso-cel may be influenced in part by these changes. Table 56.1 summarizes the characteristics of selected CD19 CAR T-cell products in B-cell malignancies.

Table 56.1 Characteristics of Selected CD19 CAR T-Cell Products in B-Cell Malignancies

	Axicabatagene ciloleucel	Tisagenlecleucel	Lisocabtagene maraleucel
Approved indications	LBCL/PMBCL	LBCL, B-ALL*	N/A
Anti-CD19 target (scFV)	FMC63	FMC63	FMC63
Costimulatory domain	CD28	4-1BB	4-1BB
Viral vector	Retrovirus	Lentivirus	Lentivirus

B-ALL, B-cell acute lymphoblastic leukemia; LBCL, large B-cell lymphoma; PMBCL, primary mediastinal B-cell lymphoma; scFV, single-chain variable fragment. *≤25 years of age.

Source: Data from Locke FL, Ghobadi A, Jacobson CA, et al. Long-term safety and activity of axicabtagene ciloleucel in refractory large B-cell lymphoma (ZUMA-1): A single-arm, multicentre, phase 1–2 trial. *Lancet Oncol.* 2019 Jan;20(1):31–42. doi: 10.1016/S1470-2045(18)30864-7; Maude SL, Laetsch TW, Buechner J, et al. Tisagenlecleucel in children and young adults with B-cell lymphoblastic leukemia. *N Engl J Med.* 2018;378(5):439–448; Schuster SJ, Bishop MR, Tam CS, et al. Tisagenlecleucel in adult relapsed or refractory diffuse large B-cell lymphoma. *N Engl J Med.* 2018;380:45–56.; Abramson JS, Palomba ML, Gordon LI, et al. Pivotal safety and efficacy results from Transcend NHL 001, a multicenter phase 1 study of Lisocabtagene Maraleucel (liso-cel) in relapsed/refractory (R/R) large B cell lymphomas. *Blood.* 2019;134(Supplement_1):241–241.

▓ POTENTIAL PRACTICE-CHANGING CLINICAL TRIALS

ZUMA-7 is a phase 3 randomized, multicenter, open-label trial opened in December 2017 that is evaluating the efficacy of axi-cel compared to standard of care in subjects with relapsed/refractory DLBCL. Patients with high-risk DLBCL who are primary refractory or relapsed after one line are randomized to salvage chemotherapy (current standard of care) versus axi-cel. Patients randomized to salvage chemotherapy are treated with a platinum-based therapy, which is then followed by an autologous stem cell transplant in responders. More than 300 patients have enrolled, with an estimated study completion date of January 15, 2023. Primary outcome measures are event-free survival. Pending the trial results, this could change the current practice from offering CAR T-cells after failure of first-line therapy.

A pivotal trial which recently expanded the indications for CD19 CAR T from LBCL to other lymphomas is ZUMA-2. It was recently U.S. FDA approved in July of 2020 as brexucabtagene autoleucel. This is a phase 2, multicenter study evaluating efficacy of KTE-X19 in subjects with relapsed/refractory mantle cell lymphoma (MCL). All patients were previously treated with a Bruton Tyrosine Kinase (BTK) inhibitor prior to enrollment. KTE-X19 uses the same CAR construct as axi-cel, but manufacturing differs in that a T-cell selection step is included in the KTE-X19 manufacturing process. Patients received a lymphodepletion regimen of fludarabine and cyclophosphamide prior to CAR infusion. Seventy-four patients were enrolled, with 68 patients being infused at a cell dose of 2×10^6.[5] ORR was 85%, with CR attained in 59%. At 12 months, estimated PFS and OS were 61% and 83%, respectively. CRS of Grade ≥ 3 was reported in 15% of patients, and neurotoxicity Grade ≥ 3 occurred in 31% of patients. Brexucabtagene autoleucel is the first gene-engineered cellular therapy for MCL.

Unfortunately, patients who relapse after CAR T-cell therapy continue to have poor outcomes. Clinical trials are underway to address these challenges as well as expand the standard use of CAR T-cells beyond LBCL and B-ALL.

▓ REFERENCES FOR SUPPLEMENTAL READING

1. Locke FL, Ghobadi A, Jacobson CA, et al. Long-term safety and activity of axicabtagene ciloleucel in refractory large B-cell lymphoma (ZUMA-1): A single-arm, multicentre, phase 1–2 trial. *Lancet Oncol*. 2019 Jan;20(1):31–42. doi: 10.1016/S1470-2045(18)30864-7

2. Maude SL, Laetsch TW, Buechner J, et al. Tisagenlecleucel in children and young adults with B-cell lymphoblastic leukemia. *N Engl J Med*. 2018;378(5):439–448.

3. Schuster SJ, Bishop MR, Tam CS, et al. Tisagenlecleucel in adult relapsed or refractory diffuse large B-cell lymphoma. *N Engl J Med*. 2018;380:45–56.

4. Abramson JS, Palomba ML, Gordon LI, et al. Pivotal safety and efficacy results from transcend NHL 001, a multicenter phase 1 study of lisocabtagene maraleucel (liso-cel) in relapsed/refractory (R/R) large B cell lymphomas. *Blood*. 2019;134(Supplement_1):241–241.

5. Wang M, Munoz J, Goy A, et al. KTE-X19 CAR T-cell therapy in relapsed or refractory mantle-cell lymphoma. *N Engl J Med*. 2020;382(14):1331–1342.

57 Cytokine Release Syndrome and Other Toxicities Associated With Novel Cellular Therapies

Jennifer M. Logue, Estelle Cervantes,
Christina A. Bachmeier, and Marco L. Davila

▓ INTRODUCTION

Immune effector cell (IEC) therapies, including chimeric antigen receptor (CAR) T-cells and bi-specific T-cell engagers (BiTEs), such as blinatumomab, have toxicities caused by profound T-cell proliferation and cytokine release following T-cell activation or engagement. The two most common toxicities include cytokine release syndrome (CRS) and neurological toxicities. The incidence and severity of these toxicities vary, depending on the construct of the cellular therapy and the disease state. The American Society for Transplantation and Cellular Therapy (ASTCT) defines CRS as "a supraphysiologic response [in which] symptoms can be progressive, must include fever at the onset, and may include hypotension, capillary leak (hypoxia) and end organ dysfunction."[1] Associated constitutional symptoms are typically flulike, including fevers, arthralgias, and myalgias. Elevations in cytokines, including interferon (IFN)-γ, tumor necrosis factor (TNF)-α, interleukin (IL)-10, IL-6, IL-8, IL-2, IL-1β, and GM-CSF, are seen. C-reactive protein (CRP) and ferritin elevations are also common but less specific.

Neurologic toxicity, also known as immune effector cell-associated neurotoxicity syndrome (ICANS), is a spectrum that can include encephalopathy, delirium, lethargy, difficulty concentrating, headache, anxiety, sleep disorder, dizziness, tremor, or agitation. ICANS is defined by the ASTCT as "a disorder characterized by a pathologic process involving the central nervous syndrome [in which] symptoms or signs can be progressive and may include aphasia, altered level of consciousness, impairment of cognitive skills, motor weakness, seizures, and cerebral edema."[1] The exact pathophysiology of ICANS remains unclear, but possibly endothelial activation, blood-brain barrier disruption, pro-inflammatory cytokines, and myeloid cells may be involved.

Aside from cytokine-associated toxicity, autoimmune toxicity also occurs with cellular therapies. Such toxicities are related to "on-target, off-tumor" effects and include B-cell aplasia, hypogammaglobulinemia, and infections. As future novel cellular therapies are developed, there will likely be an entire spectrum of these types of "on-target, off-tumor" toxicities specific to the antigen of target.

Prolonged cytopenias also occur, but the exact mechanism of this is unknown.

▓ DIAGNOSIS: CYTOKINE RELEASE SYNDROME

Several different grading systems have been developed for the assessment of CRS due to IEC, including Common Terminology Criteria for Adverse Events (CTCAE) versions 4.03 and 5.0 (National Cancer Institute), Lee criteria,[2] Penn criteria,[3] Memorial Sloan Kettering Cancer Center (MSKCC) criteria (NEJM 2018), and CAR-T-cell-therapy-associated Toxicity (CARTOX) criteria.[4] As a result of differences among these classifications, it is difficult to compare CRS rates and severity across studies from different institutions. In order to standardize grading of IEC toxicities, the ASTCT published consensus recommendations (Table 57.1).[1] CRS grade should be determined each time vital signs are recorded, and other causes of fever, hypotension, hemodynamic instability, and/or respiratory distress should be excluded, especially infection. Hemophagocytic lymphohistiocytosis/macrophage activation syndrome (HLH/MAS) has similar clinical and laboratory findings to CRS and should also be considered, though it is often difficult to draw a distinction between these disease states due to substantial overlap. There should be a reasonable temporal relationship to the administration of the cellular therapy in order to diagnose a patient with CRS, as early as within 24 hours, but most commonly between days 7 and 14 after infusion. Once fever has been treated, grading of

Table 57.1 ASTCT CRS Consensus Grading

	Grade 1	Grade 2	Grade 3	Grade 4
Fever	Temperature ≥38°C	Temperature ≥38°C	Temperature ≥38°C	Temperature ≥38°C
Hypo-tension	None	Not requiring vasopressors	Requiring a vasopressor with or without vasopressin	Requiring multiple vasopressors (excluding vasopressin)
Hypoxia	None	Requiring low-flow nasal cannula (≤6 L/min) or blow-by	Requiring high-flow nasal cannula (>6 L/min), facemask, nonrebreather mask, or venturi mask	Requiring positive pressure (e.g., CPAP, BiPAP, intubation, and mechanical ventilation)

Lee et al. *BBMT*. 2019.[1] ASTCT, American Society for Transplantation and Cellular Therapy; BiPAP, bilevel positive airway pressure; CPAP, continuous positive airway pressure; CRS, cytokine release syndrome.

CRS no longer requires fever and is instead driven by hypotension or hypoxia. Organ toxicities associated with CRS may be graded according to CTCAE v5.0, but such toxicities do not influence CRS grading. Grading is always determined by the more severe event. Grade 5 CRS is death due to CRS in the absence of another principle cause.

PROGNOSIS

Fulminant CRS can be life threatening when such complications as cardiac dysfunction, adult respiratory distress syndrome (ARDS), renal failure, liver failure, or disseminated intravascular coagulation (DIC) occur.[5] Fortunately, most cases of CRS are mild and typically reversible. Risk factors for CRS include disease burden, degree of T-cell proliferation, cellular dose, and lymphodepletion. The inflammatory markers CRP and ferritin are monitored during treatment. Because IL-6 up-regulates hepatic CRP production, CRP is seen to increase after the onset of CRS and return to baseline once CRS has ended.

TREATMENT

Grading of CRS is used to guide treatment. Grade 1 CRS is managed supportively, and further intervention is considered for patients with Grade 2 or higher. IL-6 levels are known to peak during maximal T-cell proliferation, and IL-6 receptor blockade by the recombinant humanized anti-IL-6 receptor monoclonal antibody tocilizumab has been shown to result in dramatic reversal of life-threatening CRS.[1-5] For patients at least 30 kg, tocilizumab is given 8 mg/kg intravenously (IV) over 1 hour and can repeated every 8 hours, for a maximum of 4 doses total. A dose of 12 mg/kg is used for patients <30 kg. Fever typically resolves within a few hours after tocilizumab administration, but other features of CRS can take longer to resolve. A second dose of tocilizumab should be considered if a patient does not stabilize after the first dose. Corticosteroids are also used; however, their potential to dampen the effectiveness of cellular therapies remains a concern. More severe CRS may require intensive care unit (ICU) admission with use of vasopressors and/or mechanical ventilation. Resolution of CRS is defined as resolution of fever, oxygen, and pressor requirements, unless another cause of fever, hypoxia, or hypotension is present. The overall goal of CRS management is to prevent life-threatening complications while preserving the antitumor effects of the cellular therapy.

▦ DIAGNOSIS: NEUROLOGIC TOXICITY

Neurologic toxicity is the second-most-common toxicity associated with CAR T-cell therapy. Although this toxicity was previously considered to be part of the constellations of CRS symptoms, ICANS is now considered a separate event with distinctive timing and treatment. The onset varies and can occur concurrently with CRS symptoms, after CRS has resolved, or rarely 3 to 4 weeks after cellular infusion.

The ASTCT simultaneously published a consensus grading system for neurologic toxicities of IEC in order to harmonize the definitions offered by the multitude of previously published grading systems (Table 57.2).[1] First, the patient must be assessed for the Immune Effector Cell-Associated Encephalopathy (ICE) score. This score comprises

Table 57.2 ASTCT Consensus Grading of ICANS for Adults

	Grade 1	Grade 2	Grade 3	Grade 4
ICE score	7–9	3–6	0–2	0 (patient is unarousable and unable to perform ICE)
Depressed level of consciousness	Awakens spontaneously	Awakens to voice	Awakens only to tactile stimulus	Patient is unarousable or requires vigorous or repetitive tactile stimuli to arouse. Stupor or coma
Seizure	None	None	Any clinical seizure focal or generalized that resolves rapidly or nonconvulsive seizures on EEG that resolve with intervention	Life-threatening prolonged seizure (>5 min) or repetitive clinical or electrical seizures without return to baseline in between
Motor findings	None	None	None	Deep focal motor weakness, such as hemiparesis or paraparesis
Elevated ICP/cerebral edema	None	None	Focal/local edema on neuroimaging	Diffuse cerebral edema on neuroimaging, decerebrate or decorticate posturing, cranial nerve VI palsy, papilledema, or Cushing's triad

ASTCT, American Society for Transplantation and Cellular Therapy; EEG, electroencephalogram; ICANS, immune effector cell-associated neurotoxicity syndrome; ICE, immune effector cell-associated encephalopathy; ICP, intracranial pressure.

Source: Adapted from Lee DW, Santomasso BD, Locke FL, et al. ASTCT consensus grading for cytokine release syndrome and neurologic toxicity associated with immune effector cells. *Biol Blood Marrow Transplant*. 2019;25(4):625–638.

orientation to year, month, city, and hospital (4 points); ability to name 3 objects (e.g., point to clock, pen, button; 3 points); ability to follow simple commands (e.g., "Show me 2 fingers"; 1 point); ability to write a standard sentence (1 point); and ability to count backward from 100 by 10 (1 point). Once the ICE score is calculated, the patient is assessed for depressed level of consciousness, seizure, motor findings, and cerebral edema. Like with CRS, neurotoxicity is graded by the most severe event not attributable to another cause. All other manifestations of neurologic toxicity, such as tremors, can be graded according to CTCAE v5.0, but similar to CRS, they do not influence grading. Intracranial hemorrhage is not included in grading and should not change treatment. Other possible etiologies for depressed level of consciousness, such as sedating medications, should always be considered and ruled out.

PROGNOSIS
Duration of neurologic symptoms can be as short as a few hours or as long as weeks.[5] Progression to severe neurotoxicity can occur over hours to days, and severity can fluctuate, necessitating close monitoring. Symptoms are almost always reversible, and fatal cases are rare. As Santomasso et al. show, severe neurotoxicity has been seen to correlate with early systemic inflammation, with higher-peak serum cytokines, the presence and severity of CRS, high pre-treatment disease burden, higher-peak IEC expansion, and within the angiopoietin (ANG) axis higher ANG2:ANG1 ratios (Cancer Discov, 2018).

TREATMENT
Nonspecific symptoms, such as headache, tremor, myoclonus, asterixis, and hallucinations, should not trigger specific interventions; rather, they are managed symptomatically.[5] Unlike CRS, neurotoxicity typically does not respond to tocilizumab, because it does not cross the blood-brain barrier. The primary treatment is corticosteroids, which should be considered as early as Grade 2. Dexamethasone 4 to 10 mg IV or its methylprednisolone equivalent is the favored option. Steroids can be repeated every 6 hours, though this is not standardized. As with severe CRS, severe neurologic toxicity should also prompt early consideration for transfer to an ICU level of care, and intubation should be considered for airway protection. Seizure prophylaxis is also used but is institution-specific.

▧ HEMATOLOGIC TOXICITIES
B-CELL APLASIA AND HYPOGAMMAGLOBULINEMIA
Another adverse effect specific to CD19-directed T-cell therapies is the depletion of non-malignant B-cells. This "on-target, off-tumor" effect occurs due to T-cells targeting CD19 on normal and tumor B-cells alike, leading to B-cell aplasia and, subsequently, hypogammaglobinemia.

Though the depletion of non-tumor B-cells may lead to adverse effects, it is also a marker of anti-CD19 T-cell activity. Hypogammaglobinemia severity correlates with B-cell aplasia and can be managed with intravenous immunoglobulin (IVIG) replacement, but this is not standardized.

PROLONGED CYTOPENIAS

Though depletion of blood cells is common immediately following CAR T-cell treatments, prolonged cytopenias that persist for a period longer than 30 days also occur. The mechanism behind this delay in count recovery remains unclear but may be a result of prior treatment with chemotherapy. Treatment for patients faced with low blood cell counts is supportive care.

INFECTIONS

The development of B-cell aplasia, hypogammaglobulinemia, and prolonged cytopenias after CD19-directed T-cell therapies all contribute toward making these patients more susceptible to infection. In the absence of protective immunoglobulins, the reactivation of dormant viruses, such as hepatitis B, can occur. Respiratory infections and infections caused by encapsulated bacteria are the most common infections seen in the setting of B-cell aplasia. Limitation of steroid use, infusion of IVIG, and use of prophylactic antibiotics are common practices to avoid and manage infections. Kansagra et al. recommend that children treated with tisagenlecleucel maintain immunoglobulin G (IgG) levels >400 mg/mL (BBMT, 2018). In adults, IgG levels are commonly monitored over time, and IVIG is given when infection occurs and hypogammaglobulinemia is present; however, there is no standard of care. Typical antibiotic prophylaxis includes an antifungal, antiviral, and antibacterial.

▨ POTENTIAL PRACTICE-CHANGING CLINICAL TRIALS

The pathophysiology of CRS and neurotoxicity is becoming better understood as preclinical models identify mechanisms that can be further evaluated. Prospective clinical trials are needed to evaluate these mechanisms and determine optimal toxicity management. We anticipate that over the next few years, there will be trials investigating the role of inhibitors of granulocyte-macrophage colony-stimulating factor (GM-CSF), catecholamine, IL-1, and IL-6 as well as with tyrosine kinase inhibitors, such as ibrutinib and dasatinib, in CRS prophylaxis or treatment.

▨ REFERENCES FOR SUPPLEMENTAL READING

1. Lee DW, Santomasso BD, Locke FL, et al. ASTCT consensus grading for cytokine release syndrome and neurologic toxicity associated with immune effector cells. *Biol Blood Marrow Transplant.* 2019;25(4):625–638.

2. Lee DW, Gardner R, Porter DL, et al. Current concepts in the diagnosis and management of cytokine release syndrome. *Blood.* 2014;124(2):188–195.

3. Porter D, Frey N, Wood PA, et al. Grading of cytokine release syndrome associated with the CAR T cell therapy tisagenlecleucel. *J Hematol Oncol.* 2018;11(1):35.

4. Neelapu SS, Tummala S, Kebriaei P, et al. Chimeric antigen receptor T-cell therapy—assessment and management of toxicities. *Nat Rev Clin Oncol.* 2018;15(1):47–62.

5. Maude SL, Barrett D, Teachey DT, et al. Managing cytokine release syndrome associated with novel T cell-engaging therapies. *Cancer J.* 2014;20(2):119–122.

58 Cancer-Associated Thrombosis in Hematologic Malignancies

Karen Feghali, Arun Kadamkulam Syriac,

and Utkarsh Acharya

▓ INTRODUCTION

The risk of venous thromboembolism events (VTE) in cancer patients is seven times higher than the general population. While underestimated, the risk of VTE in hematologic (heme) malignancies is as common as in solid tumors. The incidence of VTE in heme malignancies varies according to the cancer type, disease stage, anticancer treatment, and the use of central venous catheters (CVC). This chapter reviews the epidemiology, therapeutic strategies, and general outcomes of VTE in leukemia, lymphoma, myeloma, and stem cell transplantation.

▓ EPIDEMIOLOGY

Prior research that focused on hematologic malignancies is limited by small sample size. A recent Danish study with a large cohort population of 32,141 hematologic cancer patients demonstrated that the 10-year absolute risk for VTE following hematologic cancer was 5.2% (*Haemostasis.* 2019; doi: 10.1111/jth.14475). This population was found to be at three times the risk for VTE when compared to the general population. This association is generally stronger in the short term, within 6 months of diagnosis, than in the long term. Additionally, several studies have evaluated both clinical and laboratory risk factors for VTE in cancer patients (Table 58.1). Among these, the Khorana risk score (KRS) was introduced in 2008 and has been validated in large cohorts of patients with a variety of malignancies (*Haematologica.* 2019;104(6):1277–1287). The KRS is calculated by assigning points for clinical parameters, including tumor site, platelet count, white blood cell (WBC) count, hemoglobin level, and body mass index (BMI). This study, although it included lymphoma patients, focused mainly on solid tumors, with limited guidance for risk stratification in all liquid tumors. This paucity of available data pertaining to the risk of VTE in hematologic malignancies hinders effective risk mitigation and therapeutic intervention.

LEUKEMIA

In leukemia, the overall risk of VTE in patients with acute lymphoblastic leukemia (ALL) and acute promyelocytic leukemia (APL) is approximately 10% at 6 months from diagnosis. Particularly

Table 58.1 Summary of Main Risk Factors Associated With Increased VTE in Different Types of Malignancy

Type of Malignancy	Main Risk Factors for Increased-Risk VTE
ALL	The use of L-asparaginase-based chemotherapy regimens
APL	Disseminated intravascular coagulation
CML	Ponatinib based treatment
Lymphoma	High disease stage, CNS involvement, high LDH, doxorubicin- or methotrexate-based chemotherapy
MM	Use of immunomodulatory drugs
Autologous SCT	Use of immunomodulatory drugs in MM
Allogenic SCT	Acute and chronic GVHD

ALL, acute lymphoblastic leukemia; APL, acute promyelocytic leukemia; CML, chronic myelocytic leukemia; CNS, central nervous system; GVHD, graft-versus-host disease; LDH, lactate dehydrogenase; MM, multiple myeloma; SCT, stem cell transplantation; VTE, venous thromboembolism events.

among ALL patients, VTE risk increases rapidly within the first year after cancer diagnosis. The risk of VTE is lowest, around 2%, with acute myelocytic leukemia (AML). In ALL, the main risk factor for developing thrombosis is the use of L-asparaginase. Other independent risk factors associated with VTE in adults with ALL include platelet count between 50,000/mcL and 99,000/mcL, presence of Philadelphia chromosome, age >40 years, and the use of CVC. APL, which constitutes around 10% of AML cases, is also strongly associated with thrombosis and bleeding due to the inherent risks associated with disseminated intravascular coagulopathy (DIC) in this population. There are limited data on the incidence of de novo thrombosis in chronic myelocytic leukemia (CML), but an increased incidence of thrombosis has been reported with ponatinib use. The etiology of increased VTE with ponatinib remains unclear, although it may be secondary to impaired vascular endothelial cell angiogenesis. In patients with chronic leukocytic leukemia (CLL), the data regarding risks of VTE are still limited but share overlapping biology with lymphoproliferative disorders.

LYMPHOMA

Lymphomas are associated with high risk of roughly 10% of developing VTE. However, lymphomas represent a heterogenous group of disorders with notable variability in disease biology, histology, sites of involvement, and tumor burden. Thus, the use of the KRS may not always be applicable, given these iterations. Therefore, novel VTE prediction models, such as the ThroLy score, are being validated (*Am J Hematol.* 91(10):1014–1019). The risk factors in this model include previous VTE, mediastinal involvement, BMI over 30, extranodal disease, neutropenia, and hemoglobin <10 g/dL. Other independent risk factors for VTE in lymphoma include female sex, high hemoglobin, high creatinine, central nervous system (CNS) involvement, high lactate dehydrogenase, and doxorubicin- or methotrexate-based chemotherapy. Additionally, studies have demonstrated that patients with high-grade lymphoma, including T-cell lymphoma, Diffuse large B-cell lymphoma (DLBCL), and Hodgkin lymphoma, have almost twice the incidence of VTE compared with patients with low-grade lymphoma, thus warranting further studies.

MULTIPLE MYELOMA

As shown in a large Danish study, the risk for VTE was highest in patients with multiple myeloma (MM). Thrombosis in MM has recently received more attention due to high rates of VTE associated with immunomodulatory drugs (IMiDs), including pomalidomide or lenalidomide. IMiDs increase factor VIII and von Willebrand factor, induce protein C resistance, and reduce thrombomodulin, thus contributing to a hypercoagulable state. Patients with MM treated with IMiDs in combination with other agents (glucocorticoids, doxorubicin, erythropoietin) have VTE rates >20%.

STEM CELL TRANSPLANT (SCT)

Despite the expected post-transplant thrombocytopenia subsequent to high-intensity chemotherapy, such patients are at higher risk of VTE as a result of hospitalizations and vascular access. Studies in MM patients having undergone autologous SCT demonstrated an incidence between 3% and 23.5% of VTE, although the higher incidence may be confounded by concurrent IMiD therapy. Allogeneic SCT recipients are also at an increased risk for VTE, confirmed by retrospective data assessing VTE risk in leukemia, lymphoma, and MM patients subsequent to their first allogenic SCT. The incidence of VTE was reported at 7.1% at 2 years. Of the studied variables, history of prior VTE was the only significant predictor, and both acute and chronic graft-versus-host disease (GVHD) were found to be independently associated with thrombosis, implying an inflammatory influence on endothelial dysfunction. Additionally, all thrombosis, except for upper extremity thrombosis, was associated with non-relapse mortality.

▓ PREVENTION AND TREATMENT

Hematologic malignancies have been underrepresented in studies evaluating prevention and treatment of VTE in cancer patients. Prospective studies evaluating thromboprophylaxis and management of VTE in heme malignancies are lacking.

PROPHYLAXIS IN HOSPITALIZED PATIENTS

In hospitalized acutely ill patients with active hematologic malignancies, American College of Chest Physicians (ACCP) and American

Society of Clinical Oncology (ASCO) guidelines recommend VTE prophylaxis during hospitalization in the absence of contraindications. This has been proven to reduce mortality (24 fewer deaths in 1,000), with no difference in major bleeding. Generally, low-molecular-weight heparin (LMWH) is used for prophylaxis in hospitalized cancer patients, and continuation of VTE prophylaxis is not recommended post discharge. In hospitalized patients undergoing major surgery, perioperative VTE prophylaxis is indicated, as the risk of postoperative VTE in patients with cancer is twice that in those without cancer. Pharmacologic thromboprophylaxis with either unfractionated heparin (UFH) or LMWH should be initiated 2 to 12 hours preoperatively and should be continued for at least 7 to 10 days. Extended prophylaxis with LMWH for up to 4 weeks postoperatively is recommended for high-risk cancer patients undergoing major abdominal or pelvic surgery.

PROPHYLAXIS IN OUTPATIENTS

General guidelines recommend against routine use of VTE prophylaxis for the outpatient cancer population except for high-risk patients. In myeloma patients treated with IMiDs, guidelines recommend the routine use of VTE prophylaxis. Additionally, based on new trials, updated ASCO guidelines from 2019 recommend outpatient prophylaxis for all high-risk patients (KRS of 2 or higher) with apixaban, rivaroxaban, or LMWN, provided there are no significant risk factors for bleeding. However, these recommendations do not categorically encompass patients with liquid tumors and thus require clinical jurisprudence.

PROPHYLAXIS IN STEM CELL TRANSPLANT RECIPIENTS

There are no firm guidelines for VTE in SCT patients, although hematologic parameters and clinical risk factors, GVHD, and veno-occlusive disease should be taken into account when considering the utility of anticoagulation in this population.

MANAGEMENT OF VTE

In the acute setting, initial anticoagulation of VTE in cancer patients may involve LMWH, UFH, fondaparinux, rivaroxaban, or apixaban. LMWH traditionally has been preferred for treatment of VTE in cancer patients. It is generally preferred over warfarin in cancer patients, as overall recurrence of VTE and bleeding is lower with LMWH. Incorporation of novel oral anticoagulants is becoming increasingly popular, given their non-inferior efficacy and favorable bleeding profiles (i.e., apixaban) when compared to LMWH in cancer patients (*N Engl J Med.* 2019;380(8):711–719). The expert consensus is to extend anticoagulation treatment beyond 6 months in all active cancer patients based on inherently increased recurrence risk. The decision regarding the type and duration of anticoagulation must be individualized and continually assessed to best discern favorable risk-benefit ratio.

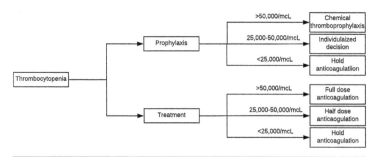

Figure 58.1 Venous thromboembolism event prophylaxis and treatment in hematologic cancer patients with thrombocytopenia.

▓ SPECIAL POPULATIONS
THROMBOCYTOPENIA

Hematologic malignancies are particularly challenging, given higher incidence of thrombocytopenia as a result of myelosuppression, marrow failure, or hypersplenism. Most recent guidelines are based on observational studies to categorically advocate for best practices regarding thromboprophylaxis or VTE treatment in this setting. Management considerations are summarized in Figure 58.1. Generally, enoxaparin, an LMWH with a short half-life, is used in these patients. There are currently no data for the use of direct oral anticoagulants in cancer patients with thrombocytopenia.

IMMUNOMODULATOR DRUGS IN MULTIPLE MYELOMA

As mentioned earlier, current guidelines recommend chemical thromboprophylaxis in MM patients receiving IMiDs. The choice of thromboprophylaxis in this setting is based on VTE risk factors and the regimen being used. If the IMiD is given as a monotherapy, then thromboprophylaxis is recommended with aspirin. If the IMiD is given with any other drug, including steroids, then the patient should be evaluated for additional VTE risk factors, including previous history of VTE, active infection, history of inherited thrombophilia, cardiac disease, diabetes, CVC or pacemaker placement, immobilization, chronic kidney disease, BMI over 30, and the use of erythropoietin. Patients with 0 or 1 risk factor should receive low-dose aspirin. Patients with more than 1 of the above risk factors for VTE are recommended to receive chemical thromboprophylaxis with LMWH or warfarin.

L-ASPARAGINASE IN ALL

As discussed above, VTE is a common complication of L-asparaginase-based regimens in ALL. It also leads to disruption of coagulation proteins, with a decrease in plasma antithrombin, fibrinogen, and

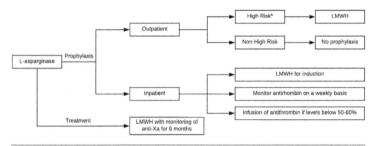

Figure 58.2 VTE prophylaxis and management in ALL patients receiving L-asparaginase-based therapy.

*High risk: inherited thrombophilia, prior history of VTE, CVC placement, active infection, immobilization, body mass index >30, cardiac disease, diabetes, chronic kidney disease. ALL, acute lymphoblastic leukemia; CVC, central venous catheters; LMWH, low-molecular-weight heparin; VTE, venous thromboembolism events.

plasminogen leading to thrombotic complications. Therefore, current guidelines by the International Society on Thrombosis and Hemostasis (ISTH) recommend active thromboprophylaxis consideration, antithrombin monitoring, and factor repletion, as summarized in Figure 58.2 (*J Thrombosis Haemostasis*, 18(2):278–284).

PROGNOSIS

Thrombotic events are the second-leading cause of death in cancer patients after death from cancer itself. There are no clear associations between VTE events in heme malignancies and disease prognoses. However, a recent study demonstrated that VTE in any type of malignancy carries an increased risk of death compared to cancer patients without VTE. Whereas anticoagulation in heme malignancies was shown to decrease incidence and recurrence of VTE, there is no evidence to date to support that it prolongs survival overall.

POTENTIAL PRACTICE-CHANGING CLINICAL TRIALS

To date, studies on VTW in hematologic malignancies are limited. Given the known association of L-asparaginase therapy with thrombosis in ALL, a trial is currently being conducted to better understand the influence of the coagulation parameters during treatment with asparaginase, with the goal of making it possible to prevent thrombosis in this setting (NCT01094392).

Immunomodulator drugs are also known to increase risk of thrombosis in MM patients, with current guidelines recommending thromboprophylaxis with aspirin, LMWH, or warfarin based on a risk stratification model. There are ongoing trials that are investigating the use of direct oral anticoagulants (DOAC) for VTE prophylaxis in this context (NCT02958969, NCT02749617, NCT03428373). The information gained from those trials will allow physicians to make more informed choices about anticoagulation strategies to manage VTE in their hematologic cancer patients.

▦ REFERENCES FOR SUPPLEMENTAL READING

1. Key NS, Khorana AA, Kuderer NM, et al. Venous thromboembolism prophylaxis and treatment in patients with cancer: ASCO clinical practice guideline update. *J Clin Oncol*. 2020;38(5):496–520. doi: 10.1200/jco.19.01461

2. Kraaijpoel N, Carrier M. How I treat cancer-associated venous thromboembolism. *Blood*. 2019;133(4):291–298. doi: 10.1182/blood-2018-08-835595

3. Samuelson Bannow BT, Lee A, Khorana AA, et al. Management of cancer-associated thrombosis in patients with thrombocytopenia: guidance from the SSC of the ISTH. *J Thrombosis Haemostasis*. 2018;16(6):1246–1249. doi: 10.1111/jth.14015

4. Kekre N, Connors JM. Venous thromboembolism incidence in hematologic malignancies. *Blood Rev*. 2019;33:24–32. doi: 10.1016/j.blre.2018.06.002

5. Kekre N, Kim HT, Ho VT, et al. Venous thromboembolism is associated with graft-versus-host disease and increased non-relapse mortality after allogeneic hematopoietic stem cell transplantation. *Haematologica*. 2017;102(7):1185–1191. doi: 10.3324/haematol.2017.164012

59 Tumor Lysis Syndrome

Mintallah Haider and Michael Jaglal

■ INTRODUCTION

Tumor lysis syndrome (TLS) is an oncologic emergency character-ized by metabolic derangements resulting from rapid cell death. Cell death can be spontaneous in the setting of rapidly dividing cancer cells or secondary to treatment targeting cancer cells. The outcome is an efflux of cellular material replete in potassium, phosphorous, and uric acid. These metabolic shifts can lead to acute renal impair-ment, cardiac arrhythmias, central nervous system (CNS) toxicity, and possible death. Due to the high morbidity and mortality of TLS, it is important to recognize patients at risk, prioritize prevention, and intervene when treatment is indicated.

■ PATHOPHYSIOLOGY

Cancer cells are rich in potassium, phosphorous, and uric acid. Hyperkalemia can affect the myocardium, resulting in devastating arrhythmias and ultimately death. Uric acid (UA), a byproduct of purine catabolism, can crystalize and obstruct renal tubule flow. Uric acid also causes endothelial dysfunction and local ischemia, result-ing in renal failure. An increase in serum phosphorous can cause increased risk of calcium phosphate precipitation in the renal tubules, and ultimately this can lead to renal injury and renal failure. Excess phosphorous binds to calcium, thus creating calcium phosphate, which can also deposit in cardiac tissue and lead to arrhythmias. The secondary decrease in serum calcium can lead to CNS toxicity and cardiac toxicity.

■ DIAGNOSIS

TLS can be classified based on laboratory criteria with or without clin-ical manifestations. The criteria defined by Cairo et al. are outlined in Tables 59.1 and 59.2. Note that lactate dehydrogenase (LDH) is not in the criteria, though it is sensitive but not specific to TLS.

■ POPULATION AT RISK

Certain malignancies and patient characteristics are associated with higher TLS risk (Table 59.3). Older age is associated with decreased renal reserve, thus theoretically predisposing older patients to TLS, though there are no data to specify an age. Patients who are volume

Table 59.1 Cairo–Bishop Laboratory Criteria for TLS

Factor	Value	Change from Baseline
Uric acid	≥8 mg/dL	25% increase
Potassium	≥6 mEq/L	25% increase
Phosphorous	≥4.5 mg/dL	25% increase
Calcium, corrected	≤7 mg/dL	25% increase

TLS, tumor lysissyndrome.

Table 59.2 Cairo–Bishop Grading for Clinical TLS

Clinical criteria	Grade 0	Grade I	Grade II	Grade III	Grade IV	Grade V
Creatinine	<1.5 × ULN	1.5 × ULN	>1.5-3 × ULN	>3–6 × ULN	>6 × ULN	Death
Cardiac arrhythmia	No	No intervention indicated	Non-urgent intervention required	Symptomatic and incompletely controlled medically or controlled with device (defibrillator)	Life-threatening arrhythmia with CHF, hypotension, syncope, or shock	Death
Seizures	No	–	One brief generalized seizure well controlled with anticonvulsant; infrequent motor seizure not interfering with ADL	Seizure activity with altered mentation; poorly controlled; breakthrough seizures despite medical intervention	Seizure that is prolonged, repetitive, difficult to control (status epilepticus or intractable epilepsy)	Death

All changes must not be attributable to chemotherapy. ADL, activities of daily living; CHF, congestive heart failure; TLS, tumor lysis syndrome; ULN, upper limit of normal.

depleted, whether secondary to symptoms of disease or treatment, are also at increased risk. Patients on chronic nephrotoxic medications, malignancies with bulky disease, high cell turnover, and cell sensitivity to treatment carry higher risk of TLS. Comorbidities,

Table 59.3 Cairo et al. TLS Risk Stratification

High risk	Advanced Burkitt's lymphoma/leukemia; ALL with WBC ≥100,000 or with LDH twice ULN; AML with WBC ≥100,000, DLBCL with LDH twice ULN and bulky disease
Intermediate risk	AML with WBC 25–100,000; ALL with WBC <100,000 and LDH less than twice ULN; early stage Burkitt's lymphoma/leukemia with LDH less than twice ULN; DLBCL with LDH twice ULN without bulky disease
Low risk	Indolent lymphoma; CLL; chronic phase CML; AML with WBC <25,000; multiple myeloma; solid tumors[a]

[a]TLS is less frequent in solid tumors, though patients with advanced or metastatic disease and those with baselinelike elevations in LDH, potassium, phosphorous, or uric acid may have a higher risk.[1]

ALL, acute lymphoblastic leukemia; AML, acute myelocytic leukemia; CLL, chronic lymphocytic leukemia; CML, chronic myelocytic leukemia; DLBCL, diffuse large B-cell lymphoma; LDH, lactate dehydrogenase; TLS, tumor lysis syndrome; ULN, upper limit of normal; WBC, white blood cell.

Table 59.4 Dosing and Side Effects of Medications for TLS by Risk

Risk for TLS	Medication	Side Effects
Intermediate	Allopurinol up to 300 mg PO BID	Rash, renal insufficiency due to acute interstitial nephritis, elevated liver enzymes
High	Rasburicase 3–6 mg IV once, monitor uric acid	Contraindicated in glucose 6 phosphate dehydrogenase deficiency and pregnant/lactating women. High cost.

BID, twice daily; IV, intravenous; PO, oral; TLS, tumor lysis syndrome.

including renal disease, cardiac disease, and diabetes, can increase risk of TLS. More recently, the use of docetaxel has been recognized to increase risk of TLS in solid tumors, and patients with elevated UA, bulky tumors, or dehydration require monitoring with treatment.

■ PREVENTION

Patients at high or intermediate risk for TLS should be well hydrated and have prevention therapy as detailed in Table 59.4. Urine alkalinization has not been shown to be superior to normal saline. Intermediate-risk patients should be treated with allopurinol for at least 24 to 48 hours prior to initiating therapy. Feboxustat is also available and has been compared to allopurinol, with similar efficacy but at a much higher cost. High-risk patients or those with uric acid >7.5 mg/dL should be treated prophylactically with rasburicase 3 to 6 mg IV, with 3 mg being as efficacious in addressing uric acid levels up to 12 mg/dL.

TREATMENT

Unless anuric, administer aggressive IV hydration with goal urine output 2 mL/kg/hr combined with loop diuretic if volume overload is a concern. Each metabolic derangement, including hyperkalemia, hyperphosphatemia, hypocalcemia, should be treated as clinically indicated. Elevated uric acid should be treated with rasburicase 0.2 mg/kg IV daily or twice daily until normal. Although off label, a fixed dose of rasburicase 6 mg IV is the most commonly utilized regimen for treatment; however, studies have shown that a fixed dose of 3 mg IV can be as effective for patients with baseline uric acid level up to 12 mg/dL and is cost-effective. Hemodialysis or renal replacement is indicated in patients with anuria, refractory hyperkalemia, and symptomatic hypocalcemia.

For those patients who cannot tolerate allopurinol, have an inadequate response with allopurinol, or are without access to rasburicase, another oral selective inhibitor of xanthine oxidase, febuxostat, can be administered. In a meta-analysis comparing rasburicase and febuxostat, both medications had similar response rates, effects on uric-acid levels, and adverse events. The latter does not require dose adjustments for mild/moderate renal impairment, has fewer drug interactions, but does need to be used with caution in the setting of cardiovascular disease.

REFERENCES FOR SUPPLEMENTAL READING

1. Cairo MS, Bishop M. Tumor lysis syndrome: new therapeutic strategies and classification. *Br J Haematol*. 2014;127:3–11.

2. Alakel N, Middeke JM, Schetelig J, et al. Prevention and treatment of tumor lysis syndrome, and the efficacy and role of rasburicase. *Onco Targets Ther*. 2017;10:597–605.

3. Kraus SK, Burdalski CE, Timlin C, et al. A comparison of single dose rasburicase 3 Mg versus 6 Mg for the management of tumor lysis syndrome. *Blood*. 2015;126(23):4511.

4. Bhardwaj S, Varma S. Rare incidence of tumor lysis syndrome in metastatic prostate cancer following treatment with docetaxel. *J Oncol Pharm Pract*. 2018;24(2):153–155.

5. Bellos I, Kontzoglou K, Psyrri A, et al. Febuxostat administration for the prevention of tumour lysis syndrome: a meta-analysis. *J Clin Pharm Ther*. 2019;44(4):525–533.

60   Thrombotic Microangiopathy

Jonathan R. Day, Ljiljana V. Vasovic,
and Ruchika Goel

▓ INTRODUCTION

Thrombotic microangiopathy (TMA) encompasses several overlapping clinical syndromes with different etiologies, based on a common pathologic lesion defined by thrombosis of small-caliber blood vessels (i.e., arterioles and capillaries), resulting in endothelial cell damage. The consequent findings include but are not limited to (a) consumptive thrombocytopenia with purpuric capillary bleeding; (b) microangiopathic hemolytic anemia (MAHA), Coombs negative hemolytic anemia due to increased high shear stress with apparent schistocytes; (c) wide distribution of tissue ischemia with or without neurologic symptoms, including change of mental status and seizures; (d) renal involvement ranging from minimal to acute oliguric renal failure; and (e) fever. The aforementioned five features, collectively known as the "classical pentad," are characteristic of fully developed clinical presentation, nowadays are rarely seen together, and are not required for the diagnosis of TMA. Thrombocytopenia and MAHA alone should raise a clinical concern and initiation of diagnostic testing and empirical therapy. It is important to note that while TMAs almost always cause MAHA, not all MAHAs are due to TMA. By definition, the classic TMAs are hemolytic uremic syndrome (HUS) and thrombotic thrombocytopenic purpura (TTP). Other conditions with TMA include atypical HUS, disseminated intravascular coagulation, sepsis, scleroderma renal crisis, malignant hypertension, pre-eclampsia/HELLP (hemolysis, elevated liver enzymes, low platelet) syndrome, antiphospholipid antibody syndrome, cancer associated TMA, stem cell transplant, drug-induced/toxicity (immune mediated vs. toxicity) (e.g., quinine vs. calcineurin inhibitor toxicity), and cobalamin C defect.

Due to the mortality rate of untreated TMA of >90%, urgent treatment is required and must be tailored to the etiology. As a result, a systematic algorithmic approach is adopted for concurrent management and to distinguish a number of possible and challenging differential diagnoses. Early recognition and low threshold for treatment of TTP is critical for identifying the so-called diad (thrombocytopenia and MAHA) and, with the addition of renal failure, form the "triad" of TMA. A thorough systematic review of preceding symptoms, such as diarrhea, other infectious etiologies, medication history, and obtaining relevant tests promptly facilitate appropriate treatment while possibly avoiding unnecessary and harmful therapy.

▓ PRIMARY TMA SYNDROMES

Primary TMA syndromes include hereditary and acquired specific disorders, including TTP and HUS. With the improving understanding of disease etiology, the classification and nomenclature are continuing to evolve. The histologic findings of TMA include numerous fibrin thrombi and/or platelet aggregates obstructing lumens of capillaries and arterioles. In the case of specific organ involvement, thickening of arteriolar and capillary walls, endothelial swelling/detachment, and subendothelial accumulation of proteins and cell debris are pronounced after endothelial damage due to toxins or complements in HUS.

THROMBOTIC THROMBOCYTOPENIC PURPURA

TTP is a clinical diagnosis supported by finding ≤10% activity of a disintegrin and metalloproteinase with a thrombospondin type 1 motif, member 13 (ADAMTS13). Deficiency of ADAMTS13 leads to accumulation of ultra-large von Willebrand factor (ULVWF) multimers that bind platelets and form microthrombi that initially semi-occlude arterioles, creating high shear stress produced MAHA. The downstream embolization of platelet-von Willebrand factor (vWF) microthrombi in the capillary network perpetuates the pathophysiologic cycle with ischemic change and capillary burst presenting as a purpura, not limited to skin but virtually present in all organs. Deficiency of ADAMTS13 can be hereditary (Upshaw–Schulman syndrome) or acquired as a result of inhibition of ADAMTS13 activity by an autoantibody. TTP usually presents in an acute stetting of profound thrombocytopenia and widely disseminated thrombosis. TTP typically has more systemic manifestations of organ injury than other primary TMA syndromes. In TTP, abnormalities of the central nervous system (CNS), heart, pancreas, thyroid, adrenal glands, intestinal mucosa, and other tissues may occur, typically sparing of the pulmonary system.

HEMOLYTIC UREMIC SYNDROME

HUS was previously broadly classified as "typical/infectious related" or "atypical" (aHUS), depending on the underlying etiology. Despite this nomenclature, there are syndromes that do not fall into this two-tiered classification of HUS and are thus designated as "idiopathic."

- **Typical HUS/Shiga toxin-mediated hemolytic uremic syndrome (ST-HUS)**
  - The typical form of HUS, often referred to as STEC-HUS (for Shiga toxin-producing *Escherichia coli* HUS), is secondary to toxin-producing organisms, such as enterotoxigenic *E. coli* (O157:H7 or O104:H4) or *Shigella dysenteriae*, and clinically

presents with a history of bloody diarrhea in the majority of cases.

- Although most cases are sporadic, large outbreaks related to sanitation issues often occur.

- Shiga toxins cause direct damage to renal epithelium, mesangium, and vascular endothelial cells, leading to oliguria, hematuria, and ultimately kidney failure.

- The typical pathologic picture includes "bloodless" glomeruli, with complete closure of the capillary lumina, endothelial swelling and detachment, and subendothelial accumulation of proteins and cell debris.

- **AHUS/Complement Mediated Thrombotic Microangiopathy (CM-TMA)**

  - aHUS/CM-TMA is due to dysregulation of the alternative pathway of the complement cascade.

  - A hereditary or acquired deficiency of regulatory proteins that normally serve to restrict activation of the alternative pathway of complement (e.g., complement factor H [CFH], complement factor H–related proteins [CFHRs], membrane cofactor protein [MCP, CD46]) or a hereditary abnormality of proteins that accelerate activation of the alternative pathway (e.g., complement factor B [CFB], C3) can lead to uncontrolled activation of complement on cell membranes, including the vascular endothelium and kidney cells, and lead to complement-mediated angiopathy.

- **Idiopathic HUS**

  - This category of HUS is defined by the presence of TMA and absence of a diagnosis of TTP, aHUS/CM-TMA, or any accepted secondary disease association. It is important to recognize that this is a diagnosis of exclusion.

  - This category is only used after genetic screening has ruled out aHUS/CM-TMA, and no secondary association can be identified. Mostly it is a historical diagnosis and generally avoided as more causes become known.

▒ SECONDARY TMA

Disorders such as septicemia, autoimmune disorders (e.g., systemic lupus erythematosus [SLE], antiphospholipid antibody syndrome), streptococcal infections, malignancy, chemotherapy, malignant hypertension, pregnancy/HELLP , and drugs can cause secondary TMA syndromes (*Blood*. 2017;129(21):2857–2863).

- **Drug-induced TMA:** There are two distinct categories of drug-induced TMA (DITMA).

- Immune-mediated
  - Some agents induce the formation of drug-dependent antibodies that react with platelets, neutrophils, endothelial cells, and/or other cells.
  - Ticlopidine and quinine are prototypic medications implicated in TMA that presents with severe acute kidney injury. Other agents include oxaliplatin, adalimumab, antimicrobial drugs, and quetiapine.
- Nonimmune or dose-dependent/toxicity-mediated
  - A variety of medications can cause acute or chronic dose-dependent, toxicity-induced TMA syndromes due to direct cellular damage.
  - Dose-dependent, toxicity-induced TMA is primarily caused by multiple classes of drugs, which are chemotherapeutic agents (such as gemcitabine and mitomycin), immunosuppressive agents (such as cyclosporine and tacrolimus), vascular endothelial growth factor (VEGF) inhibitors (such as sirolimus and bevacizumab), narcotics (such as oxymorphone), interferons, and illicit drugs (cocaine).
  - Gemcitabine may cause DITMA by both immune-mediated or dose-dependent, toxicity-mediated mechanisms.

- **Transplant-associated TMA**
  - TMA may occur following allogeneic or autologous hematopoietic stem cell transplant (allo- or auto-HSCT), although it is very rare after autologous transplant.
  - The etiology can include radiation during the conditioning regimen, administration of a calcineurin inhibitor for graft-versus-host disease (GVHD) prevention, and/or cytotoxic chemotherapy.
  - Patients usually present with gradual onset of MAHA with thrombocytopenia and gradually elevated serum creatinine.
  - Post-transplant TMA is a clinical diagnosis, and systemic infection (e.g., sepsis and disseminated intravascular coagulopathy [DIC]) must be excluded.
  - The consensus statement of the Bone Marrow Transplant Clinical Trials Network proposed MAHA with thrombocytopenia along with renal and/or neurologic involvement in the defining criteria.
  - Immediate discontinuation of the implicated drugs, such as calcineurin inhibitors (e.g., cyclosporine, tacrolimus), is essential.
  - The management of post-transplant TMA is largely supportive, and therapeutic plasma exchange (TPE) in post-transplant TMA is generally not effective.
  - Some patients recover following the discontinuation of calcineurin inhibitors alone, but other patients have progressive

disease with ongoing hemolysis and worsening organ dysfunction, resulting in poor overall long-term prognoses.

▦ DIAGNOSTIC EVALUATION

The basic initial evaluation of TMA is focused on confirming that the patient has thrombocytopenia and MAHA, which is suggested by the complete blood count (CBC) with the presence of thrombocytopenia and anemia and a significant amount of schistocytes on the patient's peripheral blood smear. Laboratory findings of intravascular hemolysis include an elevated plasma lactate dehydrogenase (LDH), reduced (or undetectable) plasma haptoglobin level with increased indirect bilirubin, plasma aspartate aminotransferase (AST), and plasma-free hemoglobin seen in severe cases. The direct antiglobulin (DAT), or direct Coombs test, is negative, except in *Streptococcus pneumoniae*–associated HUS (*Nephron*. 1999;82:183–184). Prothrombin time (PT) and partial thromboplastin time (PTT) are normal, and elevation might be present due to other comorbidities or point toward DIC. The blood urea nitrogen/creatinine levels and their relative rates of increase, hyperkalemia, presence of proteinuria, hematuria, and urine output must be monitored and/or evaluated. ADAMTS13 activity and inhibitor status should be ordered to confirm TTP diagnosis. It is important to remember that drawing blood for analyzing ADAMTS13 level and activity testing *must* be done prior to plasma infusion, as it is important to avoid potentially false-positive results. IgG inhibitors are found in a high proportion of ADAMTS13-deficient patients. Based on mixing studies, only 80% to 90% of autoimmune TTP patients have detectable inhibitors at presentation. However, more than 90% manifest inhibitors at some time during their clinical course. Enzyme-linked immunosorbent assay (ELISA) autoantibody assays have higher sensitivity than mixing studies but may yield false-positive results in 5% to 10% of individuals without autoimmune TTP. Detectable IgG inhibitor exists as more of a continuum, and inhibitor levels may vary in each patient.

One may also consider complement testing, though normal levels do not exclude CM-TMA (CH50, C3, C4, C4d, and other complement tests). Other testing may be ordered based on findings from history and physical, such as stool culture for *E. coli* O157:H7 or O104:H4, and Shiga toxin stool PCR if bloody diarrhea presents (*Mayo Clin Proc*. 2016;91(9):1189–1211).

After the initial workup, it is imperative to identify which TMA syndrome(s) is/are most likely present and initiate appropriate treatment. Even though the turnaround time for ADAMTS13 testing can be several days, it is essential to confirm the diagnosis of TTP. This confirmation should NOT delay plasma exchange/infusion, as it should be initiated based on a presumptive clinical diagnosis. One may calculate a PLASMIC score (see Table 60.1) to determine likelihood of severe ADAMTS deficiency in an adult. (*Lancet Haematol*. 2017;4(4):e157–e164).

Table 60.1 PLASMIC Score Calculation for Severe ADAMTS13 Deficiency in Adults

PLASMIC Score	Points
Platelet count <30 K cells/mcL	1
Evidence of hemolysis (any of the below)	1
Reticulocyte count >2.5%	
Undetectable haptoglobin	
Indirect bilirubin >2 mg/dL	
No active cancer	1
MCV <90 fL	1
INR <1.5	1
Creatinine <2.0 mg/dL	1

Interpretation: 0–4 points = Low risk of severe ADAMTS13 deficiency; 5 points = intermediate risk of ADAMTS13 deficiency; 6–7 points = High risk of ADAMTS13 deficiency.

ADAMTS13, a disintegrin and metalloproteinase with a thrombospondin type 1 motif, member 13; INR, International Normalized Ratio; MCV, Mean Corpuscular Volume.

Source: Based on Bendapudi PK, Hurwitz S, Fry A, et al. Derivation and external validation of the PLASMIC score for rapid assessment of adults with thrombotic microangiopathies: a cohort study. *Lancet Haematol.* 2017;4(4):e157–e164.

Importantly, not all MAHA is caused by TMA. Other disorders to consider in the differential diagnosis that may manifest similar TMA findings include myelofibrosis, a metastatic malignancy infiltrating bone marrow; mechanical heart valve effect; extracorporeal membrane oxygenation (ECMO); dialysis; and malignant hypertension. If MAHA is not present, other acute systemic illnesses associated with pancytopenia must be considered (e.g., aplastic anemia, hemophagocytic lymphohistiocytosis [HLH], paroxysmal nocturnal hemoglobinuria [PNH], and SLE in adults).

The following clinical features can be used as distinguishing features among the primary TMA syndromes:

- **Patient age**
  - Infants/young children: Coagulation and metabolism-mediated TMAs typically present in infants. Children more commonly present with ST-HUS, *S. pneumoniae* associated HUS (SP-HUS), complement-mediated TMA (hereditary or acquired), hereditary TTP, or hereditary metabolism mediated. Acquired TTP is rare in infants and young children.
  - Adults: Adults can be affected with any of the acquired or hereditary TMA syndromes. However, adults more commonly present with acquired TTP, DITMA, and hereditary complement-mediated TMA.

- **Kidney injury**
  - All the primary TMAs can be associated with some kidney injury.
  - However, the degree/severity of injury may be a helpful distinguishing feature.
    - Minimal to no kidney injury: Typically supports a diagnosis of hereditary or acquired TTP.
    - Sudden, severe kidney injury: Sudden onset acute kidney injury, especially when associated with anuria, supports DITMA.
    - Slow progressive kidney injury: Following several days of abdominal pain and diarrhea is characteristic of ST-HUS, complement-mediated TMA, or metabolism-mediated or coagulation-mediated TMA.
    - Very gradual onset of kidney injury: Over weeks to months may be seen in patients with DITMA caused by toxic chemotherapeutic or immunosuppressive drugs.
- **Other factors**
  - Change in mental status, myocardial infarction (MI), petechiae on the skin, and other systemic presentations are most common in TTP and other TMA compared to HUS.

TREATMENT

THROMBOTIC THROMBOCYTOPENIC PURPURA

Initiating empiric and urgent TPE treatment for suspected TTP is of paramount importance. The decision to treat is based on clinical judgment, because ADAMTS13 results are often not available for several days. Urgent plasma infusion should be initiated while preparations are underway for TPE. To avoid potential false-positive results, blood for ADAMTS13 levels and activity should be drawn prior to any plasma infusion. TPE has advantage over plasma infusions by providing a large amount of ADAMTS13 and concurrently removing the inhibitor. Optimal therapy for TTP is still based on TPE by using at least one plasma volume (PV) exchange with fresh frozen plasma over a 5- to 7-day course until platelet count reaches above 150×10^9/L for 2 consecutive days. LDH and hemoglobin levels should be substantially normalized for several days. Inhibitor strength may affect initial response to TPE, but the titer does not necessarily define prognosis (i.e., time to remission and/or relapse), because it may change over time. While TPE is the backbone, most patients are also treated with steroids. Additional therapies vary greatly by institutional practice; some may also receive rituximab upfront or as treatment for refractory disease, and high-risk cases may receive caplacizumab. Rituximab upfront in combination with steroids, when studied against historical controls, had lower remission rates and shorter hospitalizations. Rituximab as treatment for refractory disease showed higher rates of recovery and lower relapse rates. Timing of rituximab administration should be considered, as 60% to 70% are removed by TPE. Caplacizumab is a an anti–von Willebrand factor humanized, bivalent variable-domain-only immunoglobulin fragment, which inhibits interaction between von Willebrand factor multimers and platelets. Use of caplacizumab may be considered based on the recent HERCULES trial showing a faster normalization of platelet count; 74% lower risk of a composite of TTP-related death, recurrence, or a major thromboembolic event; decreased number of TPE days; and less time in the hospital (*N Engl J Med*. 2019;380(4):335–346). Other treatments currently under investigation include recombinant ADAMTS13, Anfibatide, Bortezomib, *N*-acetylcysteine, and IgG-degrading enzymes.

Standardization of disease definition, management, and response evaluation for TTP are as follows: Treatment response is defined as platelet count above 150×10^9/L for 2 consecutive days, accompanied by normal or normalizing LDH and stable or improving neurologic deficits. Durable treatment response is defined as treatment response that lasts at least 30 days after discontinuation of plasma exchange. Exacerbation is defined as recurrent disease within 30 days after reaching treatment response. Relapse is recurrent disease 30 days or longer after reaching treatment response. Refractory disease occurs when there is no treatment response by day 30 and/or no durable treatment response by day 60. For known hereditary TTP, infusion of plasma alone is sufficient treatment. If it is not known, TPE also replaces ADAMTS13 and should not be withheld. Future treatments may include recombinant ADAMTS13 infusions, which have shown promise in vitro and in mouse models.

AHUS/CM-TMA

The treatment of aHUS is broadly divided into plasma therapy or eculizumab. Plasma therapy (plasma exchange/infusion) was essentially the primary and only therapy available for a long time for aHUS. TPE delivers normal levels of CFH, complement factor I (CFI), and C3 and also removes mutant CFH, CFI, CFB, C3, and anti-CFH antibodies via apheresis. The treatment of aHUS/CM-TMA has changed drastically with the addition of eculizumab (C5-targeted monoclonal antibody [mAb] inhibiting terminal complement activation) to the armamentarium of agents and is now first line for treatment of aHUS/CM-TMA (*N Engl J Med*. 2013;368(23):2169–2181). The recommended schedule is initial weekly induction therapy, which transitions to every other week. Effectiveness of Eculizumab in aHUS both before end-stage renal disease (ESRD) and after kidney transplantation has been recognized. Eculizumab prevents the recurrence of TMA during treatment, improves renal function, allows discontinuation of chronic TPE/

plasma infusion, and is well tolerated. Some data suggest that eculizumab may be discontinued in patients with favorable responses and reinitiated if relapses occur; risk of relapse is higher in patients with CFH and CD46 mutation. The major concern with eculizumab treatment is the risk for infection with encapsulated bacterial organisms, particularly *Neisseria meningitidis*, as a result of terminal complement blockade. Therefore, patients must receive meningococcal vaccination before being treated with eculizumab (and covered with appropriate antibiotics for 14 days if there is not enough time to wait for the immune response). Ideally, patients should also receive the pneumococcal and *Haemophilus influenzae* vaccinations before dosing. The worldwide use of anti-C5 mAb continues to be limited by its very high price.

If eculizumab is not readily available, plasma therapy should be initiated within 24 hours of a presumed diagnosis of aHUS and is proposed to be only about 70% effective in achieving hematologic remission. Renal remission is less predictable and may depend on the time lapse from disease onset to initiation of therapy. As genetic testing is typically not available at initial presentation, plasmapheresis may be started. Plasma infusions or exchange should be performed daily until the platelet count, LDH, and hemoglobin levels are substantially improved or even normalized or until an alternate treatment strategy has been decided upon. Renal function is an important marker to follow during the use of plasma therapy, especially in the setting of acute kidney injury. However, care must be taken to not use the serum creatinine level to guide plasma therapy when the patient may have irreversible renal injury. Persistence of hemolysis or lack of improvement in thrombocytopenia after 3 to 5 days of plasma therapy should be considered as nonresponse to therapy and is an indication to discontinue plasma exchange and begin eculizumab.

ARE THERE TTP OR TTP-LIKE DISORDERS WHEN TPE SHOULD NOT BE USED?

The differential diagnosis of TTP is often very challenging. However, because of the overlap in clinical presentation and high mortality among patients with TTP, there are some conditions where early initiation of TPE is ineffective and possibly harmful. TMA patients without severe ADAMTS13 deficiency do not benefit from TPE. For example, Shiga-toxin-associated HUS (STx-HUS) has not been shown to respond to TPE; thus, it should not be attempted in these patients. MCP deficiency does not respond to TPE, because MCP protein is not a plasma protein. Importantly, In DAT+, SP-HUS, plasma can be harmful and washed red blood cells (RBCs) should be provided. Thus, it is important to recognize TMA and rapidly initiate appropriate laboratory testing to aid in the diagnosis.

◼ REFERENCES FOR SUPPLEMENTAL READING

1. George JN, Nester CM. Syndromes of thrombotic microangiopathy. *N Engl J Med*. 2014;371(7):654–666.

2. Kremer Hovinga J, Coppo P, Lämmle B, et al. Thrombotic thrombocytopenic purpura. *Nat Rev Dis Primers*. 2017;3:17020. doi: 10.1038/nrdp.2017.20

3. Scully M, Cataland S, Coppo P, et al. Consensus on the standardization of terminology in thrombotic thrombocytopenic purpura and related thrombotic microangiopathies. *J Thromb Haemost*. 2017;15(2):312–322. doi: 10.1111/jth.13571

4. Sarode R, Bandarenko N, Brecher ME, et al. Thrombotic thrombocytopenic purpura: 2012 American Society for Apheresis (ASFA) consensus conference on classification, diagnosis, management, and future research. *J Clin Apher*. 2014;29(3):148–167.

5. Masias C, Vasu S, Cataland SR. None of the above: thrombotic microangiopathy beyond TTP and HUS. *Blood*. 2017;129(21):2857–2863. doi: 10.1182/blood-2016-11-743104

Therapeutic Apheresis Indications

Ljiljana V. Vasovic, Jonathan R. Day,
and Ruchika Goel

▨ INTRODUCTION

Therapeutic apheresis is a medical procedure in which whole blood is withdrawn from a patient and separated extracorporeally to remove a pathologic component, and remaining blood components are returned to the patient with an appropriate replacement to maintain euvolemia. In hematologic emergencies necessitating the procedure, the appropriate compartments may be removed, including white blood cells (WBCs), leukocytapheresis, red blood cells (RBCs), erythrocytapheresis, platelets thrombocytapheresis, or plasma plasmapheresis/therapeutic plasma exchange (TPE). Common indications for apheresis in hematologic malignancies are categorized according to the American Society for Apheresis (ASFA) 2019 recommendations, as outlined in Table 61.1.

▨ THERAPEUTIC APHERESIS INDICATIONS IN HEMATOLOGIC MALIGNANCIES

HYPERLEUKOCYTOSIS

Hyperleukocytosis occurs when peripheral WBC or leukemic blast counts are >100 × 10^9/L, putting patients at risk for leukostasis in small vessels. This is seen in cases of patients with acute myelogenous leukemia (AML) with blast counts >100 × 10^9/L and in acute lymphoblastic leukemia (ALL) with blast counts >400 × 10^9/L. The higher counts in ALL are tolerable due to the smaller size, more deformability, and less "sticky" and pro-inflammatory properties of lymphoblasts than myeloblasts. The myelomonocytic and monocytic/monoblastic subtypes of AML have an increased risk of leukostasis, making leukocytapheresis potentially indicated when blast counts are >50 × 10^9/L. Leukostasis presents clinically as central nervous system (CNS) and/or pulmonary disturbances, including dizziness, confusion, somnolence, headache, visual disturbances, coma, respiratory distress, hypoxemia, pulmonary infiltrates, or parenchymal hemorrhage. Hyperleukocytosis in AML is initially treated with temporary cytoreductive agents, such as hydroxyurea/cytarabine, along with IV hydration, electrolyte correction, urine alkalization, and allopurinol to lower plasma uric acid. Coagulopathies must be managed as appropriate. Packed RBC transfusion should be avoided, as it may worsen hyperviscosity. Hyperleukocytosis in AML or ALL "with symptoms" of leukostasis is a Category I indication for leuko-cytapheresis. If blast counts are high, but no symptoms are present, the indication becomes Category III. However, in AML cases with

Table 61.1 Hematologic Malignancy-Related Therapeutic Apheresis Emergencies

Disease Entity	Therapeutic Apheresis Modality	Disease Condition	Category*	Grade†
Hyperleuko-cytosis	Leukocytapher-esis	1. Symptomatic leukostasis	II	2B
		AML blast count >100 × 10⁹/L		
		ALL blast count >400 × 10⁹/L		
		2. Prophylaxis	III	2C
Thrombocy-tosis	Thrombocyta-pheresis	1. Symptomatic with platelets >1,000–1, 500 × 10⁹/L	II	2C
		2. Prophylaxis or Secondary	II	2C
Polycythe-mia vera and eryth-rocytosis	Erythrocyta-pheresis	Polycythemia vera	I	1B
		Secondary erythrocytosis	III	1C
Hypervis-cosity in monoclonal gammopa-thies	TPE	1. Symptomatic	I	1B
		2. Prophylaxis for rituximab	I	1C
Cryoglobu-linemia	TPE	Symptomatic/ severe	II	2A
	IA	Symptomatic/ severe	II	2B
Thrombotic thrombo-cytopenic purpura	TPE	Microangiopathic hemolytic anemia	I	1A
Thrombotic microan-giopathy, drug-associated	TPE	Ticlopidine	I	2B
	TPE	Clopidogrel	III	2B
	TPE	Gemcitabine/ Quinidine	IV	2C

(continued)

Table 61.1 Hematologic Malignancy-Related Therapeutic Apheresis Emergencies (continued)

Disease Entity	Therapeutic Apheresis Modality	Disease Condition	Category*	Grade†
Thrombotic microan-giopathy, HSCT- asso-ciated	TPE	Refractory/salvage therapy	III	2C

*ASFA Category: I, apheresis is accepted as first-line therapy; II, apheresis is accepted as second-line therapy; III, optimum role of apheresis therapy is not established; IV, apheresis may be ineffective or harmful. †ASFA grade recommendation: 1, strong recommendation; 2, weak recommendation. Evidence quality: A, high-quality evidence; B, moderate-quality evidence; C, low-quality or very low-quality evidence.

ALL, acute lymphoblastic leukemia; AML, acute myeloid leukemia; HSCT, hematopoietic stem cell transplant; IA, immunoadsorption; TPE, therapeutic plasma exchange.

Source: Modified from *ASFA Therapeutic Apheresis—Guidelines 2019*.

rapidly increasing blast counts >100 × 10^9/L and in myelomonocytic and monocytic subtypes, apheresis may be beneficial regardless of lack of leukostasis symptoms, given the high risk of these groups for precipitating complications. One procedure typically decreases the WBC count by up to 60%. The procedure is repeated daily until leukostasis symptoms resolve and blast count is <50 × 10^9/L in AML patients and <400 × 10^9/L in ALL patients.

THROMBOCYTOSIS

Thrombocytosis occurs either in the primary setting of myeloproliferative disorders (MPDs) or in the secondary setting as a reactive process to another underlying condition. Unlike in secondary/reactive processes, primary thrombocytosis is due to abnormal platelet clones with compromise of their normal function, thus leading to risk for thrombotic/hemorrhagic events. Although all MPDs can exhibit primary thrombocytosis, essential thrombocythemia (ET) is the most frequent presenting primary cause and is associated with rates of thromboembolism of 1.9% to 3% per patient per year. These events include cerebral vascular accidents, myocardial infarcts, and first-trimester pregnancy loss. Mucocutaneous bleeding is also seen in one-third of ET patients due to defects in platelet aggregation, and acquired von Willebrand syndrome may occur in patients with very high platelet counts >1,500 × 10^9/L. Nonemergent management of thrombocytosis in ET is handled by low-dose aspirin, hydroxyurea, or interferon-α/anagrelide in pregnant patients. Thrombocytapheresis is indicated in extreme thrombocytosis of >1,500 × 10^9/L and hemorrhage or acute thromboembolism in addition to the previously mentioned initial acute treatments and thus, is used as an adjuvant therapy (Category II). It is also indicated when antiplatelet agents are ineffective, in cases of extreme rebound thrombocytosis status postsplenectomy, in high-risk pregnancy with history of recurrent fetal loss, or in pregnant women in whom hydroxyurea is contraindicated and who are refractive to alternative cytoreductive agents. If emergent surgery is needed in a patient with primary thrombocytosis, thrombocytapheresis can also be utilized to rapidly return platelet levels to normal for prevention of postsurgical bleeding risk and rebound thrombocytosis. Treatment should be performed daily until the platelet counts normalize in addition to the cytoreductive agents. Usually, 1.5 to 2 times the total blood volume (TBV) is processed, and one procedure can reduce platelets up to 60%. Saline replacement fluid is used with the citrate anticoagulant, while heparin should be avoided to prevent ex vivo platelet clumping.

HYPER-PARAPROTEINEMIA

Monoclonal gammopathies can lead to hyperviscosity, particularly in Waldenström macroglobulinemia, with Immunoglobulin M (IgM) paraproteins ≥3 g/dL in the plasma. It can also be seen in multiple myeloma, with monoclonal Immunoglobulin G_3 ≥3 g/dL and Immunoglobulin A ≥6 to 7 g/dL. While serum viscosity >4 centipoise (cp) is considered to be a risk factor for hyperviscosity (normal: 1.4–1.8 cp), the actual manifestation of in vivo viscosity is more variable. However, viscosity >6 cp has been shown to be associated with hyperviscosity symptoms more consistently. These symptoms are similar to the previously mentioned cases of rheologic compromise with CNS and pulmonary compromise, retinal vessel changes, congestive heart failure (CHF), and coagulopathic changes. The rise in viscosity leads to a logarithmic rise in shearing stress on small vessel walls. While patients with Waldenström macroglobulinemia may be simply monitored if there is a low level of involvement by lymphoplasmacytic lymphoma in the marrow, those with hematologic aberrancies and constitutional symptoms are treated with cytoreductive agents, including rituximab. When these patients also show hyperviscosity symptoms, they should undergo plasmapheresis, or TPE, prior to cytoreductive medications. Because up to 50% of patients falling in the latter group experience a "flare" increase of IgM in the first 4 weeks following rituximab initiation as compared to their baseline level, prophylactic TPE may be helpful to avoid precipitating hyperviscosity symptoms. When IgM ≥5 g/dL, TPE should be performed prior to initiating rituximab. Due to the nonlinear relationship of the amount of monoclonal immunoglobulins to in vivo blood viscosity, TPE may be performed at relatively lower volumes as compared to other indications, with 1.0 to 1.5 total plasma volume (TPV) recommended. There is a significant viscosity decrease with as little as one procedure, with reversal of retinal changes reported in many studies. TPE can be performed daily until acute symptoms abate and then weekly for up to 4 weeks as a bridge to a more definitive treatment of the underlying condition. Immunoglobulin levels and clinical symptoms should be monitored to assess the efficacy of treatment. Serum viscosity studies can be followed to assess the level at which patients are no longer are hyperviscous.

OTHER EMERGENT INDICATIONS

Emergent red blood cell exchange, or erythrocytapheresis, is indicated in patients with sickle cell disease who present with acute stroke (Category I) and acute chest syndrome (Category II). Thrombotic thrombocytopenic purpura is a Category I indication for TPE with plasma as replacement fluid. However, hematopoietic stem cell transplant–associated thrombotic microangiopathy (TMA) is a Category III indication. These conditions and their corresponding treatments are discussed in Table 61.1 and in further detail in their respective chapters.

▓ PRACTICAL CONSIDERATIONS

The first consideration upon considering apheresis is contacting the apheresis team to schedule the procedure, order blood components, and evaluate vascular access, processes that commonly are the rate-limiting steps in beginning treatment. Two lines of access are required, one for withdrawal and one for fluid return, either peripheral usually antecubital veins or dual lumen catheters. These must be rigid, with Hickman and most dialysis-type catheters meeting this requirement. Central venous catheters can also be utilized. Femoral lines should only be used for short course procedures due to a higher risk of bacterial contamination. Subclavian or internal jugular veins are typically preferred for procedures requiring several weeks, and tunneled catheters are better for long-term or indefinite procedures. If available, arteriovenous fistulas may be used by experienced personnel. In general, two-thirds of any substance are removed per apheresis procedure; however, this amount varies, depending on the intravascular/extravascular distribution of a substance and other factors. Hence, usually 1.5 to 2 times the patient's blood or plasma volume are removed in procedures, with 85% to nearly 100% of the volume replaced with appropriate blood products or colloid fluid to maintain hemodynamic stability. For leukocytapheresis, an erythrocyte sedimenting agent, such as 6% hydroxyethyl starch, can be added to help separate WBC from RBC, but it is not required. Laboratory testing for the amount of pathologic component present should be evaluated prior to the initial exchange procedure in order to establish a baseline and allow for accurate monitoring of treatment efficacy. Medications that are mostly protein bound may be significantly diminished after apheresis. The subtherapeutic levels of drugs can be very harmful (e.g., precipitate seizures in the case of anticonvulsants or allograft rejection in the case of immunosuppressants in post-transplant patients). Thus, it is prudent to administer all scheduled medications "after" a plasma exchange procedure.

ADVERSE EFFECTS

The majority of side effects are related to citrate, the main anticoagulant in replacement fluid. Citrate chelates calcium, leading to hypocalcemia presenting as perioral/acral paresthesia, occasionally nausea, and rarely tetany and arrhythmias. These symptoms can be alleviated or prevented with supplemental calcium in the form of oral tablets or IV infusion of 10% calcium gluconate in normal saline. In some patients, heparin may be the anticoagulant of choice. In some cases, plasma is needed as a colloidal replacement rather than 5% albumin. This is particularly the case in some emergent conditions, such as thrombotic thrombocytopenic purpura, in which factors within the replaced plasma are needed to alleviate the disease sequelae, and in patients with coagulopathies, such as hepatic dysfunction. Aside from needing time to obtain ABO-compatible plasma from the blood bank, other concerns with using plasma include increased chance of allergic reactions and anaphylaxis in patients on angiotensin-converting enzyme (ACE) inhibitors due to bradykinin accumulation. In the latter case, patients should discontinue ACE inhibitors up to 3 days prior to treatment if possible, and in emergent cases, patients should be pretreated with antihistamines and possibly steroids. Most allergic reactions are mild, presenting as urticarial reactions, and pretreatment with IV diphenhydramine will suffice in patients with histories of reaction during apheresis procedures.

REFERENCES FOR SUPPLEMENTAL READING

1. Davenport RD. Therapeutic apheresis. In: Fung MK, Grossman BJ, Hillyer CD, eds. *Technical Manual.* 18th ed. AABB Press; 2014:645–664.

2. McLeod BC, Szczepiorkowski ZM, Weinstein R, et al., eds. *Apheresis: Principles and Practice.* 3rd ed. AABB Press; 2010:229–262.

3. Simon TL, Snyder EL, Solheim BG, et al., eds. *Rossi's Principles of Transfusion Medicine.* 4th ed. Wiley-Blackwell; 2009:629–662.

4. Porcu P, Cripe LD, Ng EW, et al. Hyperleukocytic luekemias and leukostasis: a review of pathophysiology, clinical presentation and management. *Leuk Lymphoma.* 2000;39:1–18.

5. Padmanabhan A, Connelly-Smith L, Aqui N, et al. Guidelines on the use of therapeutic apheresis in clinical practice—evidence-based approach from the writing committee of the American Society for Apheresis: the Eighth Special Issue. *J Clin Apher.* 2019;34(3):171–354. doi: 10.1002/jca.21705

62 Challenging Case Vignettes With Follow-Up Questions

▨ INTRODUCTION

As evidenced throughout this second edition, critical in the diagnostic workup is morphological assessment, even in the setting of
advanced molecular techniques. In an effort to solidify knowledge
from key chapters in this handbook as well as provide additional high-
resolution pathologic figures, we have included the following 10
cases. Importantly, questions also focus on critical next steps in
management, with board-style questions. As novel cellular therapy
with chimeric antigen receptor T-cells has brought forth a paradigm change in hematologic malignancies, we also have included
a case evaluating cytokine release syndrome, which is the most significant and frequent adverse event observed with these therapies.
Additionally, please see https://connect.springerpub.com/content/
book/978-0-8261-4977-0, where access to additional cases covering
the majority of chapters can be found from the first edition.

■ CASE 1

CASE PRESENTATION

A 57-year-old female with a past medical history of hypothyroidism is referred to your clinic by her primary care physician after her blood work was notable for leukopenia during a routine physical exam.

Laboratory data are notable for a WBC 2.9 L/mcL (ANC of 493), hemoglobin of 10.1 g/dL, and platelets of 116 k/mcL.

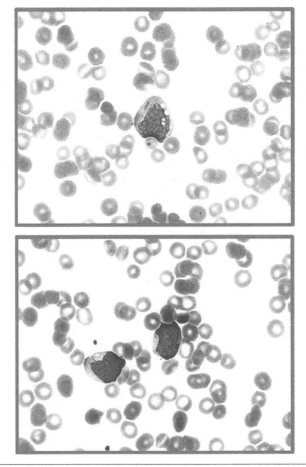

Figure 62.1 Peripheral smear is as shown. Flow cytometry on peripheral blasts is positive for CD13, CD33, CD34, CD117, HLA-DR.

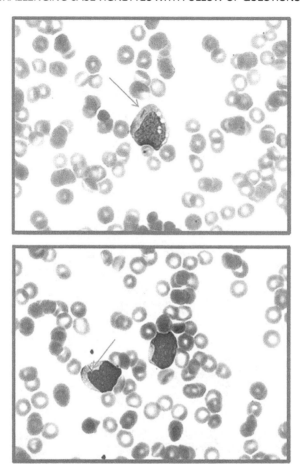

Figure 62.2 Peripheral smear is as shown with arrows.

1. **Based on the flow cytometry and above peripheral smear findings, what is the most likely diagnosis?**
   A. Acute lymphoblastic leukemia
   B. Chronic myelogenous leukemia
   C. Chronic lymphocytic leukemia with Richter's transformation
   D. Large granular lymphocytic leukemia
   E. Acute myeloid leukemia

   Explanation **E**. On flow cytometry, AML blasts most commonly express CD13, CD33, CD34, CD117, and HLA-DR. Review of peripheral blood is notable for Auer rods (blue arrows), which are azurophilic granules in the cytoplasm of leukemic blasts. They are commonly seen in acute myeloblastic leukemia with maturation (FAB M2) and acute promyelocytic leukemia (FAB M3).

BONE MARROW ASPIRATE AND BIOPSY

2. **Based on the FAB (French-American-British) classification, what subtype of AML is most consistent with the findings in Figure 62.3?**

   A. M2 (Acute myeloblastic with maturation)
   B. M3 (Acute promyelocytic leukemia)
   C. M4eos (Acute myelomonocytic leukemia with eosinophilia)
   D. M5 (Acute monocytic leukemia)
   E. M6 (Acute erythroid leukemia)

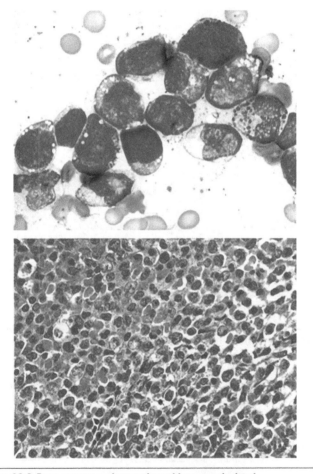

Figure 62.3 Bone marrow aspirate and core biopsy are depicted.

Explanation C. Bone marrow aspirate and biopsy are notable for numerous mye-loblasts admixed with eosinophils consistent with acute myelomonocytic leukemia with eosinophilia (M4eos). Top Panel: The Wright-Giemsa stained bone marrow aspirate smear consists of many large blasts, some containing azurophilic cytoplas-mic granules (myeloblasts), and some displaying convoluted or folded nuclei. Lacy chromatin and cytoplasmic vacuoles (monoblasts and promonocytes) are admixed with eosinophils, including dark or basophilic rough granules, mixed basophilic and eosinophilic granules, or red to orange granules in their cytoplasm, respec-tively. This indicates a different stage of maturation, characteristic of acute myelo-monocytic leukemia with eosinophilia (×1,000). Bottom Panel: A section of bone marrow biopsy shows sheets of nonocleated immature precursors/blasts with fine chromatin and high N:C ratio as well as many eosinophils and their precursors, rich in orange color cytoplasmic granules (H&E ×600).

3. **Based on the WHO classification, presence of which mutation is diagnostic of AML?**

   A. t(9;11)(p22;q23); *MLLT3-MLL*
   B. t(8;21)(q22;q22); *RUNX1-RUNX1T1*
   C. t(1;22)(p13;q13); *RBM15-MKL1*
   D. t(3;3)(q21;q26.2); *RPN1-EVI1*
   E. None of the above. A diagnosis of AML requires ≥20% blasts in the bone marrow or peripheral blood.

   Explanation B. Per WHO guidelines, a diagnosis of AML requires the presence of ≥20% blasts in the bone marrow or peripheral blood. However, the presence of certain genetic abnormalities, such as t(8;21), inv(16), or t(15;17), and myeloid sarcoma are diagnostic of AML, irrespective of bone marrow findings.

4. **What is the most common genetic abnormality associated with this type of leukemia?**

   A. t(15;17) (q24.1;q21.1); *PML-RARA*
   B. t(9;11) (p22;q23); *MLLT3-MLL*
   C. t(1;22) (p13;q13); *RBM15-MKL1*
   D. t(9;11) (p22;q23); *MLLT3-MLL*
   E. t(16;16)(p13.1q22); *CBFB-MYH11*

   Explanation E. Abnormalities of inv(16) or t(16;16) are seen in approximately 5% of patients with AML. This genetic abnormality is typically found in patients with acute myelomonocytic leukemia with eosinophilia (AML, FAB M4eo) and confers a good prognosis.

A patient is noted to have a normal karyotype, and cytogenetics are notable for inv(16). Molecular studies are notable for a biallelic CEBPA mutation and *FLT3-ITD* wild-type.

5. **What is the patient's risk status based on the information above?**

   A. Intermediate risk
   B. Intermediate-1 risk
   C. Poor risk
   D. Favorable risk

Explanation **D**. Presence of a core binding factor—inv(16) or t(16;16) on cytogenetics or a biallalic *CEBPA* mutation in the absence of a *FLT3-ITD* mutation—confers a good prognosis, and those patients are classified as having favorable risk.

6. **Which of the following confers the worst prognosis in AML?**

   A. Isolated biallelic *CEBPA* mutation
   B. *NPM1* mutation in absence of *FLT3-ITD* mutation with normal cytogenetics
   C. t(15;17) (q24.1;q21.1); *PML-RARA*
   D. *FLT3-ITD* mutation with normal cytogenetics
   E. t(8;21)

   Explanation **D**. With the exception of D, all other choices are associated with good-risk AML. FLT-3 mutations tend to correlate with intermediate to adverse prognoses.

The patient received induction chemotherapy with 7 + 3 (Cytarabine 100 mg/m² and Daunorubicin 90 mg/m²). Day 14 bone marrow biopsy revealed <5% blasts. Day 30 bone marrow shows a nomocellular marrow with <5% blasts. CBC shows WBC 4.8 L/mcL (ANC of 2,500), hemoglobin of 12.5 g/dL, and platelets of 130 k/mcL.

7. **What is the next step in managing this patient?**

   A. Referral for an autologous stem cell transplant
   B. Consolidation chemotherapy with Cytarabine 3 g/m² × 3–4 cycles
   C. Induction with CLAG (Cladrabine, Cytarabine, G-CSF ± Mitoxantrone) chemotherapy
   D. Referral for an allogeneic stem cell transplant
   E. Consolidation with Cytarabine 3 g/m² × 3–4 cycles followed by allogeneic stem cell transplant

   Explanation **B**. Patient had good response to induction chemotherapy, and this 30-day marrow is suggestive of complete remission (defined as bone marrow blasts <5%, absolute neutrophil count ≥1.0 × 10⁹/L, and platelet count ≥100 × 10⁹/L). Favorable-risk patients should receive consolidation with high-dose cytarabine chemotherapy and do not need a hematopoietic stem cell transplant in CR1. Allogeneic stem cell transplant is reserved for those who have high-risk disease or those with relapsed disease.

▒ CASE 2

CASE PRESENTATION

- A 60-year-old female presents with intermittent symptoms of watery diarrhea, skin rash, abdominal cramping, and facial flushing over the past year.
- An infectious workup for the diarrhea has been negative. The patient also reports a 10 lb weight loss over the past year.

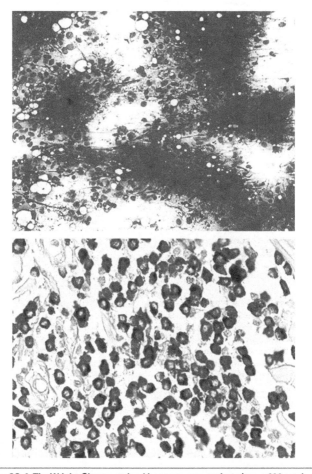

Figure 62.4 The Wright-Giemsa stained bone marrow aspirate (top, ×600 total magnification) and a toluidine blue-stained touch imprint (bottom, ×600 total magnification) highlighted many atypical spindled cells with red-purple cytoplasmic granules (metachromatic staining).

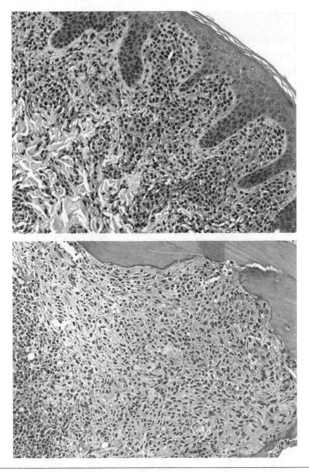

Figure 62.5 The H&E sections of the skin lesion demonstrated a diffuse cellular infiltrate in the reticular dermis (top, ×200 total magnification) as well as bone marrow involvement (bottom, ×200 total magnification). The cells display round to oval, hyperchromatic, spindled nuclei and abundant cytoplasm associated with scattered eosinophils.

- A colonoscopy was performed, with biopsies showing areas of dense mast cell aggregates.
- A CBC showed normal WBC count with mild eosinophilia (540 cells/mcL), mild anemia (10.8 g/dL), and mild thrombocytopenia (138 k/mcL).
- She undergoes a bone marrow aspiration and biopsy, and the results are as shown in Figure 62.4, in addition to her biopsy of the skin (Figure 62.5).

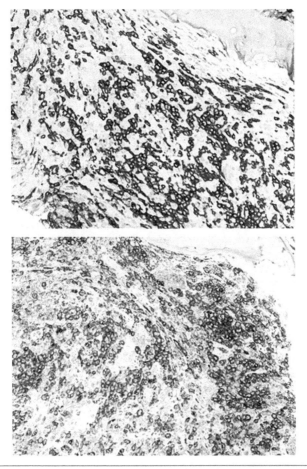

Figure 62.6 Immunohistochemical stains showed the neoplastic cells to be positive for CD117 (top, ×200 total magnification) and CD25 (bottom, ×200 total magnification).

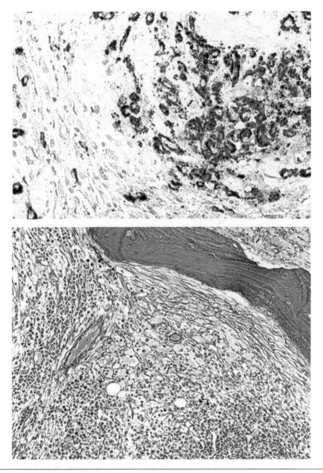

Figure 62.7 Immunohistochemical stains showed the spindled cells are positive for mast cell tryptase (top, ×600 total magnification). A reticulin stain highlighted paratrabecular and interstitial moderate-to-severe reticulin fibrosis (bottom, ×200).

1. **Which of the following is the most likely diagnosis?**
   A. Mast cell activation syndrome
   B. Serotonin syndrome
   C. Aggressive systemic mastocytosis
   D. Mast cell leukemia
   E. Urticaria pigmentosa

Explanation: **C**. The histologic and clinical findings are most consistent with systemic mastocytosis. CD117 strongly highlights mast cells in tissue and bone marrow, and mast cell tryptase positivity confirms the nature of the atypical spindled cells. CD25 is aberrantly expressed by the mast cells. The *KIT* D816V point mutation should be tested for a possible therapeutic actionable target. Aggressive systemic mastocytosis is a subtype of advanced systemic mastocytosis, characterized by at least one "C finding." C findings are evidence of organ dysfunction, while "B findings" refer to evidence of organ involvement. In this case, the patient's weight loss is due to malabsorption associated with GI involvement and not celiac disease. Mast cell leukemia is defined by ≥20% BM involvement of atypical mast cells, ≥10% circulating mast cells, or, in the rare aleukemic variant, circulating mast cells are <10% of the total leukocytes, and it typically is not associated with skin lesions.

FURTHER TESTING

- Serum tryptase level is shown to be 727 nanogram/ml. Flow cytometry is performed on the bone marrow aspirate, which confirms mast cell expression of CD117 and CD25. PCR analysis of the bone marrow aspirate shows the presence of *KIT* D816V mutation.

2. **Which cell surface marker is aberrantly expressed in mast cells of systemic mastocytosis?**

   A. CD117
   B. CD3
   C. CD34
   D. CD25
   E. CD56

   Explanation: **D**. CD25, as well as CD2, is aberrantly expressed on the mast cells of systemic mastocytosis. Mast cell tryptase can also be demonstrated by using immunohistochemistry. CD117 typically strongly highlights mast cells (among other cell types) in tissue or bone marrow, but it is a marker of normal mast cell lineage. CD34 is a vascular endothelial and myeloblast marker and typically used to assess the blast count in bone marrow core biopsies. CD3 is a pan T-cell marker.

▓ CASE 3

CASE PRESENTATION

- A 25-year-old African American male was admitted to the hospital with fever and fatigue of 1-month duration. He also reported night sweats, easy bruising on his arms, early satiety, and abdominal discomfort (LUQ). He lost approximately 15 lbs in the last 3 months. Examination was remarkable for hepatomegaly (8 cm below the costal margin) and splenomegaly (14 cm below the costal margin) without lymphadenopathy. Laboratory evaluation was notable for pancytopenia (WBC 3.8 k/mcL, Hb 10 g/dL, PLT 50 k/mcL), high LDH (800 U/L) and elevated liver-associated enzymes (AST 120 U/L, ALT 137 U/L, total bilirubin 3.0 mg/dL, direct bilirubin 2.0 mg/dL). A CT scan of the abdomen confirmed hepato-splenomegaly.

BONE MARROW BIOPSY

- This was followed by a bone marrow biopsy that revealed monotonous, medium-sized T-cells with scant pale cytoplasm, infiltrating within the sinuses of the spleen, liver, and bone marrow. Flow cytometric analysis showed the cells were CD2+, CD3+, CD7+, CD57+, γδTCR+, CD4–, CD8–, CD56–, and CD10–. Additional immunohistochemical results showed the cells were positive for the cytotoxic granules granzyme B, TIA1, and perforin. EBER-ISH (EBV-encoded RNA) was negative. PCR for T-cell receptor gene rearrangement confirmed clonality of γδ genes. Cytogenetic analysis showed isochromosome 7q and trisomy 8.

DIAGNOSTIC STUDIES

- He subsequently underwent liver biopsy that showed atypical sinusoidal lymphoid infiltrate that had the same immunophenotype as the bone marrow aspirate. Subsequently, he underwent splenectomy.

SPLENECTOMY
See Figure 62.8.

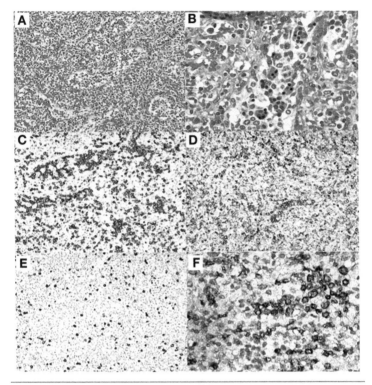

Figure 62.8 (A) Cross section of splenic parenchyma from splenectomy shows massive expansion of red pulp by atypical lymphoid cells, intermediate to large in size, dispersed chromatin, irregular nuclei, and small amount of cytoplasm (H&E ×200). (B) A high-power view highlights intrasinusoidal atypical lymphoid cells as well as increased macrophages engulfing many hematopoietic precursors (hemophagocytosis) (H&E, ×600). (C) Immunohistochemical stains highlight intrasinusoidal atypical lymphoid cells to be abnormal T-cells that are positive for CD2 (C, ×200) and CD3 (D, ×200) and negative for CD5 (E, ×200) and CD7 (image not shown). The infiltrate is TCR γ-δ subtype (F, immunoperoxidase, ×600).

DIAGNOSIS

1. **Which of the following is the most likely diagnosis?**

   A. Peripheral T-cell lymphoma, NOS
   B. Extranodal NK/T-cell lymphoma, nasal type
   C. T-cell large granular lymphocytic leukemia
   D. Hepatosplenic T-cell lymphoma
   E. Aggressive NK-cell leukemia

   Explanation **D**. Although aggressive NK-cell leukemia (ANKCL) typically presents in middle-aged patients with common involvement of the peripheral blood, bone marrow, spleen, and liver, the diagnosis should be made with great caution in EBV-negative cases (90% of ANKCL are positive for EBV). Furthermore, T-cell receptor clonality cannot be established for ANKCL, because the receptor is in germline status (see Chapter 47). Similarly, the diagnosis of extranodal NK/T-cell lymphoma, nasal type (see Chapter 48), should be questioned if the presence of EBV cannot be established. The cells of ENKTCL are CD2+, surface CD3–, cytoplasmic CD3+, CD56+, with expression of cytotoxic granules, including granzyme B, TIA1, and perforin. ENKTCL infiltrates in a diffuse or nodular pattern with extensive necrosis and apoptosis, due to angiocentric and angioinvasive behavior. Peripheral T-cell lymphoma NOS may be considered in cases of CD3+, CD56–/+ lymphoma that lack EBV positivity and cytotoxic granules.

TREATMENT

- The patient was treated with six cycles of Hyper-CVAD (fractionated cyclophosphamide, vincristine, doxorubicin, dexamethasone alternating with high dose methotrexate and cytarabine) with good response and reduction to 0.1% abnormal T-cell population.

2. What is the next line of treatment?

  A. Observation
  B. Autologous hematopoietic cell transplant (auto-HSCT)
  C. Allogeneic HCT (allo-HSCT)
  D. Consolidation chemotherapy
  E. Alemtuzumab

  Explanation C. Although there is a significant lack of prospective clinical trial data for HSTCL, the only potential for long-term survival is allo-HSCT in patients who achieve remission.

OUTCOME

- The patient undergoes pretransplant lumbar puncture, which is negative. He subsequently undergoes allo-HSCT with methotrexate and tacrolimus as GVHD prophylaxis. He is stable for 16 months when he presents with severe abdominal pain to the ED. A CT scan of the abdomen/pelvis reveals a colonic mass. He undergoes colonoscopy with biopsy.

FOLLOW-UP

- A colonoscopic biopsy shows an infiltrate composed of sheets of abnormal small lymphoid cells that on IHC staining express CD2, CD3, CD7, and CD56 and are negative for CD4, CD8, CD5, CD10, and CD30. Molecular studies identify a TCR gene rearrangement identical to the one previously characterized on both the bone marrow and liver biopsies. Staging studies shows no other sites of disease.

3. What is the treatment of this patient's relapsed disease?

  A. Pralatrexate
  B. Alemtuzumab

C. HDAC inhibitors

D. Brentuximab vedotin

E. Any of the above

Explanation **E**. All the above choices have reported activity in relapsed settings without any direct comparisons.

TREATMENT OF RELAPSED HSTCL

- There is no standard therapeutic option for patients with relapsed or progressive disease, although systemic chemotherapy using an alternative first-line regimen can be done. Allo-HSCT is suitable for individual clinical use, provided the patient does not undergo allo-HSCT after frontline therapy. However, relapsing disease is usually chemorefractory, and preference is for clinical trial, if at all possible.

- The patient recently started on single-agent Pralatrexate therapy.

PROGNOSIS

- The prognosis of HSTCL is almost uniformly poor, and no prospective trials investigating treatment approaches are reported.

- This is especially true for relapsed/refractory cases.

- However, several novel agents, such as the Aurora A kinase inhibitor alisertib and the Syk inhibitor entospletinib, are currently under investigation.

■ CASE 4

CASE PRESENTATION

A 64-year-old man with a past medical history of asthma, hypertension, and hyperlipidemia presents with symptoms of fatigue and dyspnea on exertion that have been progressive over the past 2 months. The patient denies any bleeding or recent infections. Physical exam does not identify any abnormalities. Routine lab work shows a normal CMP, with CBC showing a WBC count of 3.1 ×10^9/L (absolute neutrophil count 1,500, absolute monocyte count 450), hemoglobin of 7.4 g/dL (MCV of 104), and platelet count of 65 × 10^9/L. The rest of the lab workup, including iron studies, vitamin B12, and folic acid, is normal. The patient is referred for a bone marrow biopsy.

Conventional cytogenetics reveal the following karyotype: 45, XY, –7[14]/46, XY[6].

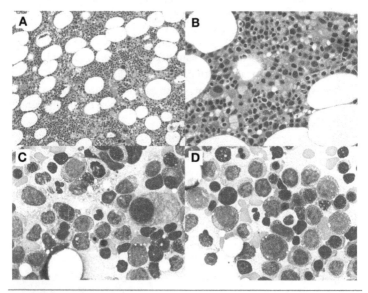

Figure 62.9 The core biopsy (images A and B) shows hypercellularity for age (~60%), hypolobated megakaryocytes, and loose clusters of immature precursors/blasts. The aspirate (images C and D) shows small, single-lobed megakaryocytes admixed with dysplastic granulocytes (hypogranulation and hyposegmentation), erythroid precursors with mild megaloblastoid maturation, and increased blasts (~17%) in clusters.

An NGS panel reveals mutations in *SRSF2* and *RUNX1*.

1. **Which of the following is the most likely diagnosis?**

   A. Acute myeloid leukemia
   B. Chronic myelomonocytic leukemia
   C. Chronic myeloid leukemia
   D. Myelodysplastic syndrome
   E. Chronic lymphocytic leukemia

   Explanation **D**. The patient has peripheral blood cytopenias, including a macrocytic anemia. Bone marrow biopsy reveals dysplasia in >10% of more than one lineage as well as increased blasts consistent with a diagnosis of MDS, supported by clonal changes identified by karyotype and NGS. There is no increase in lymphocytes, blasts are <20%, absolute monocyte count is <1,000, and cytogenetics do not reveal the Philadelphia chromosome, making other choices inappropriate.

2. **Using the Revised International Prognostic Scoring System (IPSS-R), in which risk group would this patient be categorized?**

   A. Very low
   B. Low
   C. Intermediate
   D. High
   E. Very high

   Explanation **E**. Monosomy 7 is a "poor-risk" cytogenetic change (3 points). Patient has increased blasts >10% (3 points), significant anemia of <8 g/dL (1.5 points), and moderate thrombocytopenia between 50 and 100 (0.5 points). This results in a total score of 8 points, which falls into the very high-risk category, associated with a median survival of 0.8 years.

3. **Which of the following in the most appropriate treatment option?**

   A. Epoetin alpha
   B. Lenalidomide
   C. Azacitidine (7-day schedule)
   D. Azacitidine (5-day schedule)
   E. Observation

   Explanation **C**. Azacitidine is the standard frontline treatment in high-risk MDS as a result of improved survival demonstrated in the AZA-001 study, which used a 7-day treatment regimen. While a 5-day schedule has shown efficacy in lower-risk MDS, patients with clearly high-risk disease, such as the patient here, should be treated with the standard 7-day regimen. Observation is appropriate in low-risk, asymptomatic patients with only mild cytopenias, while Epoetin alpha and lenalidomide are appropriate to treat anemia in patients with low-risk MDS.

■ CASE 5

CASE PRESENTATION

- A 25-year-old man with no significant past medical history presented with fever, worsening abdominal pain, nausea, and vomiting for the past 2 weeks. Clinical examination revealed a firm epigastric mass of 5.0 × 5.0 cm. Initial CBC and CMP were entirely within normal limits. A CT scan of the abdomen with contrast showed diffuse infiltrative lesion of the stomach wall, with multiple enlarged lymph nodes in the celiac axis and retroperitoneal region. A CT-guided biopsy of the celiac lymph node was performed. The biopsy tissue histology is reviewed below.

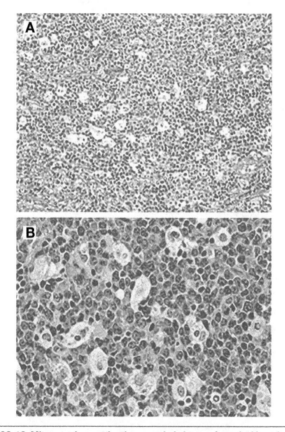

Figure 62.10 Microscopic examination revealed sheets of atypical lymphoid cells associated with increased tingible-body/phagocytizing macrophages in the background, forming a "starry sky" pattern (A, H&E, ×200). Cytologically, the atypical lymphoid cells are uniformly medium in size and exhibit a high nuclear to cytoplasmic ratio, usually more than one nucleoli and scant cytoplasm (B, H&E, ×600).

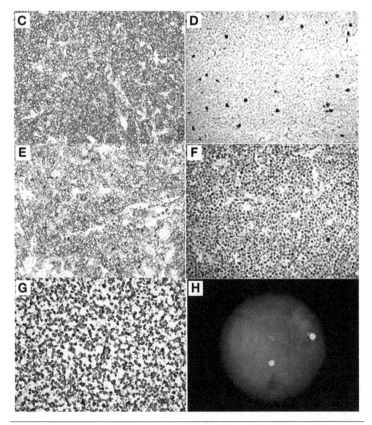

Figure 62.11 A panel of immunohistochemical staining highlights the atypical lymphoid cells to be CD20 (+) (C, ×200), BCL-2 (−) (D, ×200), CD10 (+) (E, ×200), and BCL-6 (+) (F, ×200), with a high proliferation fraction of nearly 100% (G, Ki-67, immunoperoxidase, ×200). FISH analysis using c-MYC break-apart probe identifies abnormal separated green and red signals (H).

1. **Which of the following is the most likely diagnosis?**

 A. Diffuse large B-cell lymphoma
 B. Mantle cell lymphoma, blastoid variant
 C. Burkitt lymphoma
 D. Follicular lymphoma
 E. B-lymphoblastic leukemia/lymphoma

 Explanation **C**. Both Burkitt lymphoma and diffuse large B-cell lymphoma (DLBCL) express pan B-cell antigens, including CD19, CD20, CD 22, CD79a, and PAX-5; however, they show different cytologic features. Burkitt lymphoma usually lacks CD5, BCL-2, and CD23, while mantle cell lymphoma typically expresses CD5, and nuclear staining for cyclin D1 is present in nearly 95% of cases. B-lymphoblastic leukemia/lymphoma expresses CD19, CD10, PAX-5, and TdT, with variable expression of CD20 and CD34. Follicular lymphoma shows a nodular proliferation of follicles composed of centrocytes and centroblasts and often coexpresses BCL-2, distinguishing it from Burkitt lymphoma.

2. **Which translocation of the *c-MYC* oncogene on the long arm of chromosome 8 is the most common translocation partner seen in Burkitt lymphoma on FISH studies?**

    A. Translocation of *c-MYC* with Ig heavy chain gene (*IgH*) on chromosome 14q32

    B. Translocation of *c-MYC* with kappa light chain gene (*IgK*) on chromosome 2p12

    C. Translocation of *c-MYC* with lambda light chain gene (*IgL*) on chromosome 22q11

    Explanation **A**. FISH or cytogenetic analysis is used to detect t(8;14), seen in nearly 80% of Burkitt lymphoma.

3. **The presence of which genetic rearrangement helps differentiate diffuse large B-cell lymphoma (DLBCL) from Burkitt lymphoma?**

    A. FISH for t(8;11)
    B. FISH for t(11;14)
    C. FISH for t(14;18)
    D. FISH for t(8;21)

    Explanation **C**. t(14;18) is a characteristic feature of follicular lymphoma but also a frequent translocation in DLBCL (10%–40% of cases) and absent in Burkitt lymphoma. This translocation leads to BCL-2 overexpression.

4. **The presence of which genetic rearrangement helps differentiate mantle cell lymphoma (MCL) from Burkitt lymphoma?**

    A. FISH for t(8;11)
    B. FISH for t(11;14)
    C. FISH for t(14;18)
    D. FISH for t(8;21)

    Explanation **B**. The t(11;14)(q13;32) between *IgH* and cyclin D1 is present in almost all cases of MCL.

▨ CASE 6

CASE PRESENTATION

A 60-year-old otherwise healthy man presents with a 12-month history of painful, progressive neuropathy that significantly limits his mobility. During his workup, an IgG lambda monoclonal protein is found on immunofixation. His M spike is 0.7 g/dL. His lambda free light chain is 40 mg/dL. He has no anemia, hypercalcemia, or renal dysfunction. A CT-based skeletal survey reveals no lytic bone lesions. A bone marrow biopsy reveals 5% to 10% lambda-restricted plasma cells and normal FISH and cytogenetics.

1. What would you do next?

   A. Perform a PET-CT to look for FDG avid bone lesions.

   B. Diagnose with MGUS and follow up in 12 months.

   C. Refer to Neurology to treat for MGUS-associated neuropathy.

   D. Perform a fat pad biopsy and stain his bone marrow biopsy with Congo red.

   Explanation **D**. Light chain amyloidosis should be ruled out in this patient by performing a fat pad biopsy and staining his bone marrow with Congo red. A nerve biopsy would be invasive, and these tests would establish the diagnosis in ~85% of cases.

CT-based skeletal surveys are very sensitive, and a PET-CT is not usually required to establish the diagnosis of multiple myeloma.

This patient might still have MGUS, but AL amyloidosis needs to be ruled out as a cause of his neuropathy.

Furthermore, MGUS-associated neuropathy is usually associated with an IgM monoclonal protein.

FAT PAD BIOPSY

See Figures 62.12 and 62.13.

CASE PRESENTATION CONTINUED

2. His fat pad biopsy stains positive for Congo red. What would you do next?

   A. Initiate chemotherapy for his systemic AL amyloidosis.

   B. Type the amyloid.

   C. Obtain a nerve biopsy to definitively establish the diagnosis.

   Explanation **B**. His amyloid needs to be typed with mass spectrometry (MS) or immunohistochemistry (IHC). MS is the most common method of typing in the United States, with specificity and sensitivity exceeding 98% in reference laboratories. In "good hands," IHC can have comparable outcomes, but it is more labor-intensive and can be operator-dependent.

Amyloid typing should always be performed, no matter how typical the clinical presentation. Non-AL amyloid (ATTR) can frequently be associated with MGUS, with some studies suggesting a higher incidence of MGUS in ATTR compared to that of the general population.

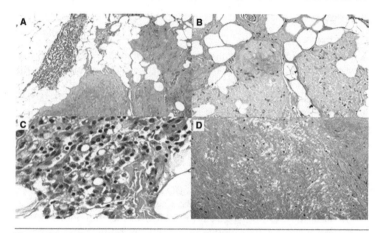

Figure 62.12 Fat pad biopsy shows extracellular depositions of pink, amorphous material in adipose tissue (A and B) and a vessel wall associated with adjacent clusters of plasma cells (C; H&E, original magnifications ×100, ×200, and ×600, respectively). Congo red stains amyloid deposition with characteristic apple-green birefringence under polarized light (D, original magnification ×200).

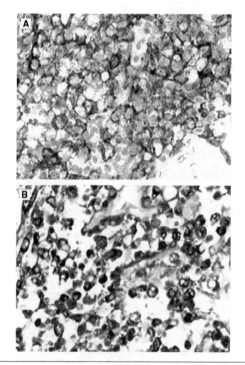

Figure 62.13 Immunohistochemical stains highlight CD138 positive (A) and lambda-restricted clonal plasma cells (B). Original magnification ×600.

Chemotherapy should ideally be initiated after the type of amyloid has been determined, but because this can take long in institutions where MS or IHC is not readily available, it is reasonable to start treatment while awaiting typing. However, typing results should be always available before an autologous transplant.

Obtaining a confirmatory organ biopsy is usually not necessary if fat and/or marrow stain positive for Congo red.

3. **MS of his fat biopsy reveals lambda light chain amyloidosis. An echocardiogram shows an ejection fraction of 60% and interventricular septum thickness of 14 mm (ULN = 12 mm). NTproBNP and troponin are 1,900 pg/ml and 0.02 ng/ml, respectively. Creatinine is 1.2 mg/dl, and 24-hour urine protein is 1,500 mg/24 hours. How would you treat him?**

   A. Refer for autologous stem cell transplant (ASCT).
   B. Initiate Bortezomib dexamethasone (Vd).
   C. Initiate Melphalan prednisone (MP).
   D. Initiate Rd.

   Explanation **A.** The most appropriate next step would be to refer the patient for an ASCT. Although this approach is not supported by phase 3 data, retrospective series suggest that carefully selected patients can have excellent long-term outcomes. Referral for appropriate candidates should be done early, because the logistics of arranging ASCT might delay this therapy by several weeks/months.

The decision to initiate treatment while waiting for ASCT evaluation and approval is a clinical one. We usually initiate treatment in patients with symptomatic cardiac involvement, rapidly progressive proteinuria/renal failure, >10% BMPCs, or who cannot be evaluated for ASCT in an expedited manner (within a few weeks from diagnosis). This is not supported by data; however, time is organ function in AL amyloidosis. Furthermore, a cycle of chemotherapy in "borderline" transplant candidates can sometimes help identify patients who would not do well with transplants (e.g., a patient doing very poorly after one cycle of CyBorD is likely to have increased morbidity and mortality, and maybe this would factor into the decision to transplant or not). And vice versa, a patient achieving an early complete remission with conventional chemotherapy might decide against ASCT.

He appears to be a possible transplant candidate, despite some cardiac involvement. He did not appear to be very symptomatic from this, because his mobility was limited by his neuropathy. This underlines the importance of thorough staging in these patients.

In this patient, we would use a triplet combination that includes an alkylator and a proteasome inhibitor, which has been shown to improve hematologic response and overall survival over MP (data presented in abstract form). However, this is not offered as an option in this vignette. Finally, we avoid immunomodulating therapies in patients with cardiac involvement, because they have been associated with cardiac decompensation.

4. **The patient declines ASCT. He would like to try upfront chemotherapy. What would you do next?**

   A. CyBorD (cyclophosphamide, bortezomib, dexamethasone)

   B. Vd (bortezomib, lenalidomide, dexamethasone)

   C. Rd (lenalidomide, dexamethasone)

   D. Melphalan, dexamethasone

   E. Clinical trial

   F. A or E

   G. All the above

   Explanation **F**. In this patient, CyBorD or a clinical trial is the best option. Triplet therapy with an alkylating agent, a proteasome inhibitor, and steroids has shown a survival benefit over an alkylator and steroid combination. We usually avoid immunomodulating drugs (IMiDs) in patients with cardiac involvement, because they are tolerated poorly in this patient population. However, if neuropathy worsens because of the bortezomib, we recommend immediate cessation of the drug, because neuropathy can be severe and life-long. In these cases, daratumumab, second-generation proteasome inhibitors (e.g., Ixazomib), or careful use of IMiDs are reasonable alternatives. In cases of advanced cardiac involvement, the addition of doxycycline can be considered. This approach is not supported by randomized data but has been shown to be safe and offer a possible benefit in this patient subgroup.

5. **CyBorD is initiated. After 4 cycles, the patient achieves CR. His neuropathy remains stable. His BNP and troponin remain stable. His proteinuria and creatinine also remain stable. What would you do next?**

   A. Stop chemotherapy.

   B. Treat for a total of 6 to 12 months.

   C. Add daratumumab.

   D. Switch to a different therapy because of the lack of organ response.

   Explanation **B**. There are no good data to support total duration of treatment in AL. We usually treat patients for a total of 6 to 12 cycles of chemotherapy and, if in VGPR or better, offer a trial of observation or maintenance therapy. If < than PR has been achieved after 2 cycles, then a switch in treatment is warranted. There are no data to support a benefit from maintenance treatment in this disease, although it is reasonable to consider on a case-by-case basis and especially in patients with >10% bone marrow plasma cells at diagnosis. Organ response lags behind hematologic response by several months. Of patients who achieve VGPR or better, median time to kidney and heart is about 6 and 12 months, respectively, with other organs (e.g., nerves) taking much longer or never responding. In this patient, who has achieved early CR, adding daratumumab or switching therapy completely will not offer a better chance for an organ response, provided there is no hematologic progression.

6. **After 6 cycles of treatment, chemotherapy is stopped, and the patient is placed on maintenance bortezomib. He remains in CR. After 12 months, his BNP is 400, troponin is <0.01 ng/mL, Cr is 1 mg/dL, and proteinuria is <500 mg/24 hours. His neuropathy has not improved. At 18 months, his immunofixation becomes positive, and his free light chains rise to 10 mg/dL. His cardiac and renal biomarkers and clinical picture are all stable. What do you do next?**

   A. Continue observation.
   B. Resume treatment.

   Explanation **B**. The patient has achieved a renal and cardiac organ response but no nerve response. At 18 months, even though he remains clinically stable and has no signs of organ involvement, he has a hematologic relapse. Unlike myeloma, where slow relapses can be observed without treatment in amyloidosis, amyloid deposition is bound to resume when a hematologic relapse occurs. Therefore, treatment should be initiated. At this point in time, the patient should strongly reconsider a transplant, because his cardiac function has improved further. In most patients with relapsed disease, we prefer a daratumumab-based regimen. Patients relapsing >2 years after their last therapy can be rechallenged with a bortezomib-based regimen. Immunomodulatory drugs can also be safer to use at this point, given his cardiac response.

◼ CASE 7

CASE PRESENTATION

A 66 year-old man with a history of hypertension and hyperlipidemia presented to the emergency department with one month of left hip pain, difficulty walking, and 20 lb weight loss. He had a fever of 39.3°C and an enlarged left axillary lymph node. Laboratory data were significant for WBC of 18×10^9/L (75% neutrophils, 18% lymphocytes), hemoglobin 11.2 g/dL, elevated erythrocyte sedimentation rate (100 mm/h; normal value <20 mm/h), and higher C-reactive protein (12.0 mg/dL; normal value <0.30 ml/dL). LDH was elevated at 294 U/L. β-2-microglobulin was 4 ug/mL. CT of thorax, abdomen, and pelvis showed enlarged left axillary lymph node (2.5 × 1.5 × 2.0 cm) and an osteolytic sacral mass (4.0 × 2.0 × 4.5 cm) invading the left sacro-iliac joint. Staging bone marrow biopsy was reportedly normal. The supraclavicular lymph node was biopsied, with H&E showing sheets of large atypical lymphoid cells with prominent nucleoli and mitotic features (see below). Immunohistochemical staining revealed the atypical cells were positive for CD3, CD30, CD45, EMA, and ALK and negative for CD20, CD34, and CD79a. Proliferative rate by Ki-67 was estimated at 62%. Human T-cell lymphotropic virus (HTLV) antibody was negative. ALK-positive ALCL was diagnosed.

1. **According to the Ann Arbor staging system, what is the stage of this patient?**
   A. Stage IIIA
   B. Stage IIIB
   C. Stage IVA
   D. Stage IVB

   Explanation **D**. Stage IVB. According to the Ann Arbor staging system, Stage IV disease is characterized by diffuse or disseminated involvement of one or more extralymphatic organs or tissues, with or without associated lymph node involvement. Fever, night sweats, or >10% weight loss is denoted by "A" for absence or "B" for presence.

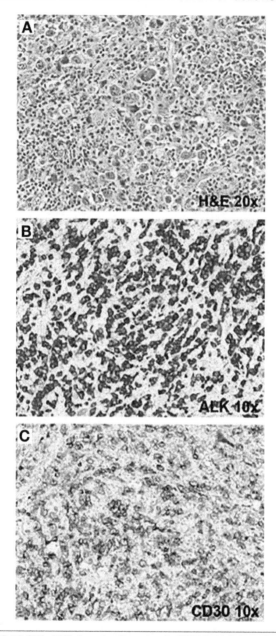

Figure 62.14 ALK+ ALCL: hematoxylin and eosin (H&E; A, 20×) shows hallmark cells with eccentric horseshoe or kidney-shaped nuclei and intermediate nuclear: cytoplasmic ratio. Tumor cells are positive for ALK and CD30 (B and C, 10×).

2. What is the recommended first-line treatment for this patient?

A. Brentuximab vedotin + CHOP × 4 cycles

B. Brentuximab vedotin + CHP × 6 cycles + involved site radiation therapy

C. Brentuximab vedotin + CHP × 6 cycles

D. Brentuximab vedotin + CHOP × 4 cycles + involved site radiation therapy

Explanation C. Brentuxmab vedotin (BV) + CHP × 6 cycles. In the ECHELON-2 trial, BV and CHP × 6 cycles were found to be superior to the previous standard of care, CHOP, in CD30-positive mature T-cell lymphomas. Vincristine (in CHOP) was omitted to avoid cumulative neurotoxicity with the addition of BV. The addition of radiation therapy is recommended for ALK-negative ALCL.

3. What confers use of Brentuximab vedotin in this patient?

A. Presence of ALK translocation

B. CD30 positivity

C. Stage of presentation

D. CD3 positivity

Explanation B. CD30 positivity. Brentuximab vedotin is an anti-CD30 drug-antibody conjugate that is approved for use in peripheral T-cell lymphomas that express CD30. These include ALK+, ALK−, and primary cutaneous ALCL (PCALCL).

▦ CASE 8

CASE PRESENTATION

- A 68-year-old man with a past medical history of hypertension presents with a 2-week history of severe fatigue. He presented to his primary care physician and was found to have an enlarged right inguinal lymph node and splenomegaly on exam.
- Laboratory evaluation revealed a WBC of 3.1 k/mcL with a normal differential, hemoglobin of 12.7 g/dL, and platelets of 87 k/mcL.
- A CT scan of the chest, abdomen, and pelvis showed extensive cervical, abdominal, and inguinal lymphadenopathy.

1. What other blood tests would you initially order in a patient with extensive lymphadenopathy and pancytopenia?

   A. HIV and EBV serology
   B. Hepatitis panel
   C. β-2 microglobulin and LDH
   D. Flow cytometry
   E. All the above

Explanation **E.** In evaluating a patient with lymphadenopathy and pancytopenia, it is important to rule out other causes of pancytopenia. In addition, in patients with lymphomas, it is important to order a hepatitis panel (especially prior to the initiation of rituximab), EBV serology, and HIV testing. In addition, elevated β-2 microglobulin and LDH are often seen in some lymphomas and can be prognostic markers.

The patient underwent an inguinal lymph node biopsy (Figure 62.15).

Flow cytometry revealed a 60% lambda-restricted clonal B-cell population with CD19 (+), CD20 (+), CD22 (+), CD5 (+), CD45 (+), FMC7 (+), CD23 (−), and CD10 (−).

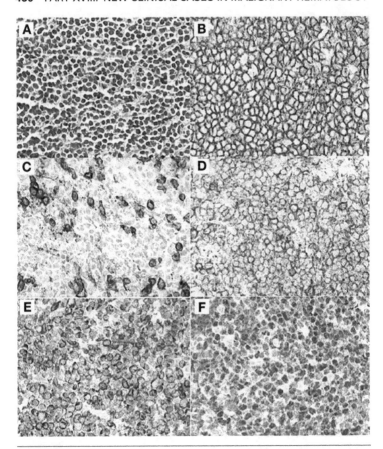

Figure 62.15 Cross section of a lymph node shows complete effacement of the normal architecture by a monotonous population of atypical small-to medium-sized lymphoid cells with round to oval nuclei, condensed chromatin, some with small visible nucleoli, and scant cytoplasm, in a background of increased vasculature (A, H&E ×600). By immunohistochemical staining, the atypical cells were positive for CD20 and negative for CD3 (B and C, immunoperoxidase, ×600). The neoplastic B cells also coexpress CD5, BCL-1, and BCL-2 (D, E, and F, immunoperoxidase, ×600).

2. Which of the following is the most likely diagnosis?

   A. Chronic lymphocytic leukemia/small lymphocytic lymphoma
   B. Diffuse large B-cell lymphoma
   C. Marginal zone lymphoma
   D. Mantle cell lymphoma
   E. Lymphoplasmacytic lymphoma

Explanation **D**. The overall histologic and phenotypic findings are diagnostic of mantle cell lymphoma. Remember that mantle cell lymphoma is a small/medium B-cell malignancy that is typically CD5+, CD10−, and CD23−. CLL/SLL expresses CD5 and CD23 and is typically CD20 dim. BCL-1 (cyclin D1) is not seen in CLL/SLL. The cells in the biopsy are predominantly small- to medium-sized, not large, as would be expected in DLBCL. Cells of marginal zone lymphoma typically are small to medium with abundant pale cytoplasm and are usually CD5- and CD10-negative. Likewise, neoplastic lymphocytes of lymphoplasmacytic lymphoma are dual CD5- and CD10-negative.

CYTOGENETICS

3. Which cytogenetic abnormality defines mantle cell lymphoma?

A. t(8;14)(q24;q32)*IgH/MYC*

B. t(11;14)(q13;q32)*IgH/CCND1*

C. t(9;22)(q34;q11)*BCR/ABL1*

D. t(14;18)(q32:q21)*IgH/BCL-2*

E. t(15;17)(q24;q21)*PML/RARa*

Explanation **B**. Mantle cell lymphoma has a specific cytogenetic abnormality, t(11;14)(q13;q32)*IgH/CCND1*, which is seen in virtually all cases of MCL. This abnormality is not positive in CLL. The translocation results in overexpression of cyclin D1, which causes abnormal proliferation of malignant cells. The other cytogenetic abnormalities are seen in other malignancies:

t(8;14)(q24;q32)*IgH/MYC* – Burkitt lymphoma

t(9;22)(q34;q11)*BCR/ABL1* – Chronic myelogenous leukemia; *BCR-ABL1* positive B-ALL

t(14;18)(q32:q21)*IgH/BCL-2* – Follicular lymphoma, DLBCL (rare)

t(15;17)(q24;q21)*PML/RARa* – Acute promyelocytic leukemia (APL)

TREATMENT

4. All the following options would be appropriate in this patient, EXCEPT

A. R-CHOP

B. Watchful waiting

C. VR-CAP

D. BR (Rituximab + Bendamustine)

Explanation **B**. This would **not** be an appropriate treatment strategy in this patient, as he has symptomatic disease (fatigue, cytopenias, splenomegaly).

▓ CASE 9

CASE PRESENTATION

A 66-year-old man with stage IV primary refractory diffuse large B-cell lymphoma (DLBCL) with liver involvement, splenomegaly, and possible bone marrow involvement presents for evaluation for treatment with anti-CD19 CAR-T cell therapy after failing two prior lines of treatment (R-CHOP, R-ICE). He has residual non-bulky disease in a hypermetabolic subcarinal lymph node measuring 4.3 × 2.8 cm. Performance status is good, with Eastern Cooperative Oncology Group (ECOG) status 0. International Prognostic Index (IPI) score is 4. The decision is made to treat with axicabtagene ciloleucel (axi-cel). He undergoes apheresis, and product manufacturing is successful. He has a baseline MRI brain with no malignancy and minimal microvascular changes. Pre-treatment CRP is elevated to 16.1 mg/L, and ferritin is 3,507 ng/mL. He receives lymphodepleting cyclophosphamide and fludarabine on days –5 through –3, and then on day 0, he receives his infusion of autologous CAR-T cells. Within 24 hours, he develops fever to 103.1°F and tachycardia to 114 bpm. He is normotensive, with 100% oxygen saturation on pulse oximetry. He is started on IV fluids, and infectious workup is initiated.

1. **What grade CRS is this patient experiencing?**
   A. Grade 0
   B. Grade 1
   C. Grade 2
   D. Grade 3
   E. Grade 4

   Explanation **B**. This is Grade 1 CRS. The patient demonstrates fever and tachycardia but no hypotension or hypoxia. Only supportive care is needed at this time.

TREATMENT

The patient is monitored vigilantly without intervention. On day 7 after cell infusion, the patient is found to be confused, states an incorrect month and year, cannot count backward from 100 to 10, and has illegible handwriting. He is lethargic but awakens to voice. Vital signs show a temperature of 103°F and heart rate of 123 bpm. He requires 2 L/min oxygen by nasal cannula and has worsening hypotension but does not currently require vasopressors.

2. **What treatment do you recommend at this time?**
   A. Tocilizumab
   B. Dexamethasone
   C. Tocilizumab and dexamethasone
   D. Topical steroids
   E. Observation

   Explanation: **C**. This patient has now developed Grade 2 CRS in addition to Grade 2 neurotoxicity. Tocilizumab and dexamethasone are needed to treat both of these syndromes adequately. Tocilizumab alone would help with CRS but not neurotoxicity. Dexamethasone alone would treat CRS and neurotoxicity but is not considered first line. Observation is not recommended, given the patient's severity of symptoms. Topical steroids have no role.

FURTHER TESTING

The next morning, the patient is back to baseline, with complete resolution of neurotoxicity. Unfortunately, he demonstrates worsening confusion, tremor, disorientation, agitation, aphasia, dysphagia, and encephalopathy over the next several days. He is placed on dexamethasone 10 mg IV every 6 hours.

3. Which of the following would be the LEAST helpful in this situation?

    A. Lumbar puncture (LP) with culture and flow cytometry
    B. Repeat MRI brain scan
    C. Electroencephalogram (EEG)
    D. Seizure prophylaxis
    E. Repeat ferritin

Explanation: **D**. Repeating the ferritin would be the least helpful. Ferritin is nonspecific and is not used to make a clinical decision regarding treatment. LP is needed to assess for infection or new central nervous system (CNS) involvement with lymphoma. Repeat MRI brain scan can show signs of stroke, evidence of new lymphoma in the brain, or cerebral edema. EEG is needed to assess for encephalopathy or seizure activity. Seizure prophylaxis should be considered, as seizure is a rare but severe manifestation of ICANS.

▧ CASE 10

CASE PRESENTATION

- A 57-year-old female with a history of follicular lymphoma status post multiple lines of chemotherapy (R-CVP, bendamustine, fludarabine, and finally chlorambucil), currently with stable disease, presented with fevers, fatigue, and cough.

- A CT scan of the chest/abdomen/pelvis at the time showed no increase in lymphadenopathy. Hence, there was no change in the care plan.

- A month later, she developed multiple skin lesions, and her examination was remarkable for a maculopapular rash noted predominantly on her face, neck, left shoulder, and scapula.

- Laboratory values at the time revealed a WBC count of 3.6 k/mcL, hemoglobin 11 g/dL, platelet count of 88 k/mcL, creatinine 0.91 mg/dL, AST 91 U/L, ALT 37 U/L, and total bilirubin of 1.9 mg/dL.

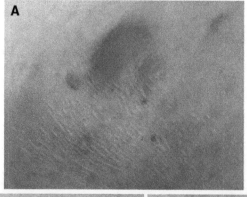

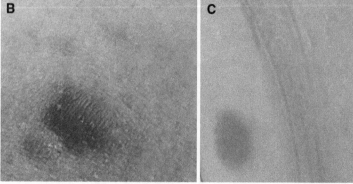

Figure 62.16 A to C: Neck, L upper shoulder, and L scapula.

SKIN RASH

Skin biopsy revealed a diffuse infiltrate of large lymphohistiocytic cells within the dermis and superficial subcutis, with an associated mixed inflammatory population of eosinophils, neutrophils, and scattered plasma cells. The cells have oval to reniform nuclei with minimal pleomorphism, occasionally polygonal and multilobated nuclei, vesicular chromatin with delicate grooves, and moderate to abundant amounts of eosinophilic (pink) cytoplasm. The neoplastic cells are positive for CD1a, CD207, S-100, CD4, CD45 (weak), and MUM-1 (focal).

HISTOLOGY AND IHC STAINING

See Figure 62.17.

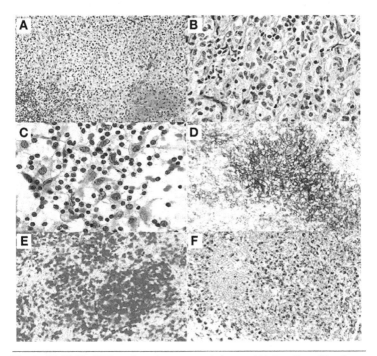

Figure 62.17 The H&E sections demonstrated abnormal histiocytic proliferation associated with an eosinophilic microabcess in a background of small lymphocytes (A, ×200), and cytologically the atypical cells showed oval to elongated and convoluted nuclei, vesicular chromatin, and abundant cytoplasm (B, ×600). Touch imprint (C, H&E, ×600) illustrated characteristic nuclear grooves in the neoplastic cells. IHC stains showed these cells to be positive for CD1a (D, immunoperoxidase, ×200) and S-100 (E, ×200). The cells were also positive for the histiocytic marker CD68 (F, ×200).

DIAGNOSIS

1. Which of the following is the most likely diagnosis?

   A. Histiocytic sarcoma
   B. Anaplastic large cell lymphoma, *ALK* positive
   C. Langerhans cell histiocytosis
   D. Recurrent follicular lymphoma
   E. Hemophagocytic lymphohistiocytosis

Explanation C. The morphologic and phenotypic features (CD1a+, CD207+ [aka Langerin], and S-100+) are most consistent with Langerhans cell histiocytosis (LCH). Although histiocytic sarcoma (HS) may have large cells, pleomorphism and nuclear irregularities are typically present, and HS is a diagnosis of exclusion; hence, the presence of LCH markers argue against this diagnosis. ALCL, *ALK* positive, by definition has large cells, but the characteristic nuclear features and LCH phenotype exclude the diagnosis. The phenotypic findings are compatible with LCH, not recurrence of the patient's original follicular lymphoma nor hemophagocytic lymphohistiocytosis. Phagocytosis of hematopoietic elements are not identified in this patient.

DIFFERENTIAL DIAGNOSIS

- LCH must be distinguished from other histiocytic and dendritic cell disorders, especially histiocytic sarcoma [HS], which is a non-Langerhans cell histiocytic disorder.

- To justify the diagnosis of HS, there is expression of one or more histiocytic markers CD163, CD68 (KP1 and PGM1), and lysozyme, and absence of Langerhans cell markers (CD1a, Langerin/CD207), among other cell types ,such as follicular dendritic cells (CD21, CD23, CD35) or myeloid markers (CD13, CD33, MPO).

HISTOLOGY AND IHC STAINING [HISTIOCYTIC SARCOMA (HS)]

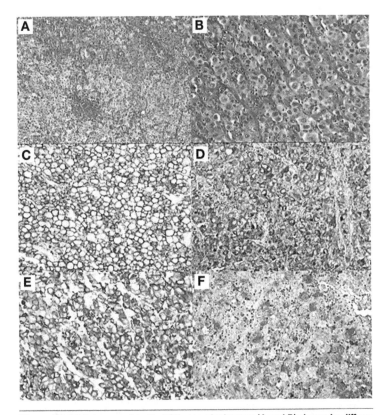

Figure 62.18 As opposed to the LCH case, the images (A and B) showed a diffuse infiltrate of large, hisitocytic-appearing cells with round to oval nuclei, distinct nucleoli, and abundant eosin ophilic or foamy cytoplasm. The neoplastic cells were positive for leukocyte common antigen, or LCA (A, CD45 (LCA), immunoperoxidase, ×600), monocytic/histiocytic markers, including CD68 (B, immunoperoxidase ×600), CD163 (C, immunoperoxidase, ×600), and partially positive for S-100 (D, immunoperoxidase ×600).

CASE PRESENTATION

- A bone marrow biopsy was negative for involvement by both FL and and LCH. MRI of the brain was normal. A repeat CT scan of the chest/abdomen/pelvis showed an increased size of lymph nodes and splenomegaly. The patient was diagnosed with multisystem LCH.

2. **Which of the following is not a "risk organ" in multisystem LCH?**

   A. Hematopoietic system
   B. Liver
   C. Spleen
   D. Skin
   E. CNS

   Explanation **D**. Other than answer choice D, all other choices are considered "risk organs" in multisystem LCH.

MOLECULAR DIAGNOSIS

3. **Mutation in which gene has been detected in just over 50% of cases of LCH?**

   A. *JAK2*
   B. *SRSF2*
   C. *MYD88 L265P*
   D. *BRAF V600E*
   E. *CALR*

   Explanation **D**. For reasons that are not entirely clear, more than half of LCH patients harbor the *BRAF* V600E mutation.

TARGETED THERAPY

- *BRAF*V600E mutation was tested on the skin biopsy specimen but was negative.

4. **Which of the following has shown activity in patients with LCH harboring the BRAF V600E mutation?**

   A. Trametinib
   B. Ipilimumab
   C. Nivolumab
   D. Vemurafenib
   E. Clofarabine

   Explanation **D**. Vemurafenib is a selective BRAF inhibitor, with significant activity observed in LCH.

CHALLENGING CASE VIGNETTE KEY	
CASE NUMBER	**SEE CHAPTER FOR MORE INFORMATION**
1	Chapter 17, Acute Myeloid Leukemia
2	Chapter 10, Systemic Mastocytosis
3	Chapter 50, Hepatosplenic T-Cell Lymphoma
4	Chapter 12, Myelodysplastic Syndromes
5	Chapter 34, Burkitt Lymphoma
6	Chapter 31, Immunoglobulin Light Chain Amyloidosis
7	Chapter 47, Anaplastic Large Cell Lymphoma
8	Chapter 37, Mantle Cell Lymphoma
9	Chapter 57, Cytokine Release Syndrome and Other Toxicities Associated With Novel Cellular Therapies
10	Chapter 51, Langerhans Cell Histiocytosis, Erdheim-Chester Disease, Rosai-Dorfman Disease, and Histiocytic Sarcoma

Appendix: Pathology Supplement

Supplemental Table 1 2008 WHO Classification of Myeloid Neoplasms and Corresponding 2016 Updates

2008 WHO Classification	Updated Classification
Myeloproliferative neoplasm	
Chronic myelogenous leukemia, *BCR-ABL1*-positive	Some diagnostic criteria are modified.
Chronic neutrophillic leukemia (CNL)**	e.g., *CSF3R* mutation is added in major diagnostic criteria in CNL.
Polycythemia vera (PV)**	Reset diagnostic criteria for PV.
Primary myelofibrosis	
Essential thrombocythemia	
Chronic eosinophilic leukemia, NOS	
Mastocytosis	→ **Mastocytosis*** (separated from MPN)
• Cutaneous mastocytosis	
• Systemic mastocytosis	
• Mast cell leukemia	
• Mast cell sarcoma	
Myeloproliferative neoplasm, unclassifiable	
Myeloid and lymphoid neoplasms with eosinophilia and abnormalities of PDGFRA, PDGFRB, or FGFR1	**Myeloid and lymphoid neoplasms with eosinophilia and abnormalities of PDGFRA, PDGFRB, or FGFR1 or with PCM1-AK2**
• Myeloid/lymphoid neoplasms with PDGFRA rearrangement	
• Myeloid/lymphoid neoplasms with PDGFRB rearrangement	• Provisional entity: Myeloid/lymphoid neoplasms with PCM1-JAK2*
• Myeloid/lymphoid neoplasms with FGFR1 rearrangement	
Myelodysplastic/myeloproliferative neoplasm (MDS/MPN)	
• Chronic myelomonocytic leukemia	

(*continued*)

Supplemental Table 1 2008 WHO Classification of Myeloid Neoplasms and Corresponding 2016 Updates (continued)

2008 WHO Classification	Updated Classification
• Atypical chronic myeloid leukemia, *BCR-ABL1* negative	
• Juvenile myelomonocytic leukemia	
• Myelodysplastic/myeloprolifera-tive neoplasm, unclassifiable	
• Provisional entity: refractory anemia with ring-sideroblasts with associated thrombocytosis (RARS-T)	→ Myelodysplastic/myeloprolifera-tive neoplasm with ring siero-blasts and thrombocytosis (MDS/MPN-RS-T)**
Myelodysplastic syndromes	
• Refractory cytopenia with uni-lieage dysplasia	→ MDS with single-lineage dysplasia**
• Refractory anemia with ring sideroblasts	→ MDS with ring sideroblasts**
	• MDS with ring sideroblasts and single-lineage dysplasia**
	• MDS with ring sideroblasts with multilineage dysplasia**
	→ MDS with multilineage dysplasia**
• Refractory cytopenia with multi-lineage dysplasia	→ MDS with excess blasts**
• Refractory anemia with excess blasts	
• Myelodysplastic syndrome with isolated del(5q)	→ MDS with isolated del(5q)**
• Myelodysplastic syndrome, unclassifiable	→ MDS, unclassifiable**
• Provisional entity: refractory cytopenia of childhood	→ The same
	Myeloid neoplasms with germline predisposition*
Acute myeloid leukemia and related neoplasms	
• AML with t(8;21)(q22;21)(q22;q22.1); *RUNX1-RUNX1T1*	
• AML with inv(16)(p13;p13.1q22) or t(16;16)(p13.1;q22); *CBFB-MYH11*	

(*continued*)

Supplemental Table 1 2008 WHO Classification of Myeloid Neoplasms and Corresponding 2016 Updates (continued)

2008 WHO Classification	Updated Classification
• Acute promyelocytic leukemia with t(15;17)(q22;q12); *PML-RARA*	→ APL with *PML-RARA***
• AML with t(9;11)(p22;q23); *MLLT3-MLL*	→ AML with t(9;11)(p22;q23); *MLLT3-KMT2A***
• AML with t(6;9)(p23;q34): *DEK-NUP214*	
• AML with inv(3)(q21q26.2) or t(3;3)(q21;q26.2); *RPN1-EVI1*	
• AML (megakaryoblastic) with t(1;22)(p13;q13); *RBM15-MKL1*	→ AML with inv(3)(q21q26.2) or t(3;3)(q21;q26.2); *GATA2, MECOM*
• AML with mutated *NPM1*	Provisional entity: AML with *BCR-ABL**
• AML with mutated *CEBPA*	→ AML with biallelic mutations of *CEBPA*
	Provisional entity: AML with mutated *RUNX1**
AML with myelodysplasia-related changes	
Therapy-related myeloid neoplasms	
Acute myeloid leukemia, NOS	
• AML with minimal differentiation	
• AML without maturation	
• AML with myelomonocytic leukemia	
• AML monoblastic and monocytic leukemia	
• Acute erythroid leukemia	
a. Myeloid/erythroid	→ The subtype no longer exists.
b. Pure erythroid	→ Pure erythroid leukemia**
• Acute megakaryoblastic leukemia	
• Acute basophilic leukemia	
• Acute panmyelosis with myelofibrosis	
Myeloid sarcoma	
Myeloid proliferations related to Down syndrome	

(*continued*)

Supplemental Table 1 2008 WHO Classification of Myeloid Neoplasms and Corresponding 2016 Updates (continued)

2008 WHO Classification	Updated Classification
• Transient abnormal myelopoiesis • Myeloid leukemia associated with Down syndrome	
Blastic plasmacytoid dendritic cell neoplasm	
Acute leukemias of ambiguous lineage	
Acute undifferentiated leukemia	
Mixed phenotype acute leukemia with t(9;22)(q34;q11.2); *BCR-ABL1*	
Mixed phenotype acute leukemia with t(v;11q23); *MLL* rearranged	
Mixed phenotype acute leukemia, B/myeloid, NOS	
Mixed phenotype acute leukemia, T/myeloid, NOS	
Mixed phenotype acute leukemia, NOS – rare	
Other ambiguous lineage leukemia	
• Natural killer (NK) – cell lymphoblastic leukemia/lymphoma	→ No longer in AML category; please see T-lymphoblastic leukemia/lymphoma
B lymphoblastic leukemia/lymphoma	
B lymphoblastic leukemia/lymphoma, NOS	
B lymphoblastic leukemia/lymphoma with recurrent cytogenetic abnormalities	
• B lymphoblastic leukemia/lymphoma with t(9;22)(q34;q11.2); *BCR-ABL1*	
• B lymphoblastic leukemia/lymphoma with t(v;11q23.3); MLL rearranged	→ B lymphoblastic leukemia/lymphoma with t(v;11q23.3); *KMT2A* rearranged
• B lymphoblastic leukemia/lymphoma with t(12;21)(p13;q22); *TEL-AML1(ETV6-RUNX1)*	

(*continued*)

Supplemental Table 1 2008 WHO Classification of Myeloid Neoplasms and Corresponding 2016 Updates (continued)	
2008 WHO Classification	**Updated Classification**
• B lymphoblastic leukemia/lymphoma with hyperdiploidy • B lymphoblastic leukemia/lymphoma with hypodiploidy (Hypodiploid ALL) • B lymphoblastic leukemia/lymphoma with t(5;14)(q31;q32); *IL3-IgH* • B lymphoblastic leukemia/lymphoma with t(1;19)(q23; p13.3); *E2A-PBX1(TCF3-PBX1)*	
	Provisional entity: B lymphoblastic leukemia/lymphoma, *BCR-ABL1*-like*
	Provisional entity: B lymphoblastic leukemia/lymphoma with iAMP21*
T-lymphoblastic leukemia/lymphoma	
	Provisional entity: early T-cell precursor lymphoblastic leukemia
	Provisional entity: natural killer cell lymphoblastic leukemia/lymphoma
*Newly proposed myeloid neoplasms listed in the revision of 2008 WHO classification, including those provisional lymphomas in 2008.	
**The diagnostic criteria of myeloid neoplasms are modified in the revision of 2008 WHO classification.	

Supplemental Table 2 2008 WHO Classification of Mature B-Cell, T-Cell, and NK-Cell Neoplasms and Corresponding 2016 Updates

2008 WHO Classification	Updated Classification
Mature B-cell neoplasms	
Chronic lymphocytic leukemia/small lymphocytic lymphoma	Monoclonal B-cell lymphocytosis*
B-cell prolymphocytic leukemia	
Splenic marginal zone lymphoma	
Hairy cell leukemia	
Splenic lymphoma/leukemia, un-classifiable	
• Splenic diffuse red pulp small B-cell lymphoma	
• Hairy cell leukemia variant	
Lymphoplasmacytic lymphoma	
Waldenström macroglobulinemia	
Heavy chain diseases	
• Alpha heavy chain disease	
• Gamma heavy chain disease	
• Mu heavy chain disease	
Plasma cell myeloma	
	Monoclonal gammopathy of unde-termined significance (MGUS), IgM*
Solitary plasmacytoma of bone	Monoclonal gammopathy of undetermined significance (MGUS), IgG/IgA*
Extraosseous plasmacytoma	Monoclonal immunoglobulin depo-sition disease*
Extranodal marginal zone lymphoma of mucosa-associated lymphoid tissue (MALT lymphoma)	In situ follicular lymphoma*
Nodal marginal zone lymphoma	Duodenal follicular lymphoma*
• Pediatric nodal marginal zone lymphoma*	
Follicular lymphoma	
Pediatric follicular lymphoma*	
Primary cutaneous follicle center lymphoma	Large B-cell lymphoma with IRF4 rearrangement*

(*continued*)

Supplemental Table 2 2008 WHO Classification of Mature B-Cell, T-Cell, and NK-Cell Neoplasms and Corresponding 2016 Updates (continued)	
2008 WHO Classification	**Updated Classification**
	In situ mantle cell lymphoma* Germinal center B-cell type* Activated B-cell type*
Mantle cell lymphoma	
Diffuse large B-cell lymphoma (DLBCL), NOS	
• T-cell/histiocyte rich large B-cell lymphoma	
• Primary DLBCL of the CNS	
• Primary cutaneous DLBCL, leg type	
EBV positive DLBCL of the elderly**	EBV positive DLBCL, NOS (not limited in elderly)*
	EBV positive mucocutaneous ulcer*
DLBCL associated with chronic inflammation	
Lymphomatoid granulomatosis	
Primary mediastinal (thymic) large B-cell lymphoma	
Intravascular large B-cell lymphoma	
ALK Positive large B-cell lymphoma	
Plasmablastic lymphoma	
Primary effusion lymphoma	
Large B-cell lymphoma arising in HHV8-associated multicentric Castleman disease**	HHV8 positive DLBCL*
Burkitt lymphoma	Burkitt-like lymphoma with 11q aberration*
B-cell lymphoma, unclassifiable, with features intermediate between diffuse large B-cell lymphoma and Burkitt lymphoma**	High-grade B-cell lymphoma with MYC and BCL-2 and/or BCL-6 rearrangements*
	High-grade B-cell lymphoma, NOS*
B-cell lymphoma, unclassifiable, with features intermediate between diffuse large B-cell lymphoma and classical Hodgkin lymphoma	

(*continued*)

Supplemental Table 2 2008 WHO Classification of Mature B-Cell, T-Cell, and NK-Cell Neoplasms and Corresponding 2016 Updates (continued)	
2008 WHO Classification	**Updated Classification**
Mature T- and NK-cell neoplasms	
T-cell prolymphocytic leukemia	
T-cell large granular lymphocytic leukemia	
Chronic lymphoproliferative disorder of NK cell	
Aggressive NK-cell leukemia	
Systemic EBV+ T-cell lymphoproliferative disease of childhood*	
Hydroa vacciniforme-like lymphoma*	
Adult T-cell leukemia/lymphoma	
Extranodal NK-/T-cell lymphoma, nasal type	
Enteropathy-associated T-cell lymphoma	
	Monomorphic epitheliotropic intestinal T-cell lymphoma* Indolent T-cell lymphoproliferative-disorder of the gastrointestinal (GI) tract*
Hepatosplenic T-cell lymphoma	
Subcutaneous panniculitis-like T-cell lymphoma	
Mycosis fungoides	
Sézary syndrome	
Primary cutaneous CD30+ T-cell lymphoproliferative disorders	
• Lymphomatoid papulosis	
• Primary cutaneous anaplastic large cell lymphoma	
Primary cutaneous gamma-delta T-cell lymphoma	
Primary cutaneous CD8+ aggressive epidermotropic cytotoxic T-cell lymphoma	
	Primary cutaneous acral CD8+ T-cell lymphoma*

(*continued*)

Supplemental Table 2 2008 WHO Classification of Mature B-Cell, T-Cell, and NK-Cell Neoplasms and Corresponding 2016 Updates (continued)

2008 WHO Classification	Updated Classification
Primary cutaneous CD4+ small/medium T-cell lymphoma	
Peripheral T-cell lymphoma, NOS	Follicular T-cell lymphoma*
Angioimmunoblastic T-cell lymphoma	Nodal peripheral T-cell lymphoma with TFH phenotype
Anaplastic large cell lymphoma, ALK positive	
Anaplastic large cell lymphoma, ALK negative*	
	Breast implant–associated anaplastic large cell lymphoma*
Post-transplant lymphoproliferative disorders (PTLD)	
Plasmacytic hyperplasia	
Infectious mononucleosis-like PTLD	
Polymorphic PTLD	
Monomorphic PTLD (B-and T-/NK-cell types)	Florid follicular hyperplasia PTLD
Classical Hodgkin lymphoma type PTLD	
Hodgkin lymphoma	
Nodular lymphocyte predominant Hodgkin lymphoma	
Classical Hodgkin lymphoma	
• Nodular sclerosis	
• Mixed cellularity	
• Lymphocyte-rich	
• Lymphocyte-deplete	

*Newly proposed lymphomas listed in the revision of 2008 WHO classification, including those provisional lymphomas in 2008.

**The types of lymphomas are modified in the revision of 2008 WHO classification.

Supplemental Table 3 Key Gene Mutations That Predict Overall Patient Prognosis in Myeloid and Lymphoid Neoplasms

Gene Name	Location	Protein Class	Associated Disease(s)	Prognostic Impact
FLT3/ITD	13q12.2	Growth factor receptor tyrosine kinase	MDS, AML	- Adverse
FLT3/TKD		Signal transduction		- None in APL
NPM1	5q35.1	Nuclear and cytoplasmic protein shuttling	AML, ALCL	Favorable (in absence or low allelic ratio of FLT3/ITD)
				Favorable in ALCL
MLL	11q23	Transcriptional regulation / Histone methyltransferase	MDS, AML	Adverse
CEBPA	19q13.1	Transcriptional regulation	AML	Favorable, when biallelic CEBPA mutated
TET2	4q24	DNA methylation	MDS, AML	Neutral
DNMT3A	2p23	DNA methylation	MDS, AML	Neutral
IDH1/2	2p33.3 and 15q26.1	DNA methylation	MDS, MPN, AML	Neutral/Adverse
ASXL1	20q11	Chromatin/histone modification	MDS, MDS/MPN	Adverse
EZH2	7q35-q36	Chromatin/histone modification	MDS, MDS/MPN	Adverse
RUNX1	21q22.3	Transcriptional regulation	MDS, AML	Adverse
BCOR/BCORL1	Xp11.4	Transcriptional regulation	MDS, AML	Adverse
ETV6	12p13	Transcriptional regulation	MDS, AML	Adverse
SETBP1	18q12.3	Transcriptional regulation	MDS, MDS/MPN	Adverse
TP53	17p13.1	DNA repair/tumor suppressor	Various myeloid and lymphoid malignancies	Adverse

(continued)

Supplemental Table 3 Key Gene Mutations That Predict Overall
Patient Prognosis in Myeloid and Lymphoid Neoplasms (continued)

Gene Name	Location	Protein Class	Associated Disease(s)	Prognostic Impact
JAK2	9p24.1 V617F codon	Signal transduction	MPN, MDS	Neutral
CBL	11q23.3	Signal transduction	MDS, MDS/MPN	Adverse
SRSF2	17q25.1	RNA splicing	MDS	Adverse
SF3B1	2q33.1	RNA splicing	MDS, CLL	Favorable (MDS)
MYD88	3p22	NF-kB activation	LPL/WM (>90%), CLL (10%), DLBCL, ABC type (8%)	Adverse in DLBCL
ATM	11q23-q23	DNA repair Tumor suppressor	CLL/SLL, MCL, T-PLL	Adverse
BRAF	V600E codon	Signal transduction	Hairy cell leukemia	Driver mutation, may respond to BRAF inhibitors

ALCL, anaplastic large; AML, acute myeloid leukemia; CLL, chronic lymphocytic leukemia; ITD, internal tandem duplication; MCL, mantle cell lymphoma; MDS, myelodysplastic syndrome; MDS/MPN, myelodysplastic/myeloproliferative neoplasm; TKD, tyrosine kinase domain.

◼ REFERENCES

1. Jaffe ES, Campo E, Harris NL, et al. *WHO Classification of Tumours of Haematopoietic and Lymphoid Tissues.* WHO Publications Center; 2008.

2. Estey EH. Acute myeloid leukemia: 2014 update on risk-stratification and management. *Am J Hematol.* 2014;89(11):1063–1081.

3. Orazi A, Foucar K, Knowles DM, eds. Flow cytometry in the assessment of hematologic disorders. In: *Knowles' Neoplastic Hematopathology.* 3rd ed. Wolters Kluwer; 2013:110–145.

4. Craig FE, Foon KA. Flow cytometric immunophenotyping for hematologic neoplasms. *Blood.* 2008;111(8):3941–3967.

5. Johansson U, Bloxham D, Couzens S, et al. Guidelines on the use of multicolor flow cytometry in the diagnosis of haematological neoplasms: British Committee for Standards in Haematology. *Br J Haematol.* 2014;165(4):455–488.

6. Pernick N. *CD markers. Secondary CD markers.* http://www.pathologyoutlines.com/cdmarkers.html

7. Grim KE BT, O'Malley DP, Weisee LM. Immunophenotypic markers useful in the diagnosis and classification of hematopoietic and lymphoid neoplasms. In: Orazi A, Foucar K, Knowles DM, eds. *Knowles' Neoplastic Hematopathology.* Wolters Kluwer; 2013:91–118.

8. Chan A, Enwere E, Johnson G, et al. Stains and molecular markers. Secondary stains and molecular markers. 2016. http://www.pathologyoutlines.com/stains.html

9. Foucar K, Reichard, K, Czuchlewski D. *Bone Marrow Pathology.* 3rd ed. American Society for Clinical Pathology; 2010.

10. Nihal M, Mikkola D, Wood GS. Detection of clonally restricted immunoglobulin heavy chain gene rearrangements in normal and lesional skin: analysis of the B cell component of the skin-associated lymphoid tissue and implications for the molecular diagnosis of cutaneous B cell lymphomas. *J Mol Diagn.* 2000;2(1):5–10.

11. Elenitoba-Johnson KS, Bohling SD, Mitchell RS, et al. PCR analysis of the immunoglobulin heavy chain gene in polyclonal processes can yield pseudoclonal bands as an artifact of low B cell number. *J Mol Diagn.* 2000;2(2):92–96.

12. Leonard DGB. *Molecular Pathology in Clinical Practice: Genetics.* Springer US; 2008:311.

13. Boehm TL, Werle A, Drahovsky D. Immunoglobulin heavy chain and T-cell receptor gamma and beta chain gene rearrangements in acute myeloid leukemias. *Mol Biol Med.* 1987;4(1):51–62.

14. Lee SC, Berg KD, Racke FK, et al. Pseudo-spikes are common in histologically benign lymphoid tissues. *J Mol Diagn.* 2000;2(3):145–152.

15. Caspersson T, Zech L, Johansson C. Differential binding of alkylating fluorochromes in human chromosomes. *Exp Cell Res.* 1970;60(3):315–319.

16. Jaffe ES, Harris NL, Vardiman JW, et al. Cytogenetic analysis and related techniques in hematopathology. In: *Hematopathology.* 1st ed. Elsevier Saunders; 2011:1058.

17. Streubel B, Simonitsch-Klupp I, Mullauer L, et al. Variable frequencies of MALT lymphoma-associated genetic aberrations in MALT lymphomas of different sites. *Leukemia.* 2004;18(10):1722–1726.

18. O'Keefe CL, Tiu R, Gondek LP, et al. High-resolution genomic arrays facilitate detection of novel cryptic chromosomal lesions in myelodysplastic syndromes. *Exp Hematol.* 2007;35(2):240–251.

19. Kallioniemi A, Kallioniemi OP, Sudar D, et al. Comparative genomic hybridization for molecular cytogenetic analysis of solid tumors. *Science.* 1992;258(5083):818–821.

20. Palanisamy N, Abou-Elella AA, Chaganti SR, et al. Similar patterns of genomic alterations characterize primary mediastinal large-B-cell lymphoma and diffuse large-B-cell lymphoma. *Genes Chromosomes Cancer.* 2002;33(2):114–122.

21. Joos S, Menz CK, Wrobel G, et al. Classical Hodgkin lymphoma is characterized by recurrent copy number gains of the short arm of chromosome 2. *Blood.* 2002;99(4):1381–1387.

22. Jinming S, Haipeng S. SNP array in hematopoietic neoplasms: a review. *Microarrays*. 2016;5(1):1. doi: 10.3390/microarrays5010001

23. Okamoto R, Ogawa S, Nowak D, et al. Genomic profiling of adult acute lymphoblastic leukemia by single nucleotide polymorphism oligonucleotide microarray and comparison to pediatric acute lymphoblastic leukemia. *Haematologica*. 2010;95(9):1481–1488.

24. Mardis ER. Next-generation sequencing platforms. *Annu Rev Anal Chem*. 2013;6:287–303.

25. Chin EL, da Silva C, Hegde M. Assessment of clinical analytical sensitivity and specificity of next-generation sequencing for detection of simple and complex mutations. *BMC Genet*. 2013;14:6.

26. Swerdlow SH, Campo E, Pileri SA, et al. The 2016 revision of the World Health Organization (WHO) classification of lymphoid neoplasms. *Blood*. 2016;127(20):2375–2390. doi: 10.1182/blood-2016-01-643569

27. Arber DA, Orazi A, Hasserjian R, et al. The 2016 revision to the World Health Organization (WHO) classification of myeloid neoplasms and acute leukemia. *Blood*. 2016;127:2391–2405.

28. Darzynkiewicz Z, Halicka HD, Zhao H. Analysis of cellular DNA content by flow and laser scanning cytometry. *Adv Exp Med Biol*. 2010; 676:137–147.

INDEX